MEDICOLEGAL PRIMER

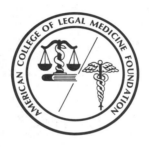

First Edition, 1991

Published by the

AMERICAN COLLEGE OF LEGAL MEDICINE FOUNDATION
1200 Centre Avenue
Pittsburgh, PA 15219

AMERICAN COLLEGE OF LEGAL MEDICINE FOUNDATION

MEDICOLEGAL PRIMER

First Edition, 1991

First Printing

Library of Congress Catalogue No. 91-072225

ISBN #0-9629575-0-X

Printed in the United States of America by

Associates Litho, Inc.
Pittsburgh, Pennsylvania

Published by the

AMERICAN COLLEGE OF LEGAL MEDICINE FOUNDATION

Editors: Cyril H. Wecht, M.D., J.D.
Harold L. Hirsh, M.D., J.D.

**Editorial
Assistant:**   Mrs. Maribeth Blettner

Officers:

Cyril H. Wecht, M.D., J.D.
President

James G. Zimmerly, M.D., J.D.
Secretary-Treasurer

**Board of
Trustees:**

Salvatore F. Fiscina, M.D., I.D.
Richard F. Gibbs, M.D., J.D.
Harold L. Hirsh, M.D., J.D.
Francis I. Kittredge, Jr., M.D., J.D.
Monroe E. Trout, M.D., J.D.

CONTRIBUTORS

James R. Bartimus, Esquire
Emidio A. Bianco, M.D., J.D.
Edwin E. Breitenbach, M.D., J.D.
James B. Couch, M.D., J.D.
Edward David, M.D., J.D.
Walter S. Feldman, M.D., J.D.
Bernard J. Ficarra, M.D., Sc.D., LL.D.
Salvatore F. Fiscina, M.D., J.D.
Jason Geiger, M.D.
Richard F. Gibbs, M.D., J.D.
Allan Gibofsky, M.D., J.D.
Donald Gilmer, M.D.
Andrew H. Greenhill, M.D.
Jay A. Gold, M.D., J.D.
Lee S. Goldsmith, M.D., LL.B.
Walter G. Gunn, M.D., J.D.
Kenneth D. Hansen, M.D., J.D.
Harold L. Hirsh, M.D., J.D.
Paul D. Hirsh, M.D.
Edward E. Hollowell, J.D.
John J. Howard, M.D., J.D.
John C. Hunsaker, III, M.D.
Mark J. Jaffe, M.D.
Paul F. Kavanaugh, Esquire

Julius Landwirth, M.D., J.D.
Theodore R. LeBlang, J.D.
Richard J. Lescoe, M.D., J.D.
William J. Mangold, Jr., M.D., J.D.
Corey H. Marco, M.D., J.D.
Valentino D.B. Mazzia, M.D., J.D.
R. Konane Mookini, M.D., J.D.
William J. Morton, M.D., J.D.
Donal D. O'Sullivan, M.D., J.D.
Julius S. Piver, M.D., J.D.
Peter A. Plumeri, D.O., LL.M.
Stewart R. Reuter, M.D., J.D.
Robert L. Sadoff, M.D.
S. Sandy Sanbar, M.D., Ph.D., J.D.
Sergio Schwartzman, M.D.
William M. Thompson, J.D., M.D.
Monroe E. Trout, M.D., J.D.
Richard Tyler, M.D., J.D.
Harvey F. Wachsman, M.D., J.D.
Cyril H. Wecht, M.D., J.D.
Victor W. Weedn, M.D., J.D.
Richard S. Wilbur, M.D.
James G. Zimmerly, M.D., J.D.

DEDICATION

This book is dedicated to those individuals who have devoted their professional careers to the practice and teaching of legal medicine. There are many facets and subdivisions of this broad field that constitute the interface of law and science in a democratic society as technologically advanced as the United States. Without the special competence and continuous efforts of various kinds of medicolegal experts, it would not be possible to achieve the optimal levels of health care, medical research, and justice in both the civil and criminal legal systems.

It is our earnest hope that this innovative Primer will provide important, practical, and timely information for large numbers of physicians and other health care professionals, and assist them in pursuing and accomplishing their professional objectives with a better understanding and appreciation of the myriad of potential legal pitfalls and problems that are inherent in our society.

PREFACE

There is no dearth of textbooks and various other kinds of publications that deal with legal medicine generally or some particular subdivision within this immense body of knowledge and practice. However, there is no book that is specifically designed for physicians who are embarking upon their postgraduate training and practicing medicine as members of a hospital or other health care institution. This *Medicolegal Primer* has been especially tailored for that large group of physicians, with the hope and expectation that the more information and knowledge they possess concerning relevant legal concepts, principles, and rules, the more effective and productive they can be as medical practitioners.

The nature and frequency of legal problems confronting physicians continue to expand in modern day society and will undoubtedly multiply in future years. It simply is not possible to practice medicine with wisdom, sensitivity, and total concern for patients' welfare and safety unless the physician is cognizant of basic legal rules and generally accepted mandates. There is no logical or justifiable reason to remain ignorant of and hostile to the legal system, which is an integral and essential part of our government. Physicians, like all other citizens, are obliged to function within the parameters of civil and criminal law, and they should feel comfortable and safe in doing so as they pursue their medical careers.

While it is not possible to cover every aspect of legal medicine in one book, we have attempted to touch upon and highlight all those areas of professional endeavor in a health care institution that constitute potential pitfalls and problems of a legal nature. The field of legal medicine is extremely broad and far-reaching with literally new developments of a significant nature occurring constantly. Interested readers are urged to seek out additional information from appropriate textbooks and journals for lengthier discussions of a particular subject. Knowledge of the information set forth in this *Primer*, coupled with a genuine, ongoing effort to exercise due diligence and concern for the best interests of patients' health, welfare, and safety, can provide an increased degree of peace of mind and a diminution of fear and antipathy toward attorneys and the legal system. If this goal can be achieved with even a small number of the readers of this *Primer*, the objectives and aspirations of the ACLM Foundation will have been realized.

Preface

The ACLM Foundation, a non-profit organization comprised of physician-attorneys, was established several years ago to help foster and develop better relationships between doctors and lawyers, and to expand medicolegal education throughout the United States. This book represents the culmination of the combined efforts of dozens of medicolegal experts who have given unselfishly of their time and talent as a special contribution in behalf of the Foundation. We are deeply grateful for their efforts, cooperation, and interest, without which this project could not have been undertaken and completed. Although this *Primer* will be revised and updated many times in the future, this initial endeavor will always be considered as the keystone and major project for the aims we initially set forth.

The editors would like to acknowledge the extraordinary efforts of Maribeth Blettner, who has served as editorial assistant of this literary endeavor from its inception. Her tireless work, personal interest, and perseverance were essential to the fruition of this ambitious undertaking.

We should also like to express our appreciation to Ms. Kathleen Kelly for her expert assistance in compiling the index for this book.

Cyril H. Wecht, M.D., J.D.
Harold L. Hirsh, M.D., J.D.

TABLE OF CONTENTS

Contents

I.
MEDICAL

ALLERGY AND IMMUNOLOGY

Introduction

Allergists and immunologists are among the blessed medical specialists relative to malpractice; they are not beset with that problem. One reason is that they are exposed to less situations that may result in litigation. Those that do exist can be avoided by adherence to established standards of care. As with all medical care, prophylaxis beats malpractice, and appropriate informed consent is one of the best preventatives.

Immunotherapy

Immunotherapy has the potential for resulting in a suit for malpractice, because the physician is actually injecting a known allergen. If it is not done cautiously and properly, a fatal anaphylaxis is more likely to occur. Before commencing immunotherapy, the physician should explain and consider alternative approaches such as environmental control and medications. Whether the injections are given in the allergist's office or by another physician at his office, a written standard protocol should be available to the provider, usually a nurse, and the patient. The instructions should contain all pertinent information. The risks inherent in immunotherapy should be clearly identified.

There is more to reactions than giving adrenaline. A specific protocol for handling reactions in the physician's office should be established. The patient should always remain in the office after an injection. A physician should always be available, even in the presence of an adequately trained office staff. A plan of management should be made available, so that the staff can promptly identify a problem and institute proper care. Treatment medications and equipment should be immediately at hand.

Sometimes, reactions occur that are not related to improper protocol. Individuals who are having increased symptoms prior to an injection are more likely to have a reaction. Increased symptoms may be secondary to recent acute exposure to an allergen, chronic increased exposure such as during pollen season, an acute viral illness, or forgetting to take a medication. Increased physical activity or exposure to higher ambient temperatures increases blood flow to the body surface and enhances the pick up of injected antigens. Therefore, during hot weather, the individual should be cool prior to an allergy injection and for several hours thereafter. Strenuous physical activity should also be avoided prior to and for several hours after immunotherapy.

If the reaction takes place at home, the patient should know how to treat such a reaction. Medications such as an antihistamine and adrenaline should be taken first, and then the patient should call the physician. The patient should know where the physician or his surrogate can be reached 24 hours a day.

When desensitization is undertaken, several medications should be avoided. Beta blockers are very dangerous because they block the receptors used for treating allergic reactions. Beta agonists (epinephrine, aluret, etc.) will have no effect.

Allergy Testing

Allergy testing is another procedure potentially fraught with liability. There are two standard recognized techniques for in-vivo testing. One is the skin prick or scratch technique, the other is the intradermal method. The first is less sensitive than the second, and has the advantage of being wiped from the skin if a severe reaction occurs. Usually, scratch testing is performed to screen for reactions to specific antigens. Antigens that produce negative or insignificant scratch reactions are then used for intradermal testing. Intradermal testing is considered approximately 100 to 1,000 times more sensitive than scratch testing. The danger of intradermal testing is because of its increased sensitivity, and because the antigen is actually injected into the body. Reactions incident to the intradermal technique can be minimized by starting with lower concentrations and gradually increasing them.

Medications

Some medications that allergists use may aggravate other medical conditions. Medications containing epinephrine or other cardiovascular stimulants should not be prescribed in the presence of hypertension, heart disease, thyroid disease, or prostatic hypertrophy with urinary difficulties. Anticholinergics may also aggravate urinary tract problems. Antihistamines, decongestants, beta agonists or other cardiovascular stimulants should not be given to patients taking antihypertensives or antidepressants containing MAO inhibitors. Allergens given to a patient taking Tagamet or Erythromycin may result in a serious drug interaction, producing high fever, and even death.

Insect and Food Allergy

Insect and food allergies are potentially life-threatening. Fatalities most often occur because of circulatory collapse. Swelling of the throat may cause asphyxia. Most reactions occur away from medical assistance. For that reason, it behooves the patient to have available self-administered epinephrine in a syringe at all times. Two preparations are available. The Epi-pen is available for both adults and children in an automatic apparatus that ejects a needle and injects adrenaline when the pen is thrust against the injection site. The Ana-kit requires the patient to twist the plunger, insert the needle into the site, and inject the desired amount.

Asthma

Asthma is a potentially life-threatening condition. During the past decade, the incidence of morbidity and death from asthma has increased significantly. Asthma is defined as a state in which the bronchial tubes are over-reactive and react to stimulation by constricting, producing excessive mucus, and becoming swollen. All of the responses result in narrowing of the airway and restricting breathing. This is a very labile condition which requires diligent and vigilant monitoring. Exposure to allergens and irritants, infections, stress, anxiety, and other medical problems may exacerbate the problems.

An emergency plan should be discussed with the patient. The patient should know what to do and how to get care. Treatment should be individualized. It is important to follow asthmatics with objective standards such as pulmonary function testing. Without objective standards to monitor asthma, the physician may be at risk for negligence.

Theophylline

Theophylline is a medication with potentially dangerous properties. It has a narrow window of safety. It must be given slowly intravenously. It should be remembered that it lowers the seizure threshold. Theophylline circulates bound to serum proteins. The lower the concentration of serum proteins, the greater the free circulating Theophylline, and the higher the risk of Theophylline toxicity. In older people, who may have lowered blood globulin levels, elevated Theophylline levels are fraught with danger.

CARDIOLOGY

Standard of Care

Cardiologists, like all physicians, must adhere to established standards of care. They are best advised to be familiar with prevailing standards. A standard which is determined by common law principles is a judge-made law or statutory law. A judicially imposed standard of care means the standard is established retrospectively at the time the injury occurred, which invariably is several years earlier. This exposes the physician to a standard that has not yet been enunciated. Underlying this peril is the rapidly expanding knowledge in this medical field, which renders a uniform set of standards obsolete by the time such standards are published and disseminated.

The trend is clear. Physicians must use their best judgment in every case. Conforming to local or community standards may no longer be sufficient in deciding what is "good medicine". The great shield of "professional standards" is slowly eroding in the courts, and in some instances, the courts are setting the cardiovascular standard of care as a matter of law. For example, a judge may decide alone that an EKG should have been obtained on a patient who presents at an emergency room complaining of chest pain.

Diagnostic Modalities

Cardiac diagnoses require an accurate, complete, and exhaustive history and physical examination. Critical, however, is laboratory testing. The cardiologist must be knowledgeable and transmit this knowledge to the patient, so that he or she can participate in the management of care.

The currently available cardiovascular diagnostic techniques include, among others:

- Blood chemistries, arterial gases, and urine tests;
- Electrocardiogram (ECG), phonocardiogram, and vectorcardiogram.
- Echocardiogram, M-mode and 2-D, at rest or during exercise, with or without contrast;
- Holter ambulatory monitoring of cardiac rhythm;
- X-rays of the heart and chest, including CT chest scan, magnetic resonance imaging (MRI), and positron emission tomograms (PET);
- Nuclear (radioisotope) cardiac studies, at rest and with exercise;
- Exercise stress tolerance test (treadmill or bicyle), alone or in combination with other cardiac studies;
- Coronary arteriogram and heart catheterization, with cardiac function tests;
- Electrophysiologic studies of cardiac dysrrhythmias.

Mistakes

Cardiology is not considered an exact science, and much depends upon the physician's judgment and interpretation of many complex, and sometimes contradictory, cardiac symptoms, signs, cardiovascular test results, etc. The mere fact that a physician misdiagnosed a cardiac condition does not establish liability for cardiovascular malpractice, unless it can be proven that this misdiagnosis resulted in harm. Furthermore, an error or mistake in judgment, as contrasted to a careless or negligent judgment, is not a source of liability.

Informed Consent

A review of malpractice cases reveals that there appears to be a direct relationship between the number of lawsuits and a patient's prognosis. The poorer the prognosis, the more likely a lawsuit will be filed. It is, therefore, incumbent upon the cardiologist to identify and advise the patient of the "risk factors" which may determine his or her prognosis and fate.

The presence or absence of coronary risk factors in patients should be recorded by the physician in the medical records, and should serve as the basis for performing certain diagnostic tests and for treatment, particularly after 35-40 years of age.

For example, a totally asymptomatic 40 year old male smoker, with familial hypercholesterolemia (type IIA hyperlipoproteinemia), and positive coronary artery disease in his father who died in his 40's of myocardial infarction, should be investigated for silent myocardial ischemia by whatever diagnostic cardiovascular tests are necessary. In addition, that asymptomatic patient should be fully informed about and treated with regard to his high-risk factors, as well as educated about the complications of coronary artery disease - namely, angina, infarction, and sudden death. Failure on the part of the physician to do so may subject him to legal consequences in the event the patient develops some of those complications, and perhaps dies.

Duty to Keep Abreast

The physician's duty and responsibility is to keep abreast of modern advances of therapy of coronary artery disease, and to communicate that knowledge to the patient, who, in turn, can accept or decline a particular mode of treatment(s).

Prescribing Drugs

Drug manufacturers' package inserts and the Physicians' Desk Reference (PDR) do not recognize that they, by themselves, establish the standard of care in the prescribing of drugs; rather, they provide merely one piece of evidence.

Occasionally, a drug manufacturer's recommendations are used by the courts to establish a standard of care as a matter of law. One case held that where a drug manufacturer recommends how and when a drug should be prescribed and warns of the precautions to be taken and the inherent adverse effect, a physician's deviation from such recommendations is *prima facie* evidence of negligence. However, there must be competent medical testimony that the patient's injury was proximately (legally) caused by the physician's failure to adhere to the drug manufacturer's recommendations. Usually, whether the physician was justified or excused from his deviation is a jury question.

Duty to Recall

Traditionally, medical malpractice involves an overt act of omission or commission in treating a patient. The duty to recall arises from the continuing status of the physician-patient relationship in cases involving implantable medical devices that impose a continuing duty to inform a patient of newly discovered hazards resulting from continuing use of a particular device or medication. From a practical standpoint, the duty to recall requires physicians to maintain detailed cross-referenced medical records that are readily accessible for the life of every patient. Whenever implanted medical devices are found subsequently to be hazardous, the physician must be able to ascertain from the medical records the vulnerable patients, regardless of their relationship, and recall them if necessary.

Duty to Refer and Consult

A physician who undertakes the care of a patient, regardless of his professional status, holds himself to be capable of caring for that patient and his or her disease. The law does not dictate when a physician is required to refer or consult. Several guidelines have been established, however; when a patient requests it, or when the physician believes he is in over his head, diagnostically or therapeutically. The purpose of the referral or consultation should be established, as well as the future care of the patient - mere opinion, transfer, or a joint enterprise.

Testing

An interpretation of laboratory results by a cardiovascular physician, which differs from the interpretation of others, is not prima facie. Such a determination would depend on all the circumstances.

Physicians who undertake treatment of cardiovascular disorders may be held liable for not ordering tests and procedures that may be indicated. For example, failure to recommend or perform an arteriogram on a 30 year old patient with angina when it is medically indicated may be a basis for legal action, if the patient sustains damages, i.e., infarction or death.

The performance of expensive cardiovascular tests for the purpose of practicing defensive medicine should be avoided. Instead, the physician should generally utilize a balancing test, weighing on the one hand the necessity, accuracy, and expense of the recommended procedure against the hazards or risks of performing that particular procedure as compared with other available tests.

The physican must keep in mind that only the patient, after being fully informed, ultimately decides whether or not to undergo a particular test or procedure, except in emergency situations.

Three cardiovascular diagnostic techniques deserve special consideration because of the significant morbidity and mortality inherent in performing those procedures. They are exercise tolerance test, coronary arteriography and heart catheterization, and electrophysiologic studies.

Benefit vs. Risk Rule

When performing cardiovascular diagnostic procedures such as an arteriogram, full disclosure of the material risks and the alternatives involved is mandatory. All disclosures by the physician should be noted in the patient's medical record to protect against future allegations of lack of informed consent and negligence.

Coronary Arteriography and Heart Catheterization

Complications of coronary arteriography and heart catheterization performed simultaneously are frequent and represent substantial litigation. One reviewer has summarized the complications of coronary arteriography and heart cathetherization from numerous medical publications. Because they represent material risks, they should be appropriately communicated.

There are a multitude of complications that can occur during right heart catheterization. Certainly, operator experience is a major factor in minimizing the incidence of complications. However, the overall incidence of complications is about 25%, with serious complications in less than 5% of patients. The risk of death directly attributable to the procedure remains quite low, however, with reported mortality in the 1 to 2 in 10,000 range. With critically ill patients, mortality has been reported to be as high as 4%.

The major perils include:
- Pneumothorax - hemothorax/hydrothorax;
- Air embolus;
- Cardiac tamponade secondary to perforation of RA, RV, or SVC;
- Thromboembolic event;
- Pulmonary artery rupture and pulmonary infarctions;
- Infectious complications;
- Horner's syndrome;
- Superior vena cava syndrome;
- Arrhythmias and conduction disturbances;
- Erroneous data;
- Vasovagal reactions - nausea, hypotension, bradycardia;
- Miscellaneous, e.g., dye reaction.

The major perils or complications of coronary angiography include mortality, myocardial infarction, and cerebrovascular accidents, which are the most easily quantified.

Thromboembolism is believed to be the most frequent cause of the major complications. A less frequent cause of myocardial infarction or death is coronary artery dissection from the injection of contrast under an atherosclerotic plaque or catheter impingement when done with excessive force against the coronary artery intima. Catheter or guidewire manipulation in the arch or cranial vessels may also dislodge atherosclerotic debris, which may embolize to the brain with transient or permanent neurologic sequelae.

Several patient characteristics have been repeatedly identified which predispose to major complications. These include left main coronary artery stenosis greater than 50%, triple vessel coronary artery disease, a left ventricular ejection fraction less than 0.30, congestive heart failure, hypertension, and multiple premature ventricular ectopic beats. In addition, association functional class 4 angina has been associated with an increased risk of death.

Patients with unstable angina are at increased risk for myocardial infarction during and following coronary angiography. Critical aortic stenosis is associated with a higher incidence of sudden death following cardiac catheterization and angiography.

One registry identified ages of less than one year or greater than 60 years as high-risk groups for procedure-related mortality. However, another reported no increase in major complications in patients 65 years of age and older. The serious arrhythmias associated with coronary arteriography are ventricular fibrillation, ventricular tachycardia, and prolonged bradycardia. Local vascular complications are the most common significant risk of arterial catheterization. Potential peripheral vascular complications at the site of arterial puncture include arterial thrombosis, arterial laceration or dissection, pseudoaneurysm, hematoma, arteriovenous fistula, peripheral thromboembolism, and thrombophlebitis. Evacuation of local hematomas is rarely required.

Other local complications of the femoral artery approach include peripheral thromboembolism, pseudoaneurysm, hematoma, arteriovenous fistula, and large hematoma with vascular or nerve compromise. Retroperitoneal hemorrhage may occur following perforation of the iliac vessels. Local infection is uncommon with the femoral technique, but rare cases of septic thrombophlebitis have occurred.

Complications related to femoral vein puncture occur even when catheterization is limited to the left heart. Inadvertent femoral vein puncture attends searching for the femoral artery, and the femoral vein may also be punctured when it lies posterior to the artery.

Multiple other complications have been reported with left heart catheterization and coronary arteriography. Perforation of the heart or great vessels is uncommon and is usually associated with difficulty in catheter passage and excessive manipulation. Pulmonary edema may occur due to excess fluid administration, myocardial ischemia, or the bradycardia or negative inotropic effect of the contrast media. Hypotension may occur from the complications listed above, vasovagal reactions, anaphylactoid reactions, or contrast effects, including immediate vasodilation or late hypovolemia from osmotic diuresis. Fevers occur secondary to contrast reactions, local phlebitis or infection, or pyrogen reactions. Pyrogen reactions are caused by endotoxin contamination of resterilized catheters. Since disposable catheters are now used, pyrogen reactions occur much less frequently. Renal insufficiency can result from contrast nephrotoxicity or atheromatous emboli.

Death may result from these procedures. Additional major complications include ventricular reperfusion arrhythmias, hypotension requiring therapy, dissection of the right coronary artery, and hemorrhage requiring blood transfusion after intracoronary streptokinase. Other risks include anaphylaxis to streptokinase and hemorrhage in the area of myocardial necrosis, which may predispose to fatal cardiac rupture. The risk of bleeding from diagnostic or interventional catheterization after the administration of thrombolytic agents is also increased.

There are established guidelines of central venous and right heart catheterization:

- Be certain that the indications for catheterization are firm. If the data can be reliably obtained by other means, catheterization should be avoided.
- For catheterization of short duration, favor antecubital or external jugular routes over subclavian or internal jugular sites. Consider femoral route in patients with severe lung disease or coagulation abnormalities.
- Avoid procedures in patients who are unable to cooperate.
- If subclavian or internal jugular routes are taken, have patient in Trendelenburg position with attempt made to accentuate landmarks (e.g., towel between shoulder blades).
- Use fluoroscopic guidance whenever possible. If catheter will not readily advance, consider use of dilute contrast material.
- Perform catheterization with continuous electrocardiographic monitoring. Have defibrillation equipment in or near procedure room. Consider

prophylactic temporary pacemaker placement in patients with underlying left bundle branch block.

- Maintain strict sterility during catheter insertion and perform daily inspection of insertion site.
- Inexperienced operators must be closely supervised throughout the procedure.

In order to obtain optimal performance of percutaneous puncture, guidewire, and catheter placement, the following should be kept in mind:

- Advance a sharply beveled needle until blood is readily aspirated with a syringe. Drop the needle parallel to the axis of the vessel to facilitate guidewire passage.
- If blood is not easily withdrawn, do not attempt to advance the guidewire.
- If blood flow is pulsatile or the blood appears saturated, *do not place a sheath*. Venous or inadvertent arterial puncture can be confirmed by oximetry in most patients. Saturations less than 80% are usually venous blood.
- If the guidewire does not advance readily, assess the wire's course with fluoroscopy. In some cases, a flexible J-tip will facilitate passage of wire. Use dilute contrast injections to identify anatomy. If the guidewire cannot be readily withdrawn through the needle, withdraw the wire and needle as a unit. Failure to do so may result in shearing of the wire and particulate embolus. Following proper advancement of the guidewire, determine the wire's course if fluoroscopy is available (e.g., wire in RA or SVC and not heading cephalad in internal jugular vein or out contralateral subclavian vein with subclavian puncture). Remove the needle over the guidewire while maintaining proximal pressure on the entry site to avoid blood loss. Make a nick with a #11 blade adjacent to the guidewire, followed by initial dilation with a hemostat to facilitate dilation. Advance the dilator and sheath over the guidewire with gentle pressure and rotation at the skin. Never release the proximal end of the guidewire until it is visualized beyond the distal end of the dilator and sheath.
- Have the patient stop breathing at end expiration during guidewire and sheath exchanges. Never allow the venous system to be open to air during normal respiration. Take care to avoid flushing air bubbles into the system following initial catheter placement.
- Advance the catheter through the sheath to the desired anatomic location (e.g., SVC, RV, or pulmonary artery). If the catheter does not advance readily, confirm position under fluoroscopy.

Standard of care requirements for the management of the patient following catheter placement requires the physician to:

- Obtain a chest x-ray following the procedure to look for pneumothorax and to confirm proper catheter position. If multiple ipsilateral puncture attempts are unsuccessful (subclavian), never proceed to the contralateral side without first obtaining a chest x-ray to exclude pneumothorax.
- Ensure proper transducer height and calibration to avoid erroneous data.
- Change dressings daily. Never advance a catheter that has been in place more than a few hours.
- Do not infuse fluids through central venous catheter if blood cannot be readily withdrawn.
- Never allow a pulmonary artery catheter to remain in "permanent wedge" position. Balloon inflation may result in pulmonary artery rupture or infarction. Carefully "trouble shoot" damped tracings.
- Consider daily x-rays to confirm catheter position.

• In most cases, pulmonary artery and central venous catheters should be changed to new site every 48 to 72 hours.

Coronary arteriography and heart catheterization should be utilized only after exhaustion of *safer* diagnostic techniques. There should be a recognized medical indication for its performance, and the absence of any contraindication. Additionally, stringent hospital safety procedures and guidelines must be adhered to by the staff and technicians in the heart catheterization room. The physician arteriographer must be trained, competent, skillful, and approved by the special procedures committee of the hospital or institution for the performance of coronary arteriography and heart catheterization.

Exercise Tolerance Test

Being a provocative test, it carries a mortality rate of 1 in 10,000 exercise tests, and a morbidity rate (non-fatal complications of myocardial infarction or arrhythmia induced by exercise) of 2.5 in 10,000 tests. These complications may arise during or a few minutes after the test is completed. The physician conducting the exercise test is under a duty to perform the test only when indicated, to avoid its performance where contraindicated, and to have available all necessary instruments, drugs, and trained, preferably certified, personnel in the event of serious complications or the need for cardiopulmonary resuscitation.

Treatment of Ischemic Heart Disease

Medical treatment generally is preferred over surgery as initial therapy, except where surgery is clearly the therapy of choice. It behooves the cardiologist to contemplate the success and hazards, benefits, risks, and complications of medical treatment of coronary artery disease by invasive therapies, principally angioplasty and coronary bypass surgery.

The mortality rate from coronary angioplasty and aorto-coronary bypass surgery varies between 1 and 5-10%. The morbidity rate is higher from ensuing infarctions, arrhythmias, heart failure, strokes, etc. The mortality and morbidity rates are substantially greater when concomitant surgical procedures may be required, e.g., coronary bypass together with valve surgery and/or resection of an aneurysm of the ventricle.

In treating ischemic heart disease, consideration should be given to newer and more innovative medical procedures, including:
• Invasive and non-invasive techniques to administer thrombolytic therapy;
• Angioscopy and laser angioplasty;
• Balloon, non-surgical valvuloplasty;
• Heart transplantation;
• Sundry circulatory assist devices, and total mechanical heart.

The perils of percutaneous transluminal coronary angioplasty (PTCA) include death, non-fatal myocardial infarction, and the need for emergency surgery, as well as coronary artery occlusion and coronary artery dissection or intimal tear distal or remote to the lesion. Vascular complications include arterial thrombosis, pseudoaneurysm, hematoma, femoral arteriovenous fistula, femoral artery aneurysm, and arterial laceration. Pericardial tamponade also has been reported as a complication of PTCA from right ventricular perforation with the pacing wire, or as a rare complication of coronary artery perforation.

Catheter-induced (iatrogenic) coronary artery spasm occurs from mechanical irritation of the intima. Intracoronary contract injection has been shown to cause ventricular fibrillation and bradycardia. Thromboembolic complications have been reported. The risk of local arterial complications is real. With the transfemoral approach, the pedal pulses and the apogee of distal flow should be checked immediately after catheterization, and frequently for several hours. Immediate surgical embolectomy is indicated for femoral artery occlusion to relieve limb ischemia and to prevent propagation of the thrombus into more distal arterial branches.

Other complications include death and hemorrhage from the arterial puncture site. The introducer should remain in place until fibrinogen levels and the clotting cascade are repleted. Retroperitoneal bleeding may occur from inadvertent iliac vessel puncture, and should be suspected if the patient complains of back pain, or if bradycardia or hypotension develop. Retroperitoneal bleeding is usually self-limited following diagnostic arteriography. Evidence of continued bleeding should suggest arterial laceration and the need for surgical repair.

With the brachial cutdown approach, prevention of arterial thrombosis includes careful arteriotomy repair and routine administration of systemic Heparin at the start of the procedure. Just prior to arteriotomy repair, the proximal and distal arterial segments should be checked for free bleeding. Immediately after arteriotomy closure, the radial artery should be palpated, and the pulse amplitude should be the same as prior to the arteriotomy. If the pulse is diminished or absent, the arteriotomy should be reopened. Thrombi should be removed from the distal arterial segment by inserting a Sones' catheter for aspiration, or using a Fogarty embolectomy catheter; any intimal flaps should be resected. The radial pulse should be re-examined later the same day. If diminished or absent, arterial spasm or thrombosis has occurred. If no other signs of limb ischemia are present, the patient can be observed for return of the radial pulse on intravenous Heparin with surgery consultation. In contrast to the transfemoral approach, arterial occlusion is more common with the brachial approach, but patients can be frequently observed for the development of limb ischemia, and surgery is sometimes not required.

An uncommon local complication of transfemoral and brachial artery catheterizations is pseudoaneurysm formation from free communication between the artery and a liquifying hematoma. A pseudoaneurysm should be suspected if a pusatile mass is detected on post-catheterization followup, and should be surgically repaired because of the danger of continued enlargement and rupture.

Less frequent perils include prolonged angina, hypotension, and bradycardia.

A pitfall in left heart catheterization is an incomplete study. Studies may be incomplete because of a failure to adequately visualize all of the coronary artery branches due to poor framing, underfilling the arteries with contrast, or an insufficient number or poor choice of views. Alternatively, the procedure might be terminated early because of patient instability. There are limits to video resolution, operator experience, and patient instability or difficult anatomy, which have all resulted in incomplete studies from time to time.

Patient characteristics associated with an increased risk of major complications include main coronary artery disease, severe triple vessel disease, congestive heart failure, unstable angina, and critical aortic stenosis.

Catheter balloon valvuloplasty perils include death, femoral artery complications (one-half of which require surgery), pulmonary edema, cardiogenic shock, stroke, and cardiac tamponade. Other complications include hemorrhaging requiring transfusion, left ventricle perforation by the guidewire with cardiac tamponade requiring coronary artery bypass surgery, and aortic valve replacement for continued angina after the valvuloplasty. Embolic complications have been reported. Aortic insufficiency is mildly increased in the majority of cases.

Employability has been recommended by a group of physicians as a medical indication for ventricular aneurysmectomy and coronary bypass surgery, both of which are considered as surgical procedures.

Preventable Disorders

A physician, including a cardiovascular specialist, has a duty to know that a cardiac disorder may be prevented with appropriate care. Failure to at least attempt to prevent the disorder may subject the physician to liability if harm results. For example, prophylaxis for subacute endocarditis (SBE) in a patient with diagnosed valvular heart disease, or failure to anticoagulate a patient with a mechanical heart valve absent any contraindication for anticoagulation, may result in SBE and stroke, respectively, and liability.

Prognostic Factors

Patients with coronary artery disease frequently file malpractice lawsuits. The mortality rate of patients with clinical or arteriographically proven coronary artery disease varies between 4 to 9% annually, depending on the classification of the patients. High-risk patients with unstable angina, for example, may have an even higher mortality rate. All things being equal, patients must be given some insight as to their prognosis, so that they can adjust their lives accordingly. A diagnosis is critical.

Patients with ischemic heart disease may be classified for prognostication purposes as follows:
- Silent myocardial ischemia (Cohn's Types I, II, and III);
- Angina pectoris, stable or unstable, due to either arteriosclerotic coronary artery disease and/or coronary spasm (Prinzmetal);
- Myocardial infarction which may be old, recent, or acute, and may be either a q-wave or non-q-wave infarction;
- Heart (pump) failure, secondary to ischemic or fibrotic myocardium or ischemic cardiomyopathy;
- Cardiac dysrrhythmias, secondary to myocardial ischemia;
- Sudden death, secondary to myocardial ischemia which generally results from lethal cardiac arrhythmias.

Transplantation

One of the major legal problems that pertains to cardiac transplantation is informed consent by the donor, or by those authorized by law to speak for him or her. The donor may be an adult, a minor, a mental incompetent, or a prisoner, and may also be living or dead. Someone must provide the requisite informed consent for organ transplantation.

Inherent in the legal aspects of organ transplantion is the determination of the time of death of the donor. In criminal situations, the cause and nature of death may be critical for a successful prosecution.

Adult Donors

When the transplant donor or donee is a competent adult, his or her consent must be freely given, knowingly and voluntarily after being fully and reliably informed. The donor should be educated regarding the transplant procedure, its material risks, prognoses, and all alternative procedures. The rights of self-determination and privacy rank supreme and are fundamental. Consent must not be induced by minimizing the dangers of surgery. Psychiatric and/or psychological assessment of the donee and donor, when feasible, is advisable. The purpose of this is not only to negate possible future allegations of misrepresentation or duress, but because of the high incidence of psychiatric morbidity and suicide in transplant recipients.

Legally Incompetent Donors

When dealing with legally incompetent minors, mentally retarded patients, or psychiatric patients, a court order is always required. The consent of parents or guardians is usually required by the court. If the donor is "'brain dead'", consent must be obtained from the next-of-kin.

Cadaver Donors

For cadaver donors, the criteria determination of death should be in accordance with the laws of the particular jurisdiction. There must be a valid consent from someone who is legally capable of granting such consent, generally the next-of-kin, or the deceased individual must have exercised his or her right under the Uniform Anatomical Gift Act and signified his wish to be a donor.

The removal of organs for donation may prove difficult in those cases in which the medical examiner or coroner has jurisdiction over the body. There are certain circumstances where the donation will not be approved because the individual died violently, e.g., homicide, poisoning, industrial accident, car accident, or where there is a question as to the cause of death.

Unclaimed Bodies

Unclaimed bodies are not a source for organ donation. Statutes generally require that there has to be a waiting period of 48 hours after the death of an individual whose body is not claimed, during which time the hospital or other facility must make a reasonable search for the next-of-kin. Until a reasonable search has been completed, the body is technically *not* claimed, no consent is available, and it is almost always too late for transplantation.

Furthermore, if transplantation is still possible, the physician who wishes to use the unclaimed body in a transplant procedure is required to obtain clearance from the medical examiner or coroner. The physician must document carefully all aspects of the transplant procedure in the medical records in an attempt to avoid future liability.

Legal Aspects

There are legal perils and pitfalls for a physician who treats a patient who has designated organ donation under the Uniform Anatomical Gift Act. Under the Act, the time of death of the patient must be determined by a "treating" physician. The physician could incur liability for making an errant premature determination of the time of death of the transplant donor, resulting in premature harvesting of the heart or other organ(s).

Failure to comply with the Act is evidence of "bad faith" per se. The physician who makes an honest effort to determine the time of death based on reasonable and well-recognized medical standards, and who acts in the best interests of the patient, would probably be considered to be exhibiting good faith. Therefore, when a physician removes an organ from a donor patient in "good faith", he will probably not be liable in a civil action under the terms of the Act. The physician is probably protected from criminal liability, also. But, the physician who removes the desired organ prematurely may not be protected from a wrongful death action, even though the Act may protect the physician from the charge of mutilation or mayhem.

To date, there have been relatively few cases of medical malpractice involving heart transplant patients, because the prognosis of patients requiring transplantation is poor, and because the expectations for success are low. Furthermore, there usually has been good communication between the transplant surgeon, the patient, and relatives, and a cultivated personal relationship. The causes of action are the same in heart transplant cases as in any other medical situation - negligence, lack of informed consent, battery, invasion of privacy, fraud, abandonment, breach of fiduciary duty, etc.

Heart donors *must* be "brain dead", and may not be considered living at the time of the donation. Harvesting a heart from a "living person", i.e., one who has not been officially pronounced dead, would constitute a criminal act, and may be either intentional or negligent homicide, depending on the facts and circumstances of the donor's case.

Implantable Cardiac Devices

The implantation of heart assist devices and artificial heart valves, permanent pacemakers, defibrillators, and other cardiac devices continues to be fraught with the usual legal problems inherent in any device implantation procedure. These may include negligence for failing to implant, or for delay in implanting a cardiovascular device, or for negligently implanting a device that is not medically indicated.

All requirements for informed consent and informed refusal must be met, and care must be taken not to guarantee a specific result or cure. The patient with an implantable device usually must be followed for life. Discontinuing necessary follow-up without the patient's consent may create liability for patient abandonment. Liability for assault and battery, fraud, and misrepresentation must also be considered when implantation is not necessary. In addition, there may be liability on the part of the cardiovascular device manufacturer, based on negligence, strict liability, or breach of warranty.

Medical Device Regulation

The Medical Device Amendments of 1976 gave the Food and Drug Administration (FDA) comprehensive regulatory authority over medical devices intended for use, and also permits the FDA to require that such devices be proven safe prior to entering the marketplace.

The Consumer Product Safety Act (CPSA) of 1972, which was revised in 1981, has a medical device standard setting that is similar to the Medical Device Amendments of 1976. The CPSA was created for the purpose of protecting the public against unreasonable risks of injury associated with consumer products.

Liability of Device Manufacturers

Manufacturers of defective implantable devices may be held liable under several legal theories. First, a tort action in negligence may be brought for defective design or manufacture of the product. Recovery may be based on failure to exercise due care in design, manufacture, assembly, packaging, inspection, or testing.

Second, strict product liability. Difficulties in proving negligence led to the development of the doctrine of strict product liability, which holds the manufacturer liable for a defect, despite the exercise of all possible due care in design and manufacture of the product.

Third, warranty. Most cardiac arrest devices carry an express warranty for replacement in the event of a defect. However, the patient rarely sees the express warranty. This, coupled with the fact that the physician selects the type of implant to be used, makes it very difficult for the patient to prove reliance on the express warranty to recover in an action based on express warranty. The plaintiff must prove existence of the express warranty, scope of coverage, and reliance.

Implied warranties include warranty for fitness for a particular purpose, and warranty for merchantability. To recover under a theory of implied warranty, the plaintiff must prove that the product was defective when it was sold, that because of the defect the device did not conform to the implied warranty, and that the defect was the proximate cause of the injury.

Duty to Recall Defective Devices

The FDA "Class I recall" may be applied to manufacturers of implantable medical devices. The duty to recall extends to the physician or other health care provider, and emerges out of the physician's continuing duty to inform patients of newly discovered dangers of implantable devices and pharmaceutical drugs.

The duty to recall involves physician liability, but not in the commonly understood sense of medical malpractice.

CLINICAL PATHOLOGY LABORATORY

Introduction

For the purpose of this discussion, the term laboratory will be explored in its broadest sense as it relates to human diagnosis and therapy.

Classification

In medicine, laboratory data can be separated into two broad categories. 1) Data produced from examination of parts of the body, e.g., blood, urine, and tissues removed at surgery, are the province of the clinical pathology laboratory in the hospital. 2) On the other hand, data produced by examination of the living body as a whole can be classified into several categories: x-ray and imaging procedures with isotopes; ultrasound; physiological testing using such modalities as electrocardiography, pulmonary function tests, and thermography; psychologic testing and psychiatric evaluations, when instrument dependent.

Testing by Instruments

In testing with instruments, there are four potential sources of deviation or "error" in the results obtained. The import of each of these sources of error will vary with the test system, but each of these four considerations must be evaluated in the assessment of the meaning and significance of the laboratory data obtained. These four potential variables include the following.

The specifications of the instrument, as well as the precision with which it is made. The simplicity or complexity of the instrument will not only profoundly influence the accuracy of the test results, but also the correctness with which these results measure reality. Instruments that are constructed according to more precise specifications with redundancy and feed-back control built into the system to prevent the intrusion of instrument drift or systematic error of mechanical origin from affecting the results produced are more expensive. The manufacturer must, according to the law, have extensively tested the prototype design instrument and published the specifications to ensure reproducibility. However, the user of the instrument should also have data on hand that shows what reproducibility the instrument demonstrated in his hands. Ordinarily, the collection of this data requires weeks, if not months, of testing on site in the purchasing facility before the instrument is phased into use. In addition, the instrument should be continuously monitored during its first year of operation to determine if it continues to perform as warranted when in daily use.

The theory of operation, which is best illustrated by the following two examples. The two most common methods of determining the hemoglobin level of the blood are: 1) measuring the oxyhemoglobin content of the blood after oxidizing the hemoglobin in the blood sample; and 2) measuring the hemoglobin content by first converting it to cyancmethemoglobin. These two methods actually measure two different things. In most cases, there is no practical difference in the results obtained by the two methods. However, there are some conditions in which this difference is important. The oxyhemoglobin method does not measure carboxyhemoglobin or methemoglobin, while the cyanide method does, by combining these values with the reduced and oxygenated hemoglobin to give a total value. It is obvious that in cases in which the CO level of the blood is significant or methemoglobinemia is present, the method of analysis is of critical importance in interpreting the results.

The second example also deals with the hemoglobin level of the blood. Most such values are obtained on a blood sample drawn and subjected to laboratory analysis. In the Intensive Care Unit, however, the hemoglobin oxidation is estimated by the amount and wave lengths of reflected light from a portion of the skin in which the capillaries are close to the surface of the body. This indicates the efficiency of the patient's oxygenation mechanism. This reflectance information can be interpreted and recorded in the chart as a hemoglobin value. It is obviously important to know if the test system measures a component of the blood directly or indirectly, and to know the limits of reliability of the test method used.

The application of the test which, to some extent, overlaps with the theory of operation. The second example noted above also illustrates this problem. "Application" here refers to how the theory of the test is integrated into the test system. Reflectance analysis is a reliable biophysical method, but its precision can be increased if the basic analysand in the test substrate is directly subjected to testing, with the accuracy correspondingly reduced by the presence of an interfering substance between the test substrate and the detecting instrument, e.g., a layer of skin between the detector and the blood.

Deviations or variations also involve consideration of the testing environment. Not only are the space, light, and ambient temperature of the room within which the testing takes place important, but most significant is the quality of the personnel doing the test and the degree of knowledge and expertise they have vis-a-vis the testing process. These will influence the results. It is known, particularly by laboratory managers, that different technicians obtain different results in testing the same specimen, and that the same worker can obtain different results on the same specimen on different occasions. The amount of deviation in the test results attributable to these three variables or "errors" must be known and defined, so as to be able to report with confidence the deviation in the results from the "normal", and the significance of the deviation.

Those fallacies of laboratory testing must be understood as they apply to every type of testing. For example, the radiologist must be confident that the x-ray machines consistently produce the same amount of x-ray energy at the same settings to produce a consistent density and constant shadow pattern, which will denote the presence or absence of disease. The cardiologist must be confident that the ECG technician consistently places the chest electrodes in the same position on the chest, so that reliable interpretations can be made; for example, as to the location of foci of aberrancy in the heart, and derivatively, the probable cause of the aberration in the myocardium or coronary arteries. While interpretation of such test results is indeed part art, and less than certain, it is obvious that no physician can reliably interpret data that are sloppily or imprecisely produced.

Communication

The process of obtaining accurate laboratory data on a patient is a complex one, involving a number of steps. Any misstep can cause an error which intrudes and interferes with the production and utilization of correct and useful laboratory data.

An acceptable process, at least in hospital practice, requires:
- Comprehension of the laboratory data desired by the physician;
- Accurate communication of the order for the test by written or telephone order, and recording it on the patient's chart;
- Communication of the order to the laboratory, specifying the test desired, and identification and pickup of the specimen;
- Correct identification of the patient and specimen obtained;
- Correct identification and processing of the specimen within the laboratory;
- Timely, appropriate, and correct transmission of the test result data to the patient's chart; and
- Communication of the laboratory data to the physician with an explanation so that he will understand the meaning and significance of the data.

Only with the completion of each of these steps in sequence, and with proper advertence, will the laboratory data be of value to the patient and the physician.

Deviations

It is obvious that there are many opportunities for error, delay, and confusion in the testing process. One, a physician is distracted and fails to order the necessary test when needed. A verbal order given directly or by telephone may be misinterpreted by a nurse or other order taker, or a written order may be misinterpreted because it is illegible, vague, or ambiguous. The transmission of the order to the laboratory may not reach its destination because the hard copy requisition was mislaid or mishandled, or more likely today, the order is entered in the computer and never seen again, or entered erroneously.

Once the laboratory has the order in hand and proceeds to implement it, the wrong patient may be identified for the specimen, or the wrong specimen may be obtained for the test desired, or both. While the wrong specimen error is usually readily apparent and quickly corrected, if the specimen is obtained from the wrong patient, the error may not be discovered, and erroneous conclusions and choices are made as to diagnosis and treatment based on the misidentification error.

Assuming correct identification of the patient and specimen are made, another identification error may occur if the specimen (a test tube of blood serum, for example) is misidentified within the laboratory. In this day of multi-specimen analysers, the individual specimens are often specifically identified by position in the instrument, so that if two specimens are reversed in the order in which they are analyzed, the results of one analysis may be falsely attributed to the other patient. Recognition of this source of error has led to the development of various specific individual identification systems for specimen containers; however, such methods are not in universal use, and even this is not infallible as most laboratory installations depend on laboratory personnel to ensure correct identification of specimens and analysis data.

Misidentification

If it can be assumed that the specimen was correctly identified and analyzed, the laboratory must transmit the results to the physician via the patient's chart. This report may be transmitted by hard copy or by a computer system. In either case, the information is sent to the nursing station where the patient charts are kept. The system may call for a laboratory person to individually post each laboratory report on the chart of the patient identified on the report; or, as an alternative, the reports in bulk may be delivered to the nursing station, and the personnel at the station have the duty to place the specific reports in each patient chart. Since each of these methods ultimately depend on people for completion, an error is not only possible, but does occur. The result, at least, is delay in the availability of the report, as this type of error is usually quickly detected and corrected when the physician who ordered the test looks for the result at the time it should be available. However, there are at least two situations when this misidentification error may have serious consequences. The first occurs when the physician adverts only to the test results on the chart without noticing that his patient's name is wrong (not difficult to do with some computer printer generated reports). As a result, he makes erroneous diagnostic or therapeutic choices based on the wrong information.

The second catastrophe occurs when a consultant is called to see the patient and misinterprets the data in the chart because it does not belong to that patient. He is invariably aware that other data may be available for verification. Unfortunately, it may not be in the chart. In either case, the system has failed at the final, and probably crucial, step, i.e., the information has not been communicated to the physician accurately and in timely fashion, and he is unable to act responsibly.

Charting

A corollary of this situation is when the chart is reviewed retrospectively sometime later, as part of a utilization evaluation. Actually, at that time, the chart may appear to be complete, i.e., all the orders are on the order sheet, all the administrative papers are in place, properly made out and signed, and all the lab work that was ordered is reported in the chart. One should be able to assume that the test date and the report date on the laboratory report form accurately represents the date on which the physician received the information. Actually, the transmission of the data to the physician via the patient's chart may have occurred 24 or more hours later, or indeed never occurred and was never noted, because the test specimen had to be referred to an outside laboratory, and the report was added to the chart later in the Medical Records Department. Unless contemporaneous mention is made in the chart that the lab report is still pending, the physician will be assumed to have had the information represented on the report at the time and date of the report. Such an assumption may be very difficult to negate weeks or years later, when the physician's diagnosis and management are under attack by a peer review mechanism or by the courts.

Physician Notification

Since laboratory data has no value unless the physician who ordered the test is aware of it, there is an obligation on the part of laboratory personnel to properly communicate the results of the test to the physician. Ordinarily, this obligation is satisfied by the report system described. In extraordinary circumstances, however, this regular system may not be adequate or appropriate. It may be necessary for the laboratory to communicate directly with the physician and inform him of the results if they are unusual, abnormal, and/or represent a potentially dangerous situation for the patient.

Since the medical technologists and technicians cannot be charged with responsibility for evaluating and determining the data that are incongruent and potentially dangerous, it is the medical and legal responsibility of the laboratory director, who is a physician, to determine "panic values" for each test, which will trigger an immediate review of the test results by the director or an appropriate designate, so that a decision may be made as to whether there should be a prompt, direct communication of the results to the physician. Because of the volume of tests done, or because of the patient population served by some hospital laboratories, the system may allow, on the basis of the panic values in use, the laboratory technician or technologist, without prior review by the laboratory director, to initiate a prompt, direct report to the physician. Another modification of the system found in some hospitals is the reporting of values beyond "panic" to the nursing personnel, who have the responsibility of directly communicating with the physician. This system has the advantage of simultaneously providing the attending physician with the clinical information, and the opportunity to issue appropriate orders forthwith.

Stimulated Testing

A related consideration is the concept of stimulated testing. There are well-known patterns of disease in which abnormal test results cluster. The detection of one chemical aberrancy gives rise to the expectation of associated aberrancies in other chemical determinations, some of which may identify specific medical management problems and therapeutic solutions. As an example, the diabetic who has a high blood sugar may or may not simultaneously have ketoacidosis with associated electrolyte imbalance. Since ketoacidosis is dangerous and potentially lifethreatening, the question arises as to what is the proper laboratory response to the finding of an elevated blood sugar initially.

Panic Values

On the one hand, it would appear sensible to establish "panic values" for blood sugar that would automatically trigger measurement of the serum electrolytes and blood gases when the threshold value is exceeded (or with some procedures, if either the high or low value were passed). This approach makes sense, since the blood specimen is already in the laboratory and can have the added determination performed simply and efficaciously. The other advantage is time-saving for the patient in having a complete metabolic picture, rather than first having the sugar value reported, and then making it necessary to order the additional tests. This requires securing more blood, and finally, the reporting of all the test results. Meanwhile, the patient is in limbo.

The objections to this approach deserve serious consideration. Without automatic response to panic values, there must be an order from the physician before the hospital personnel can "assault and batter" the patient by inserting a needle in his or her vein to obtain a blood sample, or into an artery to obtain a specimen for determination of blood gases. Because originally, laboratory data was produced in a chemically restricted fashion and at relatively high cost, traditionally, the attending physician exclusively reserved the right to order each and every procedure, and the test could not be done without his specific order. The attending physician determined what, if any, laboratory data was needed to help in the diagnosis and treatment of the patient. This has changed with the imposition of "corporate" responsibility, which calls for a share-and-share alike obligation to the patient, and allows such a mechanism to implement the optimum quality of care.

An objection to this automatic procedure is that testing becomes "cookbook", and there will be over-testing based on this automatic test ordering, whether done by a computer, or indeed, even by the physician. On the other hand, some believe, despite the alleged advantages, that it is the physician who should determine what tests are needed based on the available information and his clinical judgment, and when they are to be performed.

Routine Screening

Obviously, there is a certain clinical cultural lag in this matter. In the memory of most senior practicing pathologists, initially, the availability from the early 1960's of automated testing equipment made a tremendous impact on the capability and capacity of the clinical laboratory. The equipment for the commonly ordered chemical determinations now available has a high initial cost, but a very low unit cost, for the test results produced when done on a bulk basis. About 85% of the work load of a typical hospital clinical laboratory is composed of less than 30 test procedures. The common tests are performed in high volume, whether the laboratory is automated or not. When the cost of personnel time is counted for the decision-making process and the selection of specific test patterns for individual patients and their specimens, the individual cost of broad-spectrum chemical testing, e.g., SMA-24, becomes very small. This "automatic" screening procedure produces a chemical profile of the patient that may be indicative of a disease. It is even more useful when it is normal, for then whole categories of diseases can be eliminated from consideration in the differential diagnosis. The virtue of these so-called "negative" values, developed during the initial screening process on admission to the hospital, has been well-known to pathologists for some 35 years, but has apparently been missed by many clinicians, if the recent derogatory pronouncements of the American College of Physicians on routine screening are any indication.

Cost-Effectiveness and Clinical Utility v. Physician Control

On the one hand, the cost-effectiveness and clinical utility of broad-spectrum screening is difficult to deny for the hospitalized patient. On the other hand, the desirability of physician control of the patient's care in the hospital is also difficult to deny. It is obvious that some compromise position is desirable, and such an arrangement has been established in many institutions that satisfies the particular concerns of physician-laboratorians and physician-clinicians alike. Such an intellectual accommodation is particularly desirable in any institution faced with acute clinical response problems.

Aberrant Results

An unusual and innovative approach to a comparable problem has been adopted at some institutions in which not just "panic values", but any aberrant laboratory data triggers its entry into an algorithm that leads to the ordering and performing of additional tests. This has been demonstrated to be useful in the assessment of chemical or hematological values divergent from the usual. Since the system is automatic and not dependent on clinician interaction, the net result is the rapid production of extended laboratory data for the clinician without delay or conscious effort on his part. Many of these programs are in teaching institutions, where the ultimate utility of such an approach to medical management is under evaluation. The ultimate value of this approach is yet to be determined, but some such pattern may well be the practice of the future.

Inappropriate Testing

It is a fact that laboratory tests are ordered inappropriately and used indiscriminately. While every physician will occasionally go off on a diagnostic tangent which usually, in retrospect, was not justified by the patient's condition, it is not such occasional inadvertences that produce legal consequences. It is when an inappropriate, irrational pattern of laboratory use that cannot be clinically justified is continuous. Serious consideration must be given to designating the physician an "outlier", and potentially liable for negligence based on unnecessary testing. Such a reckless and careless pattern of lab use is readily detectable by the experienced, and an explanation to his peers should be demanded and required. Frequently, the mere review by a knowledgeable, yet compassionate, considerate, and helpful, panel of respected physicians on the hospital staff, if possible, is all that is necessary to correct the aberrant pattern of behavior. In circumstances other than in the hospital, it may be necessary to establish a similar expert peer review body to try to control this practice. The local medical society is the obvious body to accomplish this task.

Stat Orders

Consideration has been given to the practice of stat orders. The word "stat" is a contraction of the Latin *statim*, meaning "immediately", and implies: "drop everything else and do it!" In practice, the interpretation of the term stat ranges all the way from "sometime today" to its intended original meaning. It is rare, however, to find stat results of any test ready in less than an hour because of the delay inherent in transmitting the order, obtaining the specimen, completing the analysis, and transmitting the report. Since the actual time required to complete a stat order would depend on the test ordered, the instrumentation available, and the personnel present, it is difficult to generalize on the reasonable expectations within a particular system. Depending on the environment and tradition of the particular test site (the hospital), there may be a pattern of immediate response and prompt reporting, or there may be something considerably less in efficiency and performance. Since the expectation is that a stat order is of great importance to the patient's well-being or survival, and the data is needed as soon as possible, the presumption also is that the physician will be on hand to receive the report as soon as it is available. It is an obvious inconsistency for the physician to order an analysis done "stat", and then not be available if the tradition of the institution is the prompt provision of such data in response to the stat order. On the other hand, it is not inconsistent if the institutional tradition is a period of delay between the issuing of the stat order and the production of the report in a manner usable by the physician.

There is a source of confusion in this matter, however. The so-called "administrative stat" is an order that reaches the laboratory marked stat, but it was not given by the physician as such. The usual explanation is that the original order was lost somewhere in the system by the ward personnel, the nurses, the laboratory personnel, or the computer. Meanwhile, the physician is making rounds, or at least awaiting the results. He expects to have the data in hand in due course. However, it was not being produced in an orderly fashion because of a system failure. Since the welfare of the patient may be significantly influenced by the absence of the data, an administrative stat order is justifiable in order to obtain the data rapidly. In that way, the patient's management may be expeditiously arranged — discharge, surgery to proceed as scheduled, IV fluids changed as needed, etc. — although the consequences for interdepartmental relations may not be salubrious. Such error-induced "stats" should be noted by way of an incident report, and the cause determined and eliminated to enhance good patient care and institutional harmony.

Peer and Utilization Review

In any evaluation or audit of the utilization of the laboratory and its data in a patient record by a third party reviewer, the central question is: "What did the physician know, and when did he know it?" Only a full consideration of the facts in the record surrounding the laboratory report will produce a reasonable and consistent evaluation, and lead to legitimate conclusions as to the quality and pertinence of the medical management and the efficiency of the institution.

Limits of Confidence (Reliability)

Experience ultimately determines when it can be confidently established what circumstances will produce a similar test result, and the probability of a disease being present when the test result is obtained. As an example, one can consider the relationship of an elevated blood sugar to the presence of diabetes mellitus. If an elevated blood sugar is found, the process of differential diagnosis is invoked. Ultimately, the value of the blood sugar in a diabetic reliably establishes the diagnosis. This is possible based on years of experience with the test and the various diseases that had to be considered. This degree of confidence in the test result and its meaning is not present with all testing modalities, however. It is, therefore, incumbent upon the test interpreter to understand the limits of reliability not only of the testing method, but also of the meaning of the test result.

Intergretation and Meaning of Laboratory Data

Once the laboratory test is done and the report made, it is the responsibility of the physician, and frequently the nurse or other practitioner such as a house officer, to interpret the data in the context of the entire case. On occasion, it falls to the court or some other branch of the judicial or administrative system to interpret the record to assess the propriety of the conduct recorded in the chart. Certain principles are necessary to properly evaluate such a record.

For those test systems of less hoary respectability than tests such as blood sugar determination, information may be available that establishes the probability of error that can be expressed in numerical terms as the confidence limits of the analysis. It is often necessary to consider alternative explanations for the actual test result and explore the extent of testing that has been done to establish the differential diagnosis for the test result. For example, the current use of the mass spectrometer/gas cromatograph (MS/GC) to test for drugs of abuse is widespread and has achieved broad acceptance as to reliability and certainty.

However, up to 1984, the chemical literature showed only 30,000 or so organic chemicals that had been defined by this method at a time when more than 65,000 organic chemicals were known to exist. Furthermore, only very limited testing of mixtures of these chemicals for effect on MS/GC results had been accomplished. Yet, this method of testing was in use for screening the urine of military personnel for a very complex mixture of organic and inorganic chemicals. The results of these tests were given compelling weight and probative value in many administrative hearings and trials of accused personnel, with resultant loss of position, pension, and career for many. This is in distinction to the type of testing that is done to detect disease, where other indicators are present. In clinical practice, laboratory testing is not used as the sole screening prccess in the absence of evidence of disease. If objective corroborative evidence is not obtained, it is very difficult to justify drawing deductive inferences from what is, in essence, an inductive scientific prccess. This is not done in medical diagnosis, but is done in the drug screening programs. Rigorous examination of any expert purporting to interpret such screening data is obviously in order in the courtroom.

Laboratory Data in a Judicial Proceeding

In the presentation of any laboratory findings in a judicial proceeding, it is necessary to employ an expert in the field to explain, evaluate, and interpret the data to the finders of fact, the judge or the jury. This expert should be qualified by training, knowledge, understanding, and experience to perform this function objectively, honestly, and without bias. This expert is not an advocate of anyone or anything but the truth. He should be prepared to present his material clearly and in such common English terminology as will illustrate rather than obfuscate. He should consider himself an instructor on behalf of the judicial body, rather than as a special pleader for one side or the other. If he succeeds in doing so, his testimony will not only be valuable to the processes of justice, but he need not fear any type or form of cross-examination. Insofar as he fails to attain such objectivity, he may indeed fear the consequences of cross-examination.

Admonitions

The side presenting the expert to the judicial body should have had adequate consultation, so that the expert will be prepared to answer questions necessary to present the material most advantageously. Adequate preparation will also equip the attorney to understand the material sufficiently to integrate the results into the presentation of the case. It will prevent the surprise that occurs when the expert testifies to scmething other than what the attorney expected. The mode of presentation of the material is critical; what may be complex and obscure when described verbally, may be greatly simplified and clarified when illustrated either by a diagram, or by a photograph or drawing. Even the presentation of the material in a pictorial outline of the topic, or as labels in a drawing that depicts the interrelationship of the concepts, can be marvelously illuminating to the judge or jury trying to understand unfamiliar material. When one is dealing with inherently pictorial material — e.g., the anatomy of the muscles of the body, or the size, relationships, and shape of the internal organs of the body - there is really no substitute for a clearly well-labeled diagram. When the witness is describing the effect of disease on these structures, reparative surgery, or trauma inflicted on the patient, the medical illustration unquestionably is the best way to demonstrate the information so that the judge or jury can best understand it. It is advisable to engage a professional medical artist. The graphic or computer printout of the testing instrument is a valuable device for the illustration of how the test results were obtained and their meaning. All demonstrative evidence should be chosen for its illustrative value in presenting factual information. It facilitates understanding. Such evidence can often be presented to the judicial body as enlarged picture boards easily seen across the room, or as projected 35 mm. slides. They can also be reproduced as large photographic prints that can be taken into a jury room for study. The enlarged boards or projections can be used as in a lecture to illustrate the points made by the expert witness and to orient the trier of facts to the nature and significance of the pertinent findings. Such illustrations should be used to present the litigant's point of view. They should never be used to distort the meaning of the test results, for the simple reason that this mechanism is also available to the other side. While demonstrative evidence is very effective in presenting the facts favorable to the presenter, it is equally effective in demonstrating attempts to disseminate or unfairly use the data and not objectively interpret it, or to skew the evidence dishonestly. The printed or pictorial readout regularly produced by the testing instrument is objective, unbiased, and inherently reliable as an expression of the results obtained. As such, it is particularly valuable in presenting the scientific facts. These objective reports can be interpreted by any knowledgeable expert for either side and, as such, are factual presentations of information.

In cross-examination, it is perfectly legitimate to inquire into the nature of the expert's qualifications. Not infrequently, the expert's bibliography is full of padding and puffery as to papers published. The extent of the expert's knowledge of the nature of the scientific matter under examination, or of the test being described, is also a source of legitimate exploration, particularly in trying to determine his knowledge as to the sources of error in the test procedure. The exploration of his knowledge of all of the possible interpretations of the test results is also legitimate; in particular, the incidence of rare and unusual causes of the results. The expert testifying in a new field or area of technology, such as thermography, should be questioned on the nature of the test system, the amount of information that is available on the scope and applicability of the test procedure, and the controversies surrounding its application. The honest expert will freely discuss the characteristics of the test system, and will justify his reliance on the test data while suitably defining the objective confidence limits that the testing method demonstrates. In any event, the cross-examiner will have to prepare for the exploration of the opposing expert's knowledge and attitudes by an in-depth study of the subject and consultation with his own expert, so as to be aware of the peculiarities of the field and the special meanings and interpretations inherent in it.

Conclusion

Laboratory or scientific data has certain characteristics that make it of material, and occasionally, compelling value to the clinician. Proper utilization depends on efficient prcduction and communication of laboratory data. In the legal process, it is essential to present such data by the use of expert testimony. An understanding of the utility and limitations of biophysical testing is necessary for the proper and just interpretation of the data in the courtroom. Scientific evidence is particularly adaptable to demonstrative techniques, which should be used at every opportunity to present informative, compelling, and useful evidence.

DERMATOLOGY

Introduction

Dermatology residency provides training in clinical dermatology, dermatopathology, microbiology, and several other aspects of clinical practice or academia. During the three year residency, unless time is spent in a private office setting, very little is learned about dermatological liability.

As a general rule, dermatology is a calm practice. For the most part, the patients are healthy and happy. They come in with problems which are usually easily diagnosed, and they are helped. There is not much "life and death" in the day-to-day practice of dermatologists.

Malpractice Environment

Medical malpractice insurance premiums are among the lowest in the field of dermatology, unless specific surgical procedures are being practiced, such as hair transplantation, dermabrasion, or plastic surgery. There should be no complacency, however. Dermatologists get sued frequently, and are often named in multiple party lawsuits.

Recent data from the Southern California Physicians Insurance Exchange (as of June 6, 1988) shows that the average settlement of a dermatology claim is approximately $30,000.00. Of 264 closed claims that were reviewed, 204 were closed with no indemnity payment, 62 cases were settled, and only one case was tried. This data may help to explain the relatively low insurance premiums for dermatologists.

The types of claims made against dermatologists helps to establish ways to attempt prevention of lawsuits. Dermatology claims fall into several categories: negligent treatment or failing to treat; adverse results; failure to diagnose; drug reactions; and miscellaneous others (e.g., slip and fall, fainting). Most claims probably stem from any of the following situations: a poor physician-patient relationship; the inability of the physician to realize the limits of his capabilities; the patient's anger; colleague interference; the delegation of duties to a non-physician staff member; or simply monetary gain incentive.

Psoriasis

An example of negligent treatment would be a patient with psoriasis, who comes to the office two or three times a week for ultraviolet light, and who might know the nurse, but rarely sees the physician. If the psoriasis is not improving, or for some reason is actually worsening and the physician is not aware of it, liability danger looms.

Scarring

An adverse result type of claim may include scarring, which should be expected after dermatological surgery. However, if the patient was not informed of this outcome, or there is a significantly different scar from what the patient was led to believe there would be, the dermatologist may be a target. For this reason, as will be reviewed below, a surgical consent pre-operatively may be helpful. Unpopular scars include keloid or hypertrophic scars, hyperpigmentation (darkening of the skin, which can occur after routine dermatologic surgery or destruction of lesions with liquid nitrogen or trichloracetic acid), persistently erythematous scars, or atrophic scars. Generally, scarring type claims should be easily avoided with both a good physician-patient relationship and pre-operative counseling.

Light Therapy Burns

Another common adverse result claim is the burning of a patient's skin during light therapy, a commonly employed treatment modality used by many dermatologists. Frequently, this is administered by staff members and not the physician himself.

Recurrences

If a lesion is surgically removed and it recurs (as can happen in a number of benign and malignant skin growths), there may be liability unless the patient was informed of this possibility and it was documented. Likewise, in inflammatory skin conditions that are apt to recur or be chronic, patients should be informed to avoid misleading them that a cure exists.

Malignant Melanoma

Failure to diagnose a malignant melanoma is the cause of the highest monetary settlements decided against dermatologists. This "mistake" may be much easier than it sounds! There are numerous ways to have this claim successfully made against a practicing dermatologist. For example, if an obviously benign type of growth, such as a wart or a skin tag, is removed from the left shoulder of a patient and not sent for pathological confirmation, and six years later, an unrelated melanoma is discovered on this patient's left shoulder, there is potential liability. Another example would be a slightly suspicious small, flat freckle that is observed during an office visit for an unrelated problem. The patient and the dermatologist decide to wait and observe the behavior of this lesion over the next 6 to 18 months. If the patient does not return for follow-up visits, and the freckle turns malignant, there are grounds for a claim. Usually, such a claim is not simply a case of a dermatologist failing to recognize a melanoma.

Drug Reactions

Drug reaction type claims against dermatologists are common. Many antibiotics are used by skin specialists for acne, skin infections, and some inflammatory conditions. Obviously, there are many side effects from antibiotics, some quite severe. Even though a reaction is not necessarily avoidable, the ensuing lawsuit may be prevented as will be discussed below. Other medications that are potentially dangerous include dapsone, a sulfone used for various bullous disorders; griseofulvin and ketoconazole used for fungal infections; and prednisone and other immunosuppressives used extensively in dermatology for various eczematous and inflammatory conditions. Adverse reactions may range from liver toxicity due to dapsone, male breast enlargement and impotence from ketoconazole, and aseptic necrosis of the hip from corticosteroids.

Office Mishaps

Miscellaneous claims include the type of lawsuit that could hit any type of business; for example, slip and fall. In the dermatologist's office, the height of examination tables, footstools, and support for a patient having light treatment are all areas that need attention. After treating a patient who has been in a reclining position, care should be taken that he or she not sit or stand too quickly. It is common for patients to have vasovagal reactions after needle sticks for blood drawing or for anesthesia. This situation should be anticipated.

Recently in my office, a patient signed in at the front desk and looked at the computer monitor that my receptionist was working with. She happened to see a list of patients with her same last name, and realized that her ex-husband's new wife was also a patient! She was obviously shaken by this realization. The legal implications of patient confidentiality started to race through my mind, although I felt better when I realized that nothing was revealed about the nature of the new wife's problem. This demonstrates, though, the fragile nature of the emotional aspect of going to a medical office.

Risk Management and Prevention

Knowing these potential legal pitfalls, the dermatologist should be able to formulate his version of risk management and prevention. First of all, as I hinted earlier, promoting a good physician-patient relationship is probably the most important aspect of risk management, not to mention the best way to make practicing medicine enjoyable. We all know stories of the medically incompetent general practitioner who never gets sued because his patients love him. Every patient should be treated as an important individual; their questions, fears, and doubts should be anticipated and answered fully. Eye contact, frequent smiling, and incorporating the patient as a partner in his or her care are all important measures.

Innovative Procedures

Knowing one's own limits is essential — using patients to try new procedures can be risky, and doing a procedure that one does not feel totally comfortable with is unwise. I have found that patients appreciate referral to a more qualified subspecialist, and almost always return to me for their next dermatological problem. Also, constant monitoring of the office staff and their work is important. I once had a medical assistant who developed her own post-operative instructions, which differed significantly from mine: A physician must know the limitations of his staff, as well as himself.

Documentation

The keys to preventative dermatological practice are similar to the guidelines for all specialties of medicine. This includes documentation, which should be adequate, complete, objective, and legible. Consent forms, or verbal consent with documentation, should be routine for any dermatological procedure. For surgery, this should include anesthetics, lab testing, and the knowledge that the type of scar cannot be determined before the operation. Photos of lesions or suspicious items should be taken if possible. When starting medications, the patient should be informed of the common side effects and potential risks.

Conclusion

In spite of all these potential pitfalls, the practice of dermatology is very rewarding. If risk management is incorporated into the daily routine of practice, the dermatologist can feel assured that he is doing everything possible to minimize liability, and therefore, can concentrate on practicing good medicine.

DRUG THERAPY

Drug Prescribing

Before any drug is prescribed, the prescribing physician should ask him/
herself a number of questions which, if answered correctly, would help prevent
the 12-17% of malpractice cases that result from drug therapy. These questions
are as follows:

1. Is the drug necessary?

In a well-known Connecticut case, a young boy was admitted for a tonsillec-
tomy and during a three day hospital stay, he received injectable vitamins and
ended up with a paralyzed arm. The court found liability because it said the vitamins were not necessary.

2. What class of drugs should be utilized for the particular patient? Are there
any less risky alternatives?

Obviously, the least potent drug is the best, and the one with the least side
effects is preferable. If aspirin is satisfactory for a patient with rheumatoid arthritis,
there is no need to begin the patient's therapy with steroids and run the risk of
serious side effects. Certainly, the medication which is efficacious and has the least
risk of side effects is the preferred one to use.

3. Has the patient been asked about previous drug allergies?

Do not ignore the patient's response to this question. In a New York case,
the physician ignored a penicillin reaction which occurred 15 years before and was
found liable for the patient's anaphylaxis. In another case, a physician was held
liable for failure to skin test before giving tetanus antitoxin. In a California case,
a patient was given penicillin for mumps, developed anaphylaxis, and died. The
physician was liable because the court said penicillin was inappropriate treatment
for mumps.

4. Is there any possibility of interactions with any other drug - potentiation
or incompatibility - which the patient may be taking at the same time (this includes
over-the-counter drugs)?

For example, one of the most frequent causes of liability is bleeding caused
by a combination of aspirin and Coumadin without appropriate warning to the
patient. Certainly, barbiturates should never be prescribed when the patient is a
known alcoholic or has been drinking heavily. Succinylchloride should not be used
in injured patients because potassium is apparently released, and with the depolar-
ization caused by succinylchloride, the patient can develop cardiac arrest.

5. Are there any secondary ingredients in the drug, such as sulphite or sodium,
which may affect particular patients?

Yellow No. 5 dye is a potent allergen, and even though it is not in the drug
per se, it may be found in the capsule. Many drugs contain sodium in varying
amounts, and physicians should be cautious in prescribing them to patients with
cardiac failure.

6. Is it necessary for laboratory tests to be performed before prescribing a
particular drug? Are those laboratory tests reliable, and have the results been
scrutinized? Should the tests be repeated after a certain period of time in order
to monitor the possible development of serious complications while the patient
continues to take that particular drug?

Complete blood counts are periodically necessary during long-term therapy
with many drugs, and eye examinations may be necessary during some therapies
such as chloroquine treatment. It is imperative for the doctor to monitor ordered
lab tests and determine whether they are reliable, and then act on them. Ear

tests, for example, are necessary for someone on long-term kanamycin or streptomycin treatment to prevent ototoxicity.

7. What dosage should be prescribed?

Under and overdosage of antibiotics are frequent causes of malpractice litigation. An overdose of drugs is the second largest category of liability cases involving medications, with analgesics leading the list, followed by hormones, antibiotics, and sedatives. Heparin has also been troubling in a number of cases. Be certain of the correct dose with the decimal point in right place.

8. What is the desired route of administration? Can the drug be administered orally? And if not, what precautions should be taken for other routes of administration?

Certainly, vitamins should never be given parenterally if the patient can tolerate oral medication. If an injection injury occurs, the courts would not look favorably upon such innocuous medications having been administered in such a manner.

9. Should the patient be warned of any adverse or toxic effects which may affect his or her driving abilities, concentration, etc.?

Antihistamines and some analgesics are notorious for their sedative properties, and patients should be warned about driving cars or operating dangerous machinery. Failure to warn the patient was used to find liability when a physician prescribed chloramphenicol, and the patient developed aplastic anemia. The injection of radio-opaques with subsequent development of adverse effects has been another problem area.

10. Can a generic form of the drug be prescribed, or is it one of the "problem" generic drugs? What are the laws in your state in regard to substitution?

Some of the problem generic drugs have been antibiotics, anticonvulsants, and digitalis preparations.

11. How can I be sure my drug orders are being carried out according to my instructions?

In a famous New York case, a doctor ordered the drug of choice for a patient with high blood pressure, but it was never given, and the patient died. The physician was held liable.

12. How long a period of time should a prescription be written for?

The physician should determine for how long the prescription should be written, and specifically state it in the orders or on the prescription form. Don't sign any open-ended prescriptions. A number of years ago, this author testified in a case where a physician gave an open-ended prescription to a patient for an analgesic, and the patient became addicted. The physician had not see the patient for three years. Normally, a prescription should not be written for more than 30 days.

Informed Consent

Informed consent in regard to drug therapy is the physician's responsibility and should not be delegated. The doctor should always be courteous and have consideration for the patient. He should present the information in an intelligible manner suitable for that particular patient's understanding. False assurances should not be given to the patient. In an emergency, the physician should explain the situation to a close relative or the legal guardian. Always make a record of what was said at the time it was said. General rules in regard to the scope of disclosure are as follows:

• The patient should be informed of his diagnosis.
• The nature of the contemplated treatment.
• The risks of that treatment.

- The prognosis if treated or not.
- Any alternative methods of treatment.

A general rule of thumb is that the more unusual the treatment, the greater the obligation of the physician to explain the therapeutic plan more thoroughly. These rules apply to all drug therapies, including recommendations by the physician for over-the-counter medicines (e.g., aspirin for a coronary patient). The rules are particularly important if the drug is experimental, or if the indication for use is not in the package insert.

Adverse Drug Reactions

According to Nelson S. Irey, M.D., a nationally renowned expert in the field of adverse drug reactions, "difficulties in evaluating drug reaction cases have arisen from the following:

- Failure to study time relationships between drugs and disease markers.
- Failure to rule out "other than drug' causes.
- Failure to use clinical laboratory data.
- Lack of communication between clinician and pathologist.

The successive steps of (1) evaluating temporal eligibility, (2) considering the points of differential diagnosis, and (3) using the various means of selecting and linking the drug to the reaction constitute a series of criteria to be met before the allegation of the drug relationship is validated."

A study was done at Johns Hopkins University several years ago, in which a research team reviewed the chart of every single patient who was admitted to the general medical service of the hospital during a three month period. Results of the Hopkins study indicated that 17% of the patients had an adverse reaction to some medication.

In a study performed by the National Association of Insurance Commissioners of over 24,000 closed claims in a single year, the greatest number of drug claims were due to allergic reactions, with antibiotics leading the list, followed by analgesics, hormones, psychotherapeutics, and agents affecting the blood, mainly anticoagulants.

The next largest group of cases in the drug category was due to overdose, with analgesics leading the list, followed by hormones, antibiotics, and sedative-hypnotics. Inadequate dose was in fifth place. The inadequate dose category was led by antibiotics.

The third largest category in the drug area was giving the patient the wrong drug, with hormones leading the list, followed by CNS depressants, agents affecting the blood, and anticonvulsants.

The fourth category was improper method of administration, with primary systemic agents followed by hormones, CNS depressants, and antibiotics. Antibiotics appear in every list. As a matter of fact, antibiotics caused three times more claims during this period of time than any other drug category.

The sixth category was giving a drug to the wrong patient, with antibiotics again at the top of the list, followed by hormones and analgesics. The next category was adverse interactions. Every single one of these claims during this period of time could have been prevented, because they were all the same. In one case, for example, the patient was on Coumadin, and the physician either forgot or neglected to tell the patient that he should not take aspirin.

The last category was prescription error, and this, again, largely involved antibiotics.

Drug Interactions

One of the frequent causes of drug reactions is the interaction of one drug with another. A drug may interfere with another drug by altering absorption, distribution, metabolism, or excretion. Absorption is usually pH-dependent and may be altered by the addition of another drug that changes the pH of the original medicine. Absorption can also be altered by surfactants or by chelation with metal ions; for example, tetracyclines with di- or trivalent metals (e.g., dicalcium phosphate).

Distribution may be affected when two or more ccmpounds compete for the same protein binding sites, since only the unbound drug is freely diffusible and active. The drug which is bound more strongly will displace the other drug. Antihistamines, for example, may displace cardiovascular agents such as norepinephrine; salicylates may displace anticoagulants such as Coumadin derivatives.

The rate of metabolism has a marked effect on the duration and intensity of drug actions. Most drugs are metabolized in the liver where they are either inactivated or converted from lipid soluble drugs into water soluble forms for excretion by the kidneys. This is accomplished either through conjugation or by enzyme induction. Any drugs that can have an adverse effect on the liver may be capable of changing the metabolism of other drugs through a possible effect on the liver microsomal enzymes. Phenobarbital, for example, may lower plasma levels of diphenylhydantoin and bishydroxycoumarin.

Excretion via the intestinal contents may be enhanced by laxatives or cathartics, and excretion via the urine by pH changes. Acidic drugs such as nitrofurantoin are excreted faster when the urinary pH is alkaline, whereas basic drugs such as amphetamines are excreted when the urinary pH is on the acidic side. Commonly-used drugs such as ammonium chloride and sodium bicarbonate are used to alter the urinary pH, or when it is necessary to enhance excretion via the urinary system. Some other factors that can affect the pharmacologic actions of the drug are: size of the crystal or particle; form of the agent - solution, salt, and so on; vehicle; coatings; degree of hydration; diluents; impurities or contaminants; viscosity; sustained release forms; solubility; container; stability; quantity of active ingredient; allergenic substances; toxicity; surface tension; storage conditions; flavoring and coloring agents; and melting point.

Conclusion

It is obvious that most malpractice cases involving drugs can be prevented. Constantly reminding oneself of several basic questions before prescribing any drug is the best prophylaxis.

EMERGENCY CARE
FLIGHT TRANSPORTATION

Pre-Hospital Care of the Patient Ground Transportation

Unique to emergency medicine is caring for the patient who is "in the field" at the scene of an accident or medical incident, or at his or her own home. It is one thing for a physician to evaluate and treat a patient who is physically present before him. It is quite another when the patient's condition is being reported via radio communications to the base hospital by EMT-paramedics. Upon this information given by a third person, the physician must make treatment decisions.

To date, there have been no nationwide standards developed governing transport of patients to the hospital from a scene. In most states, the authority to promulgate rules and regulations regarding transporting patients has been delegated to a local Emergency Medical Services Authority (EMSA). The guidelines created by the local EMSA define the scope of practice allowed EMT-paramedics in that jurisdiction. However, in most situations, the ultimate decision-making authority and responsibility have been reserved to the base hospital physician.

Anti-Dumping Rules

The Consolidated Budget Reconstruction Act (COBRA) is an attempt by Congress to describe guidelines restricting the transfer of patients for economic reasons. It requires that a patient approaching the emergency department (in person or from a scene) be evaluated for the presence or absence of an emergency, regardless of that patient's ability (or usually inability) to pay for the services. If one of the statutorily defined emergent conditions exist, the handling of the patient must conform to the law.

The anti-dumping provisions of COBRA set minimum standards for emergency medical care. This law governs hospitals with an emergency department wherein a patient with an emergency medical condition seeks medical care. If such a patient is "transferred" from the health care facility to another facility or is discharged, the patient may recover damages for "personal harm" if the condition worsens during or after such transfer or discharge. The patient must prove only that the condition was not "stabilized" at the time of transfer, and that the condition deteriorated due to transfer.

In order to avoid liability, the attending physician, or other medical personnel at the hospital, must sign a "certification that, based upon the reasonable risks and benefits to the patient, and based upon the information available at the time, the medical benefits reasonably expected from the provision of appropriate medical treatment at another facility outweigh the increased risks" of transfer. Presumably, if the patient is discharged to out-patient care at home, the benefits of these alternatives outweigh further care within the facility. In addition to the certification requirement, the transfer must also be an "appropriate transfer". Although the signed certification is a simple enough procedure for the hospital to incorporate within its medical record forms, the requirements which will satisfy the transfer being "appropriate" may not be.

The criteria required to effectuate an "appropriate transfer" include all of the following: 1) "the receiving facility. . .has available space and qualified personnel. . .has agreed to accept transfer. . .and to provide appropriate medical treatment"; 2) "the transferring hospital provides. . .appropriate medical records of (its) examination and treatment"; 3) "transfer is effected through qualified personnel and equipment"; and 4) "such other requirements as the Secretary (of Health and Human Services) may find necessary. . ." Presumably, the physician or other medical personnel who transfers the patient has the requisite knowledge of the staffing and competence of the receiving facility, and has sought agreement for acceptance by the receiving facility prior to transfer. These requirements seem applicable whether the receiving facility be an out-patient clinic, nursing home, day care program, or a more intensive treatment center.

At least 19 states have laws on the books to curb the hospital practice. This federal law seems to preempt state law which "directly conflicts with any of its requirements". It further provides for federal jurisdiction and allows the injured individual to obtain "such equitable relief as is appropriate", allowing the federal court discretion to award damages it considers to be warranted. Legal actions may be brought "two years after the date of the violation". How such provisions will be interpreted in light of tort reform legislation and shorter state statutes of limitation remains to be determined by the courts.

A patient who suffers "personal harm", resulting from violation of provisions of this law, will be entitled to those damages allowed under the state's substantive law of personal injury and wrongful death statutes. In addition to these damages, penalties of up to $25,000 per violation against the hospital and involved physician alike are applicable to provider hospitals and their employed or contracted physicians. As the penalty provision is for up to $25,000 per violation, a penalty can be quite significant if the court interprets each departure from the statute by the care provider to be a separate violation. For instance, if the receiving hospital was not notified in order to gain approval for the transfer, the medical records did not accompany the patient, and a certification was not signed, penalities may be up to $75,000 against the hospital, with a like amount imposed against the physician. Each state, however, has been left to adopt these provisions to the extent they choose, and enforce the provisions according to a mechanism of their own choosing.

Guidelines

In the pre-hospital care of a patient, the physician must be able to evaluate the unseen patient. He must also be aware of the local EMSA guidelines, and yet be flexible enough to recognize when deviations from the guidelines need to be done because it is in the patient's best interests to make the change. In essence, the base hospital physician, in evaluating and treating the unseen patient, takes the patient as if the worst case scenario existed and acts on that worst case scenario.

Police Involvement

The police may, with or without arrest, want to redirect a patient's transport to another facility. Even without making an arrest, the police may try to redirect the patient's transport. It is important for the base hospital physician to make the decision to allow or refuse the transport based on the medical risk to the patient. The police have the authority to enforce the law, but they may be exceeding that authority when they interfere with providing emergency care to an injured patient, and that interference could lead to loss of life or limb. It is the base hospital physician who should have the authority to make decisions regarding medical treatment of the patient.

The base hospital physician must know the local EMSA guidelines, so that he can recognize when a change in protocol is being requested and reply accordingly. If there is a requested change in accepted protocol, then the physician must decide that in allowing the change to be implemented, it must be to the patient's benefit, and will not increase the risk to the patient in terms of loss of life or limb.

If there is a possibility that allowing this change in protocol would harm the patient medically, the base hospital physician must notify the police that their plan of action carries an increased medical risk to the patient. The physician must be convinced that the police do understand how severe the risk is to the patient. If the police continue to insist on transporting the patient to a more distant facility (thus increasing the time before the patient is evaluated and treated in a fully-staffed emergency department), then the base hospital physician and the EMT-paramedics must make their objections known and unambiguous in both a written record and verbally where communications are recorded. However, in this stalemate, the EMT-paramedics would probably be required by police authority to transport the patient to the facility the police requested.

While transporting the patient, the base hospital physician should make it clear to the EMT-paramedics that if the patient should rapidly deteriorate, then they should detour to the nearest paramedic receiving facility and notify the police as to why they are doing so. The physician should also inform the EMT-paramedics that they are under no duty and can refuse to perform any specific intervention required by the police that is not for a medical reason, e.g., if the patient is not violent, the EMT-paramedics would not be required to restrain the patient just for police convenience. The important factors to consider in these decisions are the mechanism of injury sustained and the patient's best interests.

Multiple Injuries

In accidents which carry with them the high likelihood of multiple injuries that may not be immediately apparent, the patient should probably be stabilized at a trauma center as per protocol before being sent to a specialty center, if necessary. "Long distance" evaluation of this type of patient and careful monitoring are critical. Also, given this situation of choosing a hospital, the patient, although in pain, may be able to make an informed decision about what he or she wants to have done. The patient, if able, should have some input into this transport decision. In general, EMSA guidelines will allow for some patient input, so long as it does not jeopardize the patient or the team transporting the patient.

The base hospital physician's decision must be predicated on a careful consideration of how the patient sustained the injury, and by the patient's ability to consent for treatment. The physician must determine, and the patient must demonstrate, that he or she can make a voluntary, knowing, and intelligent decision about the situation. The patient must be able to choose.

If the patient is able to decide and demonstrates that he or she arrived at the choice in a rational manner, then the patient should be taken to the facility he or she chooses. If the patient cannot make a rational decision based on the two

choices potential "loss of limb" versus "loss of life" then the base hospital physician must authorize transport according to the patient's best interests. Here,
because the mechanism of injury suggests potential, undetected injuries which,
if left unstabilized, could be life-threatening, the physician would send the patient
to the trauma center to be stabilized initially.

Treatment of an HMO Subscriber

In an HMO, the provider has contracted with the individual patient to provide certain health care services. Here, the HMO will care for its patient, but is
requesting that the patient be transferred to its own facility. The emergency department physician must consider the decreasing probability of a successful reimplantation, given the increasing time for surgery, as against the patient bearing the
full cost of the bill, since the HMO usually will not pay for unauthorized care.

The emergency department physician's decision to authorize the transport
will be guided by the success at reimplanting, the physiologic stability of the patient,
and the patient's decision. If the patient is hemodynamically stable and other injuries have been ruled out so that the patient could tolerate the transport, and if
the patient has remained competent and can make an informed decision about
his or her care, then if the patient decides to be transported to the HMO facility,
the physician could authorize the transport. The patient would have to be well-
informed that with the increased time in transport, there is a corresponding decrease
at success in the patient's ultimate survival. The patient also needs to know that
the HMO refused to authorize treatment, and if the patient had chosen to remain
in the reimplantation center, he or she would incur the full medical costs. If the
patient cannot make a competent informed decision as to treatment, then the emergency department physician must do so.

Pre-Hospital Care of the Patient — Aeromedical Transport

Aeromedical transport by helicopter or airplane is a mode of transporting
patients needing care to a specialty care center, or to deliver available technology
to an outlying area to care for a patient. Interestingly, although there are more
than 200 hospital-based aeromedical transport programs in existence today, there
is no general medical consensus on procedures. Criteria regarding what patient
to transport and when to transport are being worked out now.

Some of the medicolegal problems inherent in these circumstances can best
be presented by virtue of a fictional case involving a 53-year-old patient who
presents to the local hospital's emergency department with a chief complaint of
chest pain. This 40 bed hospital with limited intensive care capability is in the mountains and is located 70 miles from the closest major urban center. This urban center is also across the state line. The patient is evaluated by the emergency department
physician. An EKG reveals an acute myocardial infarction, and there is no cardiology staff available. A tertiary care center located in the urban center has helicopter
services available to transport patients. This center also has tissue plasminogen
activator (TPA) capabilities. The ER physician offers to contact the tertiary care
center to accept the patient in transfer for an expanded range of care. The patient
agrees. Since the hospital is in the mountains, ground transport by ambulance
may take up to three hours. Helicopter transport will take one-third of that time.
With this range, refueling is unnecessary. The emergency department physician
contacts the hospital base physician at the tertiary care center, and that physician

agrees to the transport of the patient to them as the receiving facility. The helicopter is available and is dispatched. The flight team consists of the pilot, a nurse, and a cardiology fellow. The team arrives 45 minutes later at the outlying hospital.

At this point, any one of a number of physicians could be legally responsible for the care of the patient. The emergency department physician remains legally responsible for the patient until he transfers the patient's care to another physician. This could be the flight physician, the helicopter base physician, or the admitting physician at the receiving hospital. Here, there is a flight physician on board. The ER physician is able to transfer legal responsibility to the flight physician when he signs out to that physician upon his arrival.

In many air and ground transports, no physician travels with the transport team. In this situation, when the emergency department physician contacts the helicopter base physician, and that physician agrees to transport the patient, then the helicopter physician assumes legal responsibility for the patient when the flight team arrives at the hospital that is transferring the patient. The hospital base physician remains legally responsible during the flight and during the initial evaluation at the receiving hospital. The helicopter base physician transfers legal responsibility to the admitting physician in the receiving facility when the patient arrives and is admitted.

It has now been almost two hours since the patient began experiencing chest pain. The flight team evaluates the patient. The flight physician decides that since the optimal time to give TPA is within the first three hours, they will offer TPA now. He gets the patient to consent to the procedure.

The flight physician, who is now legally responsible for the patient's care, is also responsible for getting informed consent to TPA, not the emergency department physician. Informed consent in this setting is suspect. The patient is critically ill; the only way to optimally treat the patient is to transport immediately; the optimal time to give TPA is running out. Given the urgency of the situation, in hindsight, the patient's decision to accept or refuse treatment would appear to be made hastily and under duress. Given the clinical setting, this is the best way to increase this patient's chances of a good outcome. To refuse might be seen as an unintelligent choice.

The flight physician should explain the risks, benefits, and alternatives to treatment to the patient. The physician must document this informed consent. Unless the patient adamantly refuses and understands that he is giving up the best chance for a good outcome, the physician should proceed to give TPA.

The flight physician gives the patient TPA before the flight team takes off. When giving TPA, the physician has performed a procedure in a hospital. He may not have privileges to practice in this hospital. Today, for a physician to use a hospital facility and supplies, he needs to have privileges to practice in that hospital. In the rare situation that this flight physician does have hospital privileges, this would not be a problem. It is more usual that no one on the flight team has privileges to practice in that hospital.

In this scenario, the flight physician may also be practicing medicine without a state license. The flight team crossed state lines to transport the patient. The physician performed a procedure; that is, practiced medicine. This becomes an issue, especially with the use of shared services where a number of hospitals get together and create a helicopter service. This setup can serve a large geographic area where state lines may be crossed. Thus, the flight physician should have a license to practice in those states within the aeromedical catchment area.

These issues of practicing without privileges or without a license will come up any time anyone on the flight team, not just the flight physician, does anything to the patient, other than wheel him or her to the helicopter and take off. These same issues come up when any member of the flight team discontinues anything done to the patient by the hospital staff while the flight team remains on that facility's grounds.

Lack of hospital privileges may pose a significant problem. Certain hospitals may refuse to allow the flight team to be called at all because they have no privileges. This is even if it is in the patient's best interests to be transported and ground transport would take too long. Other hospitals may allow the team to land to transport the patient, but refuse to allow the team to do any procedures. Most hospitals, happy to have the aeromedical transport service, will allow the flight team to do what is necessary and have not considered the issue of hospital privileges.

The best situation (although it may be unreasonable) would be that any medical personnel who fly with the aeromedical transport team would obtain privileges at all hospitals that may use the service. They would also obtain a license to practice in any state to which the helicopter may fly. The other alternative would be to have the helicopter base hospital get provisional privileges or consulting staff privileges for its flight physician at all hospitals that could potentially use the service. If necessary, the privilege could be limited to those procedures medically necessary in preparing for a flight.

If the flight physician is not allowed to do a procedure which is medically necessary to safeguard the patient in flight, then he can refuse to transport the patient. Alternatively, the flight physician could comply with the rules of the hospital, but once a patient is moved to the helicopter, do the planned procedure.

The flight physician has obtained the consent of the patient to do a procedure. If he is not allowed to do it, then he could refuse to transport if the procedure was one that is necessary to keep the patient safe in flight. Or, the team could remove the patient from the hospital, and while in the helicopter, do what was planned.

EMERGENCY ROOM

Treatment Without "Consent"

In the emergency room, a physician will often need to evaluate and treat a patient where the only evidence of consent for treatment is that the patient arrived seeking to be treated. Some physicians are reluctant to treat such a patient, and they consider withholding all needed medications before getting written consent documents executed to any and all possible procedures the patient may require. An example of this is not giving pain medications to an individual with a fractured hip before trying to get written documents consenting for the needed surgical procedure. Other physicians feel that the mere presence of a patient in their emergency room gives them the tacit approval to do whatever they feel is medically indicated. This is sometimes over the patient's objections. Neither of these extremes is entirely acceptable medically or legally.

One exception to the general rule that informed consent be obtained before treating a patient is the emergency situation — a condition which threatens life or limb if not treated immediately. It is important for the physician to recognize that a true emergency does exist. Once recognized, the physician must act immediately to evaluate and treat the patient, even though no documents have been executed. If the physician does not recognize the emergency, or does not act in a timely manner, he would be negligent in not providing the basic accepted care. On the other hand, if no true emergency existed and the patient was able to give consent, and the physician evaluated and treated the patient, then he has no defense to a charge of assault, battery, or negligence.

In the emergency setting, another aspect of informed consent comes to the fore. Can a patient who is experiencing physical pain and mental anguish, and is dyspneic, diaphoretic, and hypotensive, give a valid consent to be treated or refuse to be treated? Even if the patient is alert and oriented to person, place, time, and situation, experiencing that degree of pain would make it impossible for the patient to knowingly and intelligently give consent. Or, the patient's mind may be so focused on getting rid of the noxious stimuli that any intervention that promised to relieve them would be agreeable. Consent would not be voluntary then, since the patient's will is more easily overcome. However, under the law, an adult patient who is alert and oriented to person, place, time, and situation is presumed to be competent to make treatment decisions about and for him or herself, given that no emergency exists.

In treating patients who arrive in the emergency room, the physician must obtain informed consent for treatment when it can be obtained without compromising the patient's status. The physician must recognize and act on a true emergency, even without formal written express consent being obtained before treatment, if the patient's condition, if left untreated, would lead to death or serious physical or mental disability.

In an emergency, the exception to the general rule that formal express written consent be obtained from the patient before treating would be an operative procedure.

Patients Leaving Against Medical Advice

Consider the situation where a patient is brought to the emergency room and demands to leave, despite the recommendation that he or she stay. The patient refuses to be hospitalized, or to be seen at any other facility, or for follow-up care. The patient, after being counseled as to the risks of leaving without further treatment, including hospitalization, benefits, and alternatives to treatment, continues to demand to sign out against medical advice. The patient is convinced that he or she will do well at home. An adult patient does have the right to decide on the treatment course, but the physician must determine whether the patient is legally competent to exercise that right to refuse treatment. A decision made under the influence of a narcotic, for example, cannot fairly be characterized as voluntary, knowing, or intelligent. Or, given the medical evidence of complications that occur within the first 24 hours of an acute myocardial infarction, it is not an intelligent patient that would voluntarily accept that risk. It would be different if a patient presents without excruciating pain or has not taken a narcotic. With no other external influences, that adult patient's decision might not be questioned, once the risks and benefits were explained.

However, incompetency cannot be presumed in an adult patient. To determine competency, the physician must determine that the patient can appreciate the nature and consequences of the untreated illness. The physician must also show that the patient can make a rational decision between life and death.

This situation certainly calls for much tact on the part of the physician. He must counsel the patient as to the diagnosis, prognosis, the risks of not being treated at this or any other facility, the risks and benefits of the proposed treatment course, and the alternatives to treatment. This counseling must be done so that the patient is impressed with how severe the disorder is, but not done so heavy-handedly that the patient becomes more angry, defensive, or distraught, so that the disease process is aggravated.

If the patient continues to refuse to be treated, the physician may need to approach and recruit the family, the patient's significant other, or the patient's personal physician, in the hope that they may be able to dissuade the patient from leaving against medical advice. Or, they may be able to persuade the patient to be seen promptly at another hospital. The physician is not asking that the family authorize treatment for or override the patient's competently made decision, unless he is prepared to document that the patient is incompetent and cannot consent for him or herself. Then, the family would be the surrogate decision-maker.

If this fails, and the patient continues to deny his or her medical condition, refuses all further treatment, and the family is unable to impact on the patient's decision, then given the patient's original presentation, the physician must consider one of the following options:

- The physician can place the patient under a protective hold, citing the patient as a danger to him or herself (or others), and treat the patient as an in-patient for 72 hours in a Critical Care Unit. For a protective hold to operate, the patient must be functioning under a mental disability.
- The physician can allege, for example, that a narcotic led to a drug-induced mental disability on the part of the patient. Also, the physician can demonstrate that the patient's denial of his or her present condition operates as a mental disability.

The physician can entertain this option only if he is convinced the patient is competent.

• The physician should have the patient evaluated by a second physician, who would document the history, physical exam, lab findings, diagnosis, and prognosis. This second physician, along with the initial physician, should present the patient with this information again, as well as the risks of non-treatment and the risks and benefits of treatment, together with his or her family. Both the patient and the family should sign each risk and benefit. This is far from optimal, but it is some evidence that the information was presented, and both the patient and the family chose not to act on each item.

The physician must counsel the patient on the risks and benefits of treatment and non-treatment. He must also present any reasonable alternatives to treatment. The physician is best advised not to allow the patient to sign out against medical advice and return home after being given a narcotic for pain.

If the patient refuses to be treated, the physician must find out why. If the patient gives a reason that has no basis in fact or is frivolous, then the physician should request the patient to involve his or her family or significant other in the decision. If the patient refuses to involve others, the physician must consider if the patient is competent. Even if the patient is competent, the physician may want to involve the family, significant other, or the patient's own physician.

If these people are unable to get the patient to change his or her mind and be treated, then given the initial presentation of the illness, the physician must consider placing the patient on an involuntary hold and proceed to treat him or her. The only other alternative is to document that the patient is competent, and that he or she and the family were involved together in an informed decision-making process. After being fully informed, they chose to accept the risk which could result in death.

Reporting Issues

The physician-patient relationship is a confidential relationship. The patient has a right to have certain information about him or herself be kept in confidence by the treating physician. This means that this information cannot be divulged by the physician to any third person. The information that must be kept confidential is information that is disclosed by the patient to the treating physician, so that he can evaluate and treat the patient; also, the patient must have intended that the information be kept confidential.

However, this right to confidentiality, while based on the fundamental constitutional right to privacy, is not an absolute right. This confidential information can be disclosed when the patient consents to the disclosure. It can be disclosed when the patient does not consent, but a public health reason exists for the disclosure to be made, such as when the patient is a danger to an identifiable third person, or when the patient by his or her disease or behavior creates a risk to the general public.

The issue of patient confidentiality, and the breach of that confidentiality because disclosure by reporting is required, is illustrated in the following commonly encountered emergency room scenarios.

An example of this dilemma involves a patient who presents to the emergency room after being in a barroom brawl with a chief complaint of "My hand hurts". On examination, the patient has a closed Boxers fracture. As the splint is being applied, the patient turns to the treating physician and says, "That s.o.b. John Doe. After I leave here, I'm going over to his house and blow his brains out."

The patient, speaking in anger, has made a specific threat of violence against a specified and identifiable person. Since the emergency room physician reasonably suspects that this patient is not only capable of carrying out the threat, but intends to do so, the physician must warn the potential victim of the threat made. On the other hand, if the physician does not believe that the patient would act on the threat, he must not disclose the threat.

A possible alternative to warning the threatened individual is for the emergency room physician, who believes the threat, to control the patient. He can place the patient on a 72 hour involuntary hold as being a danger to others and have him admitted to a psychiatric facility. Or, if there were a medical or surgical reason to admit the patient to the hospital, such as the patient needing surgery for the open Boxers fracture, the admission would operate as controlling the patient. If the physician puts the patient on an involuntary hold or admits him to the hospital, the physician must still consider warning the intended victim because it is believable, the individual was named by the patient, and the threat was specific.

Generally, it is when the patient identifies his potential victim that the physician should consider the threat made as real and warn the intended victim. Other factors that weigh in the decision to warn are how specific is the threat and what would be the harm to the intended victim. The emergency room physician must warn the potential victim because he was named and identifiable. Also, the threat to kill was specific and involved death as the resulting harm to the threatened individual.

In a similar situation, a young person with established schizophrenia is brought to the emergency room by the police for creating a nuisance, and the physician examines the patient. The patient rambles on about how voices from television have told him to discontinue his medications, and the voices in his head keep telling him about how the world's problems are being created by a certain well-known public official. The patient then states that the voices have told him that he should hurt this named public official.

In this situation, a schizophrenic not taking his medications has made a general threat "to hurt" an identifiable third person. There is a question of whether the physician believes that this patient understands that he made a threat and is capable of carrying out the threat. It is possible that the physician may pass this off as the ramblings of a disordered mind because the patient is so delusional. However, this threat was made against a specific and identifiable person. The physician must disclose the threat made against the potential victim.

Controlling the patient would be legally proper in this situation. The physician can place the patient on a 72 hour involuntary hold since he is potentially dangerous to himself and others while he is functioning under a mental disability. The emergency room physician is best advised to disclose the threat made to the identifiable potential victim, even if the patient is placed on an involuntary hold.

On the other hand, consider the situation where a patient is brought to the emergency room after being arrested for resisting arrest. The police want the patient medically cleared before going to jail. The patient has a variety of complaints which on evaluation disclose no injuries. Before being released to the police, the patient tells the physician, "After I get out of jail, I'm going to kill all the cops that did this to me."

The threat "to kill", although specific, is being directed against the general police population. Since there is no identifiable person to warn, the physician may not be able to disclose this patient's confidential information and warn the police. This would be a judgment call. While the physician may not disclose threats made against a general population, if he believes that this patient is capable and intent on harming members of this population, then the physician may tell the police. However, if the physician thinks that the patient was referring to the police who brought him to the emergency room, then he would have to warn those identifiable police about the threat made and the potential danger.

Suspected Child Abuse

As an example, consider a six-month-old brought to the emergency room by one parent with a chief complaint of "seems sleepy all the time" and "doesn't want to move around". No history of trauma is related by the parent. Examination reveals a lethargic child, no external injuries, a bulging anterior fontanelle, a head circumference greater than 90%, and retinal hemorrhages.

These are classic physical exam findings in the shaken baby syndrome. This syndrome is one of the various forms that child abuse can take. Under the law, a health care provider faced with these findings should be aware that they are red flags of child abuse, and he has a duty to report this by telephone and in writing to the local police authorities or to the County Welfare Department. A physician must report suspected child abuse, making sure to get and convey the following information: the name and age of the child, where the child can be located, a description of all injuries, the address of the parents if their address is different from the child's, and the names of siblings or other children living in the home.

The physician should also notify the parent who brought the child in as to his findings and suspicions of possible child abuse. The physician should also tell the parent that there is a legal requirement that this be reported, and he must try to approach the parent in a tactful, non-accusatory way, such as initiating a dialogue with the parent as a means of allowing him or her to ventilate the parent's version of the story.

If the parent, when notified that the report is being made, becomes insistent about removing the child from the emergency room, or refuses hospitalization for the child when it is warranted, then the physician must consider protective custody for the child. It does not matter how stable the child appears; it is well-known that an abused child stands only to be reinjured or killed if released back to the abusing environment. If the physician decides that the child would be in danger if removed by the parent, he may call for the local police to place the child under a protective hold.

Suspected Abuse of the Elderly

Consider the case of a 70-year-old frail patient left by an unknown party at an unknown time at the emergency room with no identification. A physical examination reveals a disoriented patient, who is moderately dehydrated.

Abandonment of an adult older than 65 years, as well as physical abuse, neglect, and abuse of a fiduciary trust relationship, constitutes elder abuse and has been made reportable by law in some jurisdictions if it is done by a person in a responsible relationship to the patient. The report must be made to the Adult Protective Services or a similar agency, depending on the jurisdiction. The local police become involved when an emergency exists, such as the elder's life is being threatened, and he or she needs to be physically removed from the environment. The physician must evaluate and treat the patient, and report the suspected elder abuse.

Alleged Sexual Assault

Consider the case of a 28-year-old patient who presents to the emergency room with a chief complaint of "I was raped." However, it is now 36 hours after the alleged attack, and the patient's main concern is about preventing pregnancy and being treated for sexually transmitted diseases. She refuses to allow consent for specimen retrieval for possible prosecution.

It is the patient's decision whether she will pursue criminal charges against her alleged assailant. In this situation, where the patient refuses to consent to the evidentiary portion of the exam, the emergency room physician is still obligated to disclose the alleged sexual assault to the police, because it involves a criminal act. However, the physician must make it clear to the patient that the time for retrieving usable specimens for a rape prosecution is limited. Since it is already 36 hours after the alleged attack, the patient's own conduct may have already compromised the specimens, including taking a shower or douching. The physician must counsel the patient that unless the specimens are retrieved now, then at some later date, she cannot change her mind and try to prosecute.

If the patient does consent to the evidentiary exam, the physician must examine the patient and obtain the required specimens in a careful and systematic manner, making certain to label the specimens correctly. In most jurisdictions, there is a defined and accepted procedure to follow. If the physician is not trained to do these things, he is best advised to yield to an expert.

In any event, the physician must examine the patient for other injuries, and attempt to rule out pregnancy, even if she relates that the date of her last normal menstrual period makes pregnancy unlikely. A urine pregnancy test is usually done. If it is positive, a quantitative beta-human chorionic gonadotropin can be performed. If the patient wants to avoid the pregnancy, the current method being offered is hormonal interception using diethylstilbestrol (DES) or an estrogen/progestin combination. The physician needs to convey the information, even though it is very unlikely, of the risks and benefits to the hormone interception method. These risks and benefits must be presented to the patient before a decision is made. Some of these risks include nausea, vomiting, irregular bleeding, known or suspected breast cancer, or other estrogen-dependent neoplasia.

A copper intrauterine device had been used as a method to interrupt a pregnancy. With its reintroduction into the United States market, it may again be offered as a post-rape contraceptive.

The physician must test for gonorrhea, chlamydia, and syphilis, and then treat the patient prophylactically. Follow-up tests are also usually performed. The physician should also offer an AIDS test to the patient during the follow-up exam. He should also provide counseling or referral for psychological reasons.

Wounds from Weapons

A representative situation involves a 36-year-old patient who presents to the emergency room with a chief complaint of "I got cut." Examination reveals a straight-edged linear laceration of the posterior right deltoid. The patient is right hand dominant. Further attempts to gather information about how the wound was inflicted yields vague answers like "fooling around in the kitchen".

Given this setting, it is likely that the wound was not self-inflicted; rather, it was inflicted by another person. Even if this information was obtained in a so-called confidential relationship, all states make the finding of a wound inflicted by a gun or knife reportable by law to the local police. It is interesting that if the wound was self-inflicted and there is a suspicion that the patient was attempting to commit suicide, it is reportable to the police, and the patient is treated under the involuntary hold laws that apply in that jurisdiction (danger to self).

Conclusion:

It is impossible to review all the common emergency room situations that have medicolegal hazards for the house officer. Many of these are covered in the other various specialty chapters.

GASTROENTEROLOGY

Introduction

Gastroenterology is a subspecialty of internal medicine dealing with the gastrointestinal tract and digestive diseases. Although data is incomplete, it appears that gastroenterologists are named in 1 to 2% of medical malpractice claims. With the advent and burgeoning application of gastrointestinal endoscopy since the late 1960's and early 1970's, gastroenterologists' legal exposure has become most related to this area of expertise.

Common causes of legal action include failure or delay in making a referral, delay in the performance of a procedure or failure to perform it entirely, failure to instruct or communicate with the patient, and complications related to therapy, most commonly medications.

Communication

The failure to effectively communicate with patients is an area of concern for physicians generally. It is a good policy to offer written instructions regarding medication use. In particular, written do's and don't's post-endoscopy should be tendered to patients. For example, an endoscopist might be liable for the damages which result from a motor vehicle accident caused by a patient given sedation three hours earlier for an endoscopy. Written instructions prohibiting driving a motor vehicle for 24 hours post-endoscopy would be an excellent defense. The notion that if the physician documented it, he did it, and if he did not document it, he did not do it, is germane.

Drug Therapy

Complications related to therapy may lead to legal exposure. Drug therapy is the most troublesome area. The most treacherous drug used in gastoenterology is Prednisone and its cogeners. Since there are a myriad of complications with this agent, especially when used long-term in patients with inflammatory bowel disease, chronic liver disease, etc., it is critical that informed consent be obtained prior to its use. The description of the drug's potential benefits, along with its risks, complications, and alternatives, should be discussed with the patient. This discussion must be memorialized in the physician's notes as a risk management technique. In this way, successful litigation arising from the use of such an agent will be minimized.

Gastric Ulcer

Errors in diagnosis are problematic, particularly a missed diagnosis of carcinoma. Certain clinical rules apply. For example, the clinical axiom that a gastric ulcer should be followed to complete healing must be heeded. Once diagnosed and treated, a gastric ulcer should be followed endoscopically or by x-ray in about eight weeks. If it does not heal, surgery should be considered. If endoscopy is the diagnostic modality, an appropriate number of biopsies (usually eight or four biopsies, plus cytology specimens) must be taken of the ulcer margin at the time of the procedure. The failure to make a timely diagnosis may lead to a malpractice claim.

Lower Gastrointestinal Tract

Medicolegal considerations involving the lower gastrointestinal tract include iatrogenic injuries in the course of invasive diagnostic and surgical procedures, and misdiagnosis resulting in failure to provide adequate treatment and increased morbidity or mortality.

Surgical Problems

Gastroenterologists commonly participate in the care of patients with surgical problems. It is important to call in surgical colleagues for both their opinions and their skills. Failure to obtain a surgical consult in a patient with variceal bleeding is remiss.

Appendicitis

Certainly, no medicolegal discussion of lower gastrointestinal disease would be complete without including appendicitis. The principal medicolegal consideration of appendicitis is in failing to make the diagnosis, resulting in the patient suffering a ruptured appendix.

The failure to recommend surgery in a 27 year old patient with an elevated white count, right lower quadrant pain, and rebound tenderness, in whom the physician suspects appendicitis, is negligent. In reality, a gastroenterologist can never be faulted for obtaining a surgical opinion, but he might often be criticized for failing to do so. This message is clear.

An appendectomy is ordinarily a straightforward surgical procedure, which conventionally requires about two days of hospitalization with very minimal risk. A ruptured appendix is a life-threatening disorder, which requires prolonged hospitalization and an extended recovery period. The problem with diagnosis of appendicitis today falls principally on hospital emergency departments, urgent care centers, and the offices of primary care physicians.

It is not the failure to make the diagnosis which is critically important from a medicolegal standpoint, but failure to obtain appropriate tests that will rule out appendicitis. More important is the failure to obtain surgical consultation.

This problem is exemplified in a case in which a third year surgical resident, while moonlighting in a hospital emergency department, treated a patient with abdominal pain. The patient had been seen by this physician on three visits, each two days apart. On the first two occasions, the patient was sent home from the hospital. When the patient came in for the third visit, he was in septic shock and renal failure.

The contention of the emergency room physician was that on the first two occasions, the patient was hydrated with intravenous fluids, he improved, and he was sent home with a diagnosis of gastroenteritis. The physician also contended that the patient bore the responsibility for not returning sooner after the second visit.

The first caveat in dealing with possible appendicitis is that any patient presenting with right lower quadrant pain in an emergency situation must be considered to have appendicitis until proven otherwise by appropriate examination and testing. Furthermore, localized pain is not a feature of gastroenteritis.

The differential diagnosis for patients presenting with localized right lower quadrant pain of relatively recent onset includes, in addition to appendicitis, in the female, pelvic problems, such as a ruptured ovarian cyst or pelvic inflammatory disease. Others include ureterolithiasis and fecal impaction. Less likely diagnoses include perforated cecal diverticulitis and terminal ileitis.

The diagnoses of terminal ileitis and Crohn's disease or granulomatous colitis (Eisenhower's disease) is occasionally made at the time of surgery for appendicitis.

A patient who presents with findings consistent with acute appendicitis, but with a history of recurrent episodes of right lower quadrant pain, must be considered for terminal ileitis. This diagnosis can usually be made by a barium enema, thus avoiding surgery.

Hurried surgery can result in an unnecessary procedure based on a misdiagnosis. A teenage male was seen in a hospital emergency department with a sudden onset of pain, localizing to the right lower quadrant. The results of a workup led to the patient being taken to surgery, where a normal appendix was found. The next day, he complained of scrotal pain, and was eventually found to have an epididymitis. Abdominal surgery can usually be avoided in these cases by proper attention to the history and physical examination. Surgical consultation must be considered in all of these situations. Basic to a diagnosis of appendicitis is an adequate history and physical examination, plus a CBC and urinalysis. Depending on the age and sex of the patient, pelvic ultrasound and barium enema examinations are important diagnostic considerations.

Once the diagnosis of acute appendicitis is entertained, additional diagnostic modalities should be considered. Treatment must proceed at a rapid pace because the golden period of time to treat appendicitis before rupture is about 24 hours. Obviously, this is not absolute, and patients may rupture in a relatively few hours, or they may go on for several days without rupture.

Another illustrative case involved a 34 year old male, who presented with localizing right lower quadrant pain for about 12 hours, and who interestingly had a similar three day episode of abdominal pain about 10 days before the onset of the present symptoms. The hospital radiologist performed a barium enema, which did not visualize the appendix. On the basis of the findings, including a 19,000 white cell blood count, surgery was performed through a right lower quadrant muscle-splitting incision, which was transformed to a rectus cutting incision when it was realized that the surgeon was dealing with a retrocecal normal appendix and an inflammatory mass involving the sigmoid colon, bladder, and omentum. The patient underwent a Hartmann procedure (excision of the inflammatory mass, closure of the distal colonic stump, and a proximal colostomy) for perforated diverticulitis. The radiologist queried post-operatively acknowledged that he had seen several sigmoid diverticula and sigmoid spasm, but the significance of these findings was obfuscated by the patient's history, physical examination, and non-filling appendix.

This patient certainly needed surgery, but through a different incision. A muscle-splitting right lower quadrant incision affords only a limited view of the abdomen. Finding a normal appendix can lead to difficulties in making the correct diagnosis and rendering proper treatment.

A ruptured ectopic pregnancy is included in the differential diagnosis of acute appendicitis in females. Pelvic ultrasound can be helpful in making the diagnosis. However, the catastrophic results from a missed diagnosis make it imperative to exhaust all diagnostic possibilities, including laparoscopy, if there is any suspicion of this diagnosis.

Another caveat is that if the patient is sent home from the emergency department, he or she must be given appropriate instructions explicitly to call or return in the event that the symptoms intensify that day or persist until the next day.

Appendicitis In Pregnancy

Abdominal pain in the course of pregnancy is not uncommon; frequently, such pain can localize in the right lower quadrant. In addition, in pregnancy, the white blood cell count will generally be elevated. Moreover, as the pregnancy progresses, the appendix will usually be elevated out of the pelvis, and it can eventually rise to the level of the gallbladder. The diagnosis of appendicitis during pregnancy can be extremely difficult. Furthermore, surgery for appendicitis can be hazardous to the pregnancy, and misdiagnosis can be catastrophic.

Fecal Impaction

It is extraordinary how many times a physician is called to the hospital emergency department to see a patient with severe abdominal pain and obstipation, which eventually turns out to be a fecal impaction. Fortunately, this problem is readily treatable with enemas. A source of speculation is how many patients are taken to surgery or undergo risky diagnostic procedures because of unappreciated fecal impaction. It is certainly something that every physician needs to be mindful of, since treatment will avoid significant diagnostic and surgical procedures fraught with complications and a great deal of expense to the patient.

Ischemic Colitis

This diagnosis can be extremely difficult to make. Often, the most useful tests are contraindicated because of the possibility of perforation of the colon. However, failure to make this diagnosis can have catastrophic results, and at times, patients need to be explored because clear-cut diagnostic information is not available. Fortunately, with plain abdominal films, the diagnosis can often be made, because a barium enema or colonoscopy may be contraindicated in the face of the potential for perforation.

Granulomatous and Ulcerative Colitis

One of the complications of chronic ulcerative colitis, particularly in long-standing disease, is cancer. The physician must be cognizant of this possibility and may need to perform bowel resection early in an attempt to avoid cancer. Toxic megacolon is also a potentially catastrophic complication of chronic ulcerative colitis. It is a constant source of concern during the course of treatment.

If terminal ileitis is found at surgery, an appendectomy can usually be performed if the cecum is not involved with the disease. However, if an appendectomy is performed in the face of such involvement, fistulization may result.

Radiation Colitis

This condition is not an infrequent complication of the treatment of pelvic carcinoma with radiation, and it can result in crippling bowel problems. Protecting the patient as much as possible in the course of radiotherapy, and acknowledging to the patient beforehand the possibility of such a complication, are important considerations for attending physicians.

Diverticulitis

The indications for surgery in a patient with diverticulitis are obstruction, perforation, and bleeding. Perforation usually results in peritonitis or abscess. Bleeding from diverticular disease is often difficult to localize, and of course, can be confused with carcinoma or other gastrointestinal bleeding at various levels of the colon and small intestine. Obstruction secondary to diverticulitis is usually a surgical emergency.

Frequently, diverticulitis presenting as a mass in the sigmoid colon is difficult to distinguish from carcinoma, and conservative treatment may be inappropriate.

For example, an elderly lady with repeated hospitalizations for diverticulitis was admitted for lower abdominal pain, nausea, and constipation. A barium enema showed a polypoid sigmoid tumor. She underwent exploratory surgery, during which a sigmoid colotomy was performed and in which no polyp was found. She had a stormy post-operative course and was readmitted to the hospital several weeks later with a pulmonary embolus. She eventually underwent sigmoid resection for obstructive disease, which proved to be benign.

This case demonstrates inadequate pre-operative and intra-operative evaluation; definitive surgery should have been performed in the initial operation. Moreover, the post-operative problems should have alerted the attending physicians to perform additional testing to make a definitive diagnosis while the patient was still in the hospital. Also, the surgeon must be mindful that diverticular disease can produce a fistula in the pelvic organs, such as the vagina and bladder, or in the small intestine.

Colonic polyps presenting as carcinoma, or perhaps converting to cancer, are a continuing hazard to procotologists and gastroenterologists. Certainly, patients with a history of polyps must be subjected to regular colonoscopic examinations, because of the distinct possibility of additional polyps and/or cancer.

Cancer of Lower Gastrointestinal (GI) Tract

Cancer of the lower GI tract presents a variety of ongoing challenges from a medicolegal standpoint.

Bleeding

One of the earliest detectable signs of cancer of the colon is occult bleeding, which can be readily detected by available laboratory tests. Any patient presenting with an alteration in bowel habits or rectal bleeding, which cannot be readily diagnosed as hemorrhoidal, must be subjected to appropriate testing to rule out the possibility of carcinoma. Flexible colonoscopy has become the most widely used diagnostic tool for this purpose, although barium enema is still frequently employed.

Life-threatening colonic bleeding can result from disease or surgery. Identification of the bleeding site can be difficult, and at surgery, the surgeon can be confronted with the dilemma of which portion and how much of the colon to remove to control the hemorrhage. An inadequate attempt at localization prior to surgery, or failure to control the bleeding, can lead to serious complications, including death.

Detection of occult bleeding has many virtues. There are some interesting recent developments. Hemoccult testing for colorectal cancer is less specific for men than for women, and for those over 60 years of age, compared with younger people.

In hemoccult screening of more than 46,000 people during the first seven years of a randomized, prospective trial, the specificity of the test was 94% for women and 92% for men. Of the 46,000 subjects, 7,230 returned at least one positive slide. Of these subjects, 183 were found to have colorectal cancers, and 22 other subjects with all negative tests were also found to have colorectal cancer.

The specificity was highest for those under 60 years of age, and decreased with increasing age. The sensivity of the test did not differ significantly between the sexes, and was 89% for the entire group. Rehydrating the slides increased the sensitivity from 81% to 92%, and decreased the specificity from 98% to 90%, resulting in a decrease in positive results. The net result was a substantial increase in diagnostic services.

Etiologic Factors

Recent studies have shed interesting information on some of the etiologic factors in the development of colon cancer. Alcohol consumption raises the risk of cancer of the sigmoid colon. This finding is based on a 17 year follow-up of more than 250,000 Japanese adults. The risk exists for both sexes, though male drinkers have a relative risk of 4.38, compared with non-drinkers. The risk for women is 1.92. Daily beer drinkers had the highest relative risk 12.57 but other alcoholic beverages also had high risks. Consumers of sake, a beverage of fermented rice, had a relative risk of 4.56, and the use of schochu, a local hard liquor, meant a relative risk of 5.90. The relative risks observed in this patient population exceed those found for other alcohol-related diseases. Daily consumers of alcohol have a relative risk of 1.66 for liver cirrhosis and 2.29 for cancer of the esophagus.

Alcohol may affect the sigmoid colon in a number of ways, including altering normal bowel movements and changing hormonal balances. Another possibility is that the contaminants of alcoholic beverages, such as mycotoxins, polycyclic hydrocarbons, N-nitrosamines, and asbestos fibers, act as carcinogens.

The idea that the active form of vitamin D offers protection against certain cancers, postulated a decade ago, has been confirmed. Since the sun is a major source of vitamin D, the findings seem to challenge the belief, held by dermatologists, that no tan is a healthy tan.

An eight year prospective study has shown that serum 25-hydroxyvitamin D (25-OHD), indeed, protects against colon cancer. Thirty-four white patients with colon cancer, who had not had a previous cancer, were matched with 67 control patients according to race, sex, and age. Their finding: the average 25-OHD concentration was lower in patients who developed colon cancer than it was in the controls (30.5 vs. 33.3 ng/ml.). The risk of colon cancer was reduced by 80% in people with concentrations between 27 and 41 ng/ml.

The association does not represent proof. The active form of the vitamin might just be a marker for calcium intake. It seems unlikely, however, that it is solely a marker, because most vitamin D in people results from exposure to sunlight. Despite the findings, the warning that no tan is a safe tan remains a valid one. The researchers are not saying that going out for 10 minutes is going to be harmful if an individual wants to make vitamin D that way. But he or she should be very careful not to expose skin with bruises and tears or skin with growths. One has to consider the risk-benefit ratio. If an individual is going to be made worse, he or she should take vitamin D supplements or drink milk.

Missed Diagnosis

Missing the diagnosis of cancer of the colon can be catastrophic, especially since such cancers are traditionally of low grade and slow growth. A high index of suspicion is critical in dealing with cancer of the colon, and routine tests for melena, i.e., endoscopic examination and barium x-rays, are essential parts of a physician's armamentarium in this situation.

Failure to Diagnose

The failure to diagnose colon cancer is increasingly an area of concern. In working up a 65 year old patient with iron deficiency anemia, visualization of the cecal area is critical. In stating that the cecum is normal in such a patient, an endoscopist must be certain to document that the cecum was visualized entirely. Photographic, video, or radiographic proof is valuable. In such a patient, the procurement of a good quality, double contrast barium study of the cecal area is prudent.

Drug Therapy

Drug therapy of colon cancer has been disappointing. There may be hope on the horizon. The results of preliminary studies on several investigative drugs are encouraging.

Colonic Surgery

Since the flora of the bowel become pathogenic upon being introduced into the abdominal cavity, any disease or surgery which results in injury to the colon can result in peritonitis and abdominal abscess. These are potentially disastrous consequences, even in this antibiotic era. Therefore, the diagnosis must be timely made, and the treatment must be vigorous.

The potential for infection is also a consideration in the performance of colon surgery on an inadequately prepared bowel, which usually occurs under emergency circumstances. The breakdown of colonic anastomoses or other suture or staple lines is also a factor in the leakage of organisms into the abdominal cavity. In these situations and when the colon tissue or repair is less than satisfactory, a temporary colostomy may avoid serious complications after surgery. Moreover, failure to make a diagnosis or provide inadequate treatment in the presence of an intra-abdominal infection (peritonitis) can result in death.

Once having undergone surgery for cancer of the colon, the patient must be subjected to a lifetime of regular colonoscopic examinations to detect any recurrence.

Surgical Injuries

Certainly, the most common injury of concern to the colon surgeon would be transection of the ureter. In surgery on either the right or left colon, it is incumbent upon the surgeon to locate the ureter and keep it in view throughout the surgical procedure.

For example, a middle-aged woman underwent elective surgery by a gynecologist for a pelvic mass, which was *not* demonstrated on pelvic scan. At surgery, the mass was found to involve the sigmoid colon, and a general surgeon was asked to participate in the operative procedure. The sigmoid colon was resected en bloc, including the ureter and adjacent vessels. The ureter was repaired and a colostomy was performed. The mass proved to be benign, i.e., diverticular disease. The patient expired in the immediate post-operative period due to bleeding and septic shock. There are a number of medicolegal problems with this case. The en bloc procedure was not warranted, especially for a benign disease. The potential for contamination and complications provided almost insurmountable risks. When in doubt, it is always better to back off and return another day.

The patient could have had an adequate bowel preparation before surgery. Moreover, a colostomy could have been performed with pelvic drainage, and diagnostic tests could have been carried out post-operatively, prior to definitive surgery.

Surgery is a matter of continuously balancing risks, and to a well-trained surgeon, the risks of performing definitive surgery in this case were unacceptable.

Colonic Fistulas

A vaginal fistula with the colon or rectum are known complications of a hysterectomy and other pelvic procedures. To that end, patients need to be warned about this potential problem before surgery.

Even with appropriate informed consent, these patients are so unhappy that they frequently resort to a lawsuit, even though there was no negligence demonstrable in the performance of the hysterectomy.

A second medicolegal problem is that repair can be extraordinarily difficult, and several surgical procedures can be required to obtain a satisfactory result.

Anal Surgery

Post-operative anal stricture or deformity that interferes with bowel movements or causes chronic pain begets a distressed patient. Surgery, particularly if it is done improperly, can result in lifelong crippling with anal incontinence or stricture.

Symptomatic hemorrhoids do not constitute a life-threatening disease. Despite this, there is a tendency to perform hemorrhoidectomies on patients with minimal symptoms, or to remove excessive anal tissue in the course of surgery. Therefore, surgery should only be performed on those patients with hemorrhoids who have symptoms that interfere with their lifestyle. Sufficient anal tissue should be left behind to produce satisfactory healing without stricture or incontinence.

Foreign Objects

The anal orifice can provide access to a variety of foreign objects, and the colon/rectum can also be the repository of ingested foreign substances. Depending upon the sharpness or size of the offending substance, the result can be obstruction, perforation, or bleeding.

Physicians recover a variety of objects from the rectum, e.g., gourds, candles, carrots, bulbs, etc. Surgeons treat patients with penetrating injuries of the lower GI tract secondary to ingested needles, pins, etc.

Avoiding one problem inherent in gastrointestinal foreign bodies is by not delaying treatment for such a serious condition, which requires a high index of suspicion and vigorous treatment once the diagnosis is established. The treatment not only involves recovering the foreign object, but treating the infection, perforation, or bleeding which has resulted.

Perirectal/Perianal Abscess

A perirectal abscess should be treated as any other abscess with immediate incision and drainage, either in the physician's office or the hospital emergency department under local anesthetic. The patient certainly does not need to be taken to the operating room and subjected to regional or general anesthesia when prompt relief and treatment can be achieved with minimal discomfort in the out-patient setting.

Injuries Due to Diagnostic Procedures

There are a variety of diagnostic procedures, such as colonoscopy, laparoscopy, and peritoneal lavage, which can result in colonic injuries.

The most common areas of malpractice for gastroenterologists are the improper performance of an endoscopic procedure, an error in diagnosis - usually failure to diagnose carcinoma - and a failure to recognize endoscopic complications.

It is mandatory that gastrointestinal endoscopists practice within reasonable standards of care. Good training and continuing medical education are mandatory. Likewise, clinical common sense and attention to detail are necessary acquired practice habits. Without these skills, endoscopic procedures will be improperly performed and lead to litigation. Examples include the attempt to remove a 3.5 cm. sessile polyp at colonoscopy, leading to a perforation; the performance of an upper endoscopy on a patient with a full stomach, leading to aspiration; and a three hour endoscopic retrograde cholangiopancreatography, leading to respiratory arrest.

Understanding the indications, as well as the contraindications, of endoscopic procedures is essential. The failure to recommend or to perform an upper endoscopy in a patient with a suspicious gastric mass is wrong. Similarly, the failure to perform a colonoscopy and polypectomy in a patient with a suspected descending colon polyp is equally incorrect.

Endoscopic complications can occur within reasonable practice. Complications such as bleeding, perforation, and infection occur within the normal scope of practice. Using a proper application of informed consent with the patient, the risks of these complications is borne by the patient. Consequently, complications should not lead to a successful lawsuit against an endoscopist.

Conversely, the failure to recognize a complication in a timely way is malpractice. Illustrative is the patient who complains of gas pains and abdominal distention post-colonoscopy. This patient should be examined and the clinical findings recorded. He or she should be observed until the clinical situation improves, i.e., the gas passes. If there is any doubt whatsoever, an abdominal film for free air should be done. Allowing the patient to go home or to eat in the interval between the procedure and the discovery of the perforation in this scenario is negligent. A gastroenterologist or an endoscopist must practice within perceived reasonable standards of care.

Perforation of the colon is a recognized complication of performing endoscopic procedures. Certainly, in the era of rigid endoscopes, there is much more likelihood of perforation. However, even with fiberoptic endoscopes being used extensively, there are still a significant number of perforations. Since this is an anticipated complication, patients need to be warned ahead of time of this possibility.

Rarely is there negligence in causing injury to the bowel, but rather in failing to make the diagnosis, with consequent delay in treatment. The consequences of colon perforation are potentially catastrophic, and the treating physician must be cognizant of this possibility at all times. Any patient complaining of abdominal pain, distention, or obstipation after endoscopic examination must be considered as a candidate for perforation. The diagnosis is established by the presence of intra-peritoneal air on plain abdominal x-rays. However, a barium enema or endoscopic examination may be necessary to make the diagnosis.

Certain patients are at a higher risk for perforation; those with chronic inflammatory conditions such as granulomatous colitis, chronic ulcerative colitis, or acute conditions such as diverticulitis. The patient must be warned about the possibility of perforation in these instances. Serious consideration must be given to this complication in deciding whether to perform the endoscopic procedure, and extra care needs to be taken in order to avoid this disastrous complication in the course of this procedure.

In an illustrative case, a middle-aged male underwent a proctoscopy, a polyp was excised with the snare, and the base of the polyp was cauterized. Two days later, the patient complained of abdominal pain. He was examined and a plain abdominal film obtained, which was reported as normal. The abdominal pain persisted, and repeat x-rays two days later showed free air. A diverting colostomy was performed. Since perforation was a known complication, when the patient showed symptoms suggestive of this complication, he was properly evaluated and healed, and the outcome was satisfactory.

Another illustrative case involved a 36 year old woman with known Crohn's disease, who underwent a laparoscopy as part of an infertility workup. Perforation of the colon occurred in the course of the procedure, and a general surgeon was immediately called in to perform a colostomy. Several surgical procedures were eventually required to obtain a satisfactory result.

In the former case, the patient was warned of the possible complication; in the latter instance, the patient insisted she had not been warned of the possibility of bowel perforation, and that she was at high risk because of Crohn's disease. Most surgeons would not avoid laparoscopy in the face of Crohn's disease. However, in both instances, the complication was handled correctly in timely fashion, minimizing exposure to liability.

In another example, a trauma surgeon performed a peritoneal lavage on a motor vehicle accident victim with a negative result. Several days later, the patient developed abdominal pain, and a CT scan showed an abscess. At surgery, it was found that in the course of the peritoneal lavage, the trocar had penetrated the left colon, producing a leak and eventual abscess. In the absence of close follow-up, this patient could have suffered a tragic result. Since the procedure was performed as an emergency, it was not possible, nor necessarily required, to apprise the patient beforehand of this possible complication.

In treating a patient with gallstones, he or she must know that in addition to surgery, there are circumstances when no specific treatment need be undertaken, or that oral preparations are available for the dissolution of the stones. Intervention can now be accomplished by a variety of procedures: lithotripsy, percutaneous cholecystolithotomy, laparoscopic cholecystectomy, and percutaneous transhepatic infusion via a catheter of methyl-tert butyl ether. Obviously, there are indications, circumstances, and material risks for each of these procedures. The therapist, including the house officer, is duty-bound to convey adequate information, so that the patient can make a knowledgeable decision.

Conclusion

This presentation is intended to introduce the physician to those areas of legal concern in the area of gastroenterology. Attention has focused on particular problematic issues related to this field of clinical practice. The discussion of medicolegal considerations of the gastrointestinal tract is intended to be selective of those diseases which provide pitfalls to the physician and surgeon, and attempts to provide a basis for avoiding or anticipating and minimizing the complications.

HIV INFECTIONS/AIDS

Duty to Treat the HIV Patient

At common law, a physician has no obligation to treat a patient until a physician-patient contract has been established. One state (Vermont) has made an exception for emergency care, and court decisions have established a duty by emergency rooms to care for those who present themselves. In addition, at least one state has found that physicians may not refuse patients on racial grounds. Still, in general, the common law rule stands in non-emergency situations.

The concern about discrimination against HIV-infected patients, however, has led to the passage of laws in some jurisdictions that would restrict the right to refuse these patients. In such areas, a physician who refuses an HIV patient may be subject not only to a civil lawsuit, but to criminal prosecution. While such laws have yet to be tested in court, it is unlikely that they would penalize a physician who did not specialize in treating the disease entity presented, provided that the physician has made reasonable arrangements for treatment elsewhere. (One such case was recently filed against a physician in New York.) Still, a physician who is presented with an HIV-positive patient, and wishes not to treat that patient, is best advised to discuss the matter with counsel familiar with that jurisdiction's laws.

Health Care Professionals

When appropriate precautionary measures are taken, health care workers are not at increased risk of HIV infection. The Centers for Disease Control (CDC) has compiled a worldwide list of 27 HIV-infected health workers with no reported non-occupational risk factors, and for whom case histories have been published in the scientific literature. In 19 of the cases, seroconversion after the point of exposure was documented. The agency is investigating 34 more cases of alleged transmission in the health care setting.

Even needlestick and similar injuries have resulted in only isolated cases of seroconversion among the hundreds of cases followed, and these seroconversions were usually in workers with either deep intramuscular penetration or significant mucus membrane contact with large amounts of blood or contaminated fluids.

Physician's Responsibility

What compels physicians to care for patients with AIDS? In essence, the law is that in the absence of a special relationship, no health care professional need treat anybody with whom he or she does not have a consensual physician-patient relationship.

The physician's responsibility to treat may transcend legal bounds. In more modern times, the AMA Ethics Code adopted in the mid-1800's attempted to present the medical community as ethically and morally bound to care for the sick. In 1957, the code was changed, however. Except in emergency situations, physicians were free to choose whom they served.

Only the "virtuous physician" model imposes on the individual physician the responsibility to care for the sick. Under this model, physicians can be held "morally accountable" for their actions. Many believe that accepting the obligation to treat the sick is not a matter for individual choice, but is an essential element of the medical profession. Because the sick need the physician, that need becomes a "moral claim" on those who are equipped to help.

Moreover, the physician's knowledge is not individually owned. Society relinquished much during the physician's educational process. In return, the physician is a partner to the "collective covenant" that acknowledges that he or she has a fidelity to the patient's interest.

In their 1986 Health and Policy Committee report, the American College of Physicians and the Infectious Disease Society of America said that all health care professionals must provide competent and humane care to all patients, including those critically ill with AIDS and AIDS-related conditions. Moreover, these organizations charged that to deny care to sick and dying patients for any reason is "unethical". The AMA Ethics Code now reflects this stand. According to the AMA, physicians who refuse to treat HIV-infected patients risk being expelled by their state medical society if its ethical and judiciary body decides that such refusal is an unethical act. Unethical behavior is grounds for expulsion from membership in most, if not all, local and state medical organizations. In light of the current atmosphere of confusion, uncertainty, and fear surrounding AIDS, such expulsion may well be controversial and even contestible, but it remains a definite risk nonetheless.

Inconsistent Pronouncements

These pronouncements on the ethical responsibility of health professionals vis-à-vis AIDS patients have not been uniformly adopted by the medical organizations which control professional conduct within each state. While some state groups have imposed a duty to treat on physicians licensed within their state, others have taken the position that physicians who decline to treat AIDS patients are not in breach of any ethical duty.

For example, the Arizona State Board of Medical Examiners has issued a statement that endorses the right of a physician to refuse to treat patients who have AIDS. Shortly after the AMA Council issued its finding, the Texas Medical Association decided that physicians ethically could refuse to treat patients with AIDS. The Texas policy permits a physician either to care for an AIDS patient, or to "refer the patient to an appropriate physician who will accept the responsibility for the care and treatment of the patient". It is not clear what the physician's duty is if such an "appropriate" physician cannot be found.

The decisions of the Texas and Arizona Medical Boards contrast with that of the New Jersey State Board of Medical Examiners, which has affirmed the AMA ethical guidelines and has suggested that physicians who refuse to treat AIDS patients may be subject to discipline. Also, the Associated Medical School of New York (a group made up of the deans of the state's 13 public and private academic health centers), as well as the Association of American Medical Colleges, affirmed the responsibility of physicians and medical students at each medical school and its affiliated hospitals to provide care for all HIV-positive patients. Moreover, these associations specifically recommend dismissal as the ultimate sanction for any students who feel that the risk of caring for AIDS patients outweighs the benefits of the learning experience, and who decline care due to varying cultural beliefs and personal values. Similarly, nursing organizations have advocated disciplinary action against members who refuse care to AIDS patients, and both clinical pathologists and morticians are expected to accord the bodies of HIV-infected persons the same fair treatment as would be given an uninfected person.

Penalties

Physicians who refuse to care for HIV-infected patients are not legally liable, because a physician's obligation to care for patients is ethical, not legal. Physicians who consider themselves unqualified, or who do not want to treat AIDS patients, can almost always refer them to other physicians. However, physicians who refuse to treat HIV-infected patients risk being expelled by their state medical society if a judiciary or administrative body decides that such a refusal is unethical.

The right of a physician not to accept a patient with AIDS, or with a positive HIV test result, can be considered equivocal. However, some local ordinances address this issue specifically, making it unlawful to deny any individual the full and equal enjoyment of goods, services, facilities, privileges, advantages, and accommodations of any establishment as a result of that person having AIDS or any of the associated conditions. A physician can be held liable for discrimination if a patient can prove that he or she refused to provide treatment solely because the patient is HIV-seropositive. Dentists, who find it particularly hard to justify not treating certain patients, are frequently the targets of such discrimination suits.

It should be noted, however, that if a patient refuses AIDS testing, a physician could conceivably exercise his or her common law right to terminate the physician-patient relationship after providing the patient with reasonable notice. This could be seen as a rational refusal to treat for non-compliance, a legally defensible action, since medical ethics and rules of professional conduct would not demand that a physician engage in, or maintain, a physician-patient relationship when the patient refuses to provide the physician with such fundamental information.

Risks

To date, the CDC has documented a number of transmitted HIV infections following casual contact. Health care professionals have been greatly concerned about nosocomial transmission of HIV. Many published studies have assessed the risk of transmission related to various activities and interactions.

The work of those who care for HIV-infected patients falls somewhere between casual contact and overt parenteral contact. The duration of their interaction is generally less than that of household members, but the frequency of their contact with bloody fluids is greater. The concentration of virus in body fluids is proportional to the number of white cells in the fluid. Therefore, HIV concentrations are highest in blood and semen, somewhat lower in vaginal secretions, and significantly lower in sweat and tears. The CDC estimates that the chance of a health care worker becoming infected with the AIDS virus after receiving a single stick from a contaminated instrument is 1% or less. Risk of seroconversion after exposure through the skin or mucous membranes, while documented, is much lower.

A study of 1,309 dentists found only one subject with HIV antibodies, despite infrequent compliance with recommended infection-control precautions, frequent occupational exposure to persons at increased risk for HIV infection, and frequent accidental inoculations with sharp instruments. Further, the risk of becoming infected is reduced to the negligible level by careful adherence to CDC guidelines, developed to prevent the transmission of AIDS between patients and health care workers.

The CDC has recommended that all patients be treated as if potentially infected, but bedside precautions often become lax in the face of such across-the-board guidelines. In this atmosphere, health care workers have a tendency to try to predict which patients are likely to be infected, and may be cautious only when dealing with them.

Although the chances of becoming infected with the AIDS virus through patient contact is low for all physicians, some are at greater risk than others. It is estimated that house staff and internists have a 0.5% annual risk of sero-converting. On the other hand, emergency department surgeons who operate on a large number of AIDS patients, and who experience frequent punctures, run a 2% annual risk of infection.

Some health care workers, e.g., surgeons, pathologists, dentists, and critical care nurses, are known to be at greater risk than the general population for contracting AIDS. Several investigators have evaluated seroconversion to HIV in a variety of clinical settings in which health care workers have prolonged or intense contact with infected patients or their moist body substances. In various reported studies of more than 2,000 such persons who were stuck by needles or experienced mucous membrane exposure, four had seroconverted. All four were subjected to needlestick injuries. No additional seroconversions occurred in the remaining study subjects, including 762 followed for longer than one year, and 432 followed for longer than two years.

The CDC has published recommended precautions for health care workers involved in invasive procedures. Because the antibody status of most patients will not be known, the recommendations summarized below apply to *all* patients:

Health care workers should take prudent measures to reduce their contact with bloody fluids from all patients. The risk from each parenteral exposure is low, but it is not insignificant.

Procedural policies should be appropriate to the risk, practical to implement, and as inexpensive as possible. They should not increase the patients' risk for an adverse outcome.

Universal Precautions

The CDC has proposed the use of universal precautions for all patient interaction involving bloody fluids. Included is the use of barrier precautions when there is likelihood of contact with blood or body fluid potentially contaminated with blood. Under universal precautions, traditional isolation practices and category isolation are still recommended, in addition to the precautions to protect personnel.

Body Substance Isolation (BSI)

Most infectious diseases are characterized by a high proportion of unrecognized or subclinical cases. Thus, nosocomial transmission of infectious agents to susceptible patients and personnel has been shown to occur repeatedly, particularly in Critical Care Units. One prominent facility has developed an isolation system in which all moist body sites and substances from all patients are handled with barrier precautions.

In contrast to traditional isolation systems, in which barrier precautions are used only for patients known to be infected, BSI directs equal attention to all patients, recognizing the role of colonized cases or infections that are otherwise undiagnosed. The increased use of barrier precautions, such as putting on clean examination gloves immediately before contact with mucous membranes and non-intact skin of all patients, reduces nosocomial transmission of infectious agents to patients, and also protects personnel from exposure to potential pathogens, including HIV. The BSI system is used instead of, not in addition to, traditional isolation and is used not only for HIV, but for all contact-spread infectious agents. The key elements of this system include the following:

• Put on clean examination gloves or sterile gloves, as the situation demands, immediately before contact with mucous membranes or non-intact skin. Wear gloves for anticipated contact with any patient's moist body substances and for cleaning soiled, reusable instruments and equipment.

• Wash hands before touching patients and immediately after any soiling.

• Wear impermeable aprons or gowns when clothing is likely to be soiled by moist body substances from a patient.

• Wear a mask, glasses, goggles, or other barriers when it is possible that your face, eyes, or mucous membranes will be splashed or soiled with moist body substances.

• Provide readily accessible mechanical resuscitation devices (such as Ambu bags and CPR pocket masks) to decrease the likelihood that health care workers will need to perform mouth-to-mouth resuscitation.

• Use private rooms for patients who soil the environment so extensively that roommates would likely have inadvertent contact with their body substances. Private rooms are also recommended for patients having an airborne communicable disease, such as tuberculosis. Otherwise, AIDS patients do not routinely need private rooms for infection control reasons.

• Place all needles, without recapping, in sturdy containers. If recapping is necessary, use a recapping device. Do not bend or cut needles. Incinerate or autoclave them before disposal.

• Securely bag all trash from patients' rooms so that it cannot leak in transit. Routine double bagging is unnecessary. This trash probably does not require incineration, autoclaving, or other special handling before disposal, even if the patient is infected; however, some states and local governments may have regulations requiring special handling. Trash handlers should wear heavy gloves to reduce the risk of punctures from needles and other sharp instruments or objects inadvertently left in wastebaskets and trash.

• Bag soiled linen so that it cannot leak in transit. Double bags or water-soluble bags are unnecessary. Laundry workers should wear heavy gloves and gowns or aprons while sorting and loading soiled linen into washing machines. Visibly soiled linen should be run through a cool rinse cycle so that stains do not set, and then washed in the usual fashion as dictated by local customs or regulations.

The reasonable preventive measures in both BSI and universal precautions have been greatly exaggerated in some facilities, where personnel wear gowns, masks, gloves, booties, and caps for routine care of infected patients. In addition, they often subject trash from these patients' rooms to expensive decontamination processes. These precautions are unnecessary and expensive, and they may significantly reduce the quality of care given to the patients.

All health care workers who perform or assist in invasive procedures must wear gloves when touching mucous membranes or non-intact skin of all patients, and use other appropriate barrier precautions when indicated, e.g., masks, eye coverings, and gowns, if aerosolization or splashes are likely to occur. In the dental setting, as in the surgical and obstetric settings, gloves must be worn for touching all mucous membranes and changed between all patient contacts. If a glove is torn or a needlestick or other injury occurs, the glove must be changed as promptly as safety permits, and the needle or instrument removed from the sterile field.

All health care workers who perform or assist in vaginal or Cesarean deliveries must wear surgical gloves and use other appropriate barrier precautions when handling the placenta or infant until blood and amniotic fluid have been removed from the infant's skin.

After use, disposable syringes and needles, scalpel blades, and other sharp items must be placed in puncture-resistant containers for disposal. To prevent needlestick injuries, needles should not be recapped, purposefully bent or broken, removed from disposable syringes, or otherwise manipulated by hand.

If an incident occurs during an invasive procedure that results in exposure of a patient to the blood of a health care worker, the patient should be informed of the incident, and previous recommendations for the management of such exposures should be followed.

Sharp Instrument Injuries

Needlesticks pose the most serious risk of blood-borne infection. Many of these accidents occur when used needles are recapped after injections. An obvious answer to this problem would be to develop safer caps, but this has not yet been done. Health care workers must handle all needles as if all patients were known to have HIV infection. This means they must avoid recapping, and they must put used syringes and unrecapped needles into a rigid, puncture-resistant container specifically designated for sharp instruments. If recapping is done, the health care provider's hand should stay behind the needle as it is covered. This can be done by using a safe recapping technique, or employing a recapping device.

When patients are thrashing or otherwise uncooperative, performing a phlebotomy or giving an injection presents a problem. In addition to wearing gloves, workers should use the new "safe" syringes, which have a sheath that pulls down to shield the needle after use. These may offer some protection in difficult situations. Injuries can also occur in surgery. The risk of acquiring HIV infection from operating on someone who is infected ranges from 1:4,500 to 1:130,000. The risk of contracting the virus from a surgical patient in a high-risk population can range from 1:100 to 10-15/10,000. Therefore, the risk of getting an HIV infection from any patient during surgery is between 1:450,000 in a high-risk population to 1-15:45,000,000 in a low-risk population.

Some surgeons advocate widespread pre-operative screening as a way of cutting that risk. They argue that if the test result is positive, they can take extra protective measures. Others see a number of problems with this approach. First, an ELISA antibody test followed by a Western Blot test can produce false-positive results. Second, testing not only invades the patient's privacy, but opens that person to discrimination. Last, the answer to taking extra care is that physicians should assume that everybody has AIDS and take care all the time.

Sharp instruments should be placed on the table, rather than being passed from hand to hand. Some authorities advocate using steel-mesh surgical gloves or thimbles while placing sutures, and the use of staples, rather than sutures, may also reduce risk. Routine use of double gloves has not been widely advocated, but it may be reasonable during long procedures, or when the gloves may become abraded or stressed.

In general, surgeons should re-evaluate any procedure involving needles and sharp objects if they regularly result in punctures or scratches. They must try to determine whether there is a safer approach.

Emergency Departments

Since many emergency department patients requiring invasive procedures are infected with the AIDS virus, the caretakers have the potential for encountering these patients. Thus, these observations reinforce the need to apply appropriate precautions to all patients ("Universal Body Substance Precautions") when providing emergency care, regardless of the patient's age or the nature of the presenting medical condition. All patients 15 years of age and older, who were triaged to the critical care area in a facility during a six week period three years ago, and who underwent any procedure related to the procurement of blood, were studied. Nine (7.1%) of the patients were shown to have unsuspected infection with HIV, compared with six (3.0%) of the patients studied a year earlier. Infected individuals were found in age groups up to 44 years old, whereas no infection was detected outside the 25 to 34 year old age range in 1986. Two of the 60 patients (3.4%), who presented with non-traumatic illnesses, were found to be infected with HIV during the survey, while there were no infections found in patients without trauma presentations one year earlier.

Although the CDC advocates flexible implementation of infection control precautions depending on the type of procedure performed, the infection control risks in the critically ill emergency department patient are difficult to predict. Therefore, it is strongly advocated that full infection control precautions — surgical gloves, gowns, masks, and eye protection — be employed by all health care personnel involved in the initial emergency care of all critically ill or injured patients.

Laboratory

Medical offices and hospitals that handle or process patient specimens should define containment procedures for handling all specimens. The personnel should observe these following procedures:

• Wear gloves when hands are likely to touch clinical specimens or surfaces, objects, or equipment contaminated by specimens.

• Wear gowns or lab coats when clothing is likely to be soiled.

• Minimize or avoid aerosols of specimens; wear masks and goggles when aerosolization is anticipated.

• Use mechanical pipetting devices; never pipette by mouth. Never smoke or eat while at the benches.

• Handle needles, slides, test tubes, and other sharp objects carefully to avoid punctures and other injuries.

• Immediately clean up spills of blood, serum, and other body substances; wear gloves and use a disinfectant.

Eye Care Professionals

Although the level of HIV in tears is low, and there has been no documented instances of HIV transmission by this fluid, transmission is theoretically possible.

Therefore, eye care professionals are advised to take appropriate precautions, including wearing gloves when possible, sterilizing or disinfecting instruments, and disinfecting contact lenses.

Dialysis

Patients with end-stage renal disease who are undergoing maintenance dialysis and who are infected with HIV or who have AIDS, can be dialyzed in hospital-based or free-standing dialysis units using conventional infection control precautions. Standard strategies for disinfection and sterilization are sufficient to prevent transmission of HIV.

Clinicians should be aware that the rate of false reactive EIAs in chronic dialysis patients was 4% in one study, much higher than the falsely reactive rate for blood donors (0.17%). When confirmed by Western Blot, the rate of truly reactives was 0.8%. The CDC is carrying out further studies to assess the prevalence of HIV among chronically dialyzed patients.

Dentistry

Dental health workers are in professional contact with a large number of patients, most of whom appear to be healthy. However, because a large proportion of persons infected with HIV do not show signs of infection, it is urgent that dental health workers take measures to protect themselves, as well as their patients, from HIV transmission. A recent report of a dentist who frequently practiced without gloves, and who apparently contracted HIV from a patient, emphasizes the importance of following infection control procedures.

The CDC has published infection control recommendations for dental health workers that may serve to prevent transmission of HIV, as well as other micro-organisms. Dentists and others in dentistry are urged to refer to the following summarized recommendations:

Gloves

• Gloves must always be worn when touching blood, saliva, or mucous membranes; when touching blood-soiled items, body fluids, or secretions, as well as surfaces contaminated with them; and when examining all oral lesions.

• All work must be completed on one patient, when possible, and the gloves removed and the hands washed and regloved before performing procedures on another patient.

• Repeated use of a single pair of gloves is *not* recommended, since such use is likely to produce defects in the glove material that will diminish its value as an effective barrier.

• Hands must be washed between patients (following removal of gloves), after touching inanimate objects likely to be contaminated by blood or saliva from other patients, and before leaving the operatory. During use, gloves may become perforated, whether or not the operator is aware of it. This allows viral contamination, as well as allowing bacteria to enter and multiply beneath the glove material. For many routine dental procedures, hand washing with plain soap appears to be adequate. For surgical procedures, an antimicrobial scrub should be used.

Protective Masks and Gloves

• Surgical masks and protective eyewear or chin-length plastic face shields must be worn when splashing or spattering of blood or other body fluids is likely, as is common in dentistry.

• Reusable or disposable gowns, lab coats, or uniforms must be worn when clothing is likely to be soiled with blood or other body fluids. If reusable gowns are worn, they may be washed, using a normal laundry cycle. Gowns should be changed at least daily, or when visibly soiled with blood.

Instruments and Surfaces

• Impervious-backed paper, aluminum foil, or clear plastic wrap may be used to cover surfaces that may be contaminated by blood or saliva, and that are difficult or impossible to clean and disinfect. These coverings should be removed (while gloved), discarded, and then replaced (after ungloving) with clean material between patients.

• Instruments that penetrate soft tissue and/or bone should be sterilized after each use. Instruments that are not intended to penetrate oral soft tissue or bone, but that may come into contact with oral tissues, should also be sterilized after each use, if possible; however, if sterilization is not feasible, the latter instruments should receive high-level disinfection.

Metal and heat-stable dental instruments should be routinely sterilized between uses by autoclaving, dry heat, or chemical vapor.

Routine sterilization of handpieces between patients is desirable. In the case of handpieces that cannot be sterilized, other complete cleaning and disinfection procedures should be followed. The same is true of ultrasonic scalers and air/water syringes.

Because water retraction valves within the dental unit may aspirate infective materials back into the handpiece and water line, these valves should be replaced with a non-aspirating method of coolant water containment.

Failed Protection

Lawsuits were filed separately by two physicians with AIDS. A house officer, who attributed her AIDS to a 1983 needlestick at King's County Hospital in New York, settled out of court for $1.35 million. She had sued the hospital and two other physicians, charging negligence and breach of confidentiality. In Baltimore, another house officer attributed his AIDS to a cut he received in 1983. A capillary tube that he was sealing broke in his hand, covering it with the contents, blood from a leukemia patient who had received at least 100 units of blood and blood products. The patient's stored serum later tested antibody-positive for HIV. He sued Johns Hopkins Hospital to defend his reputation and obtain appropriate benefits. The suit was settled three weeks before the trial date.

Guidelines

There are guidelines for a health care worker exposed to HIV-infected materials. The worker should be tested as soon as possible after exposure, and if initially seronegative, six weeks later, and periodically thereafter. The currently available tests are the enzyme-lined immunosorbent assay (ELISA) and the Western

Blot. An individual is considered seropositive if repeatedly positive ELISA tests are confirmed by a positive Western Blot assay. Because even the combination of these tests does not exclude false-positive results, the meaning of a positive test result in a physician depends on the likelihood that he or she is infected and the joint false-positive rate in the laboratory where the test is performed.

To Screen or Not to Screen

There is no controversy about whether HIV testing should be done when it is indicated for a patient's medical evaluation. However, screening solely to provide information for health care workers remains controversial. Those who advocate screening all hospital or office patients argue that the risk to health care workers outweighs the cost of screening. Furthermore, a negative HIV test might lead health care workers to lower their guard in treating such patients or handling their specimens, paradoxically increasing their risk for infection.

No existing evidence shows that health care workers reduce their risk for HIV infection when they know that a patient is HIV-positive. In fact, they may actually increase the risk of contamination by using precautions only with patients who are HIV-positive. Therefore, regardless of whether screening is done, precautions should be used for all patients in order to interrupt transmission and make the work place safer.

The question posed by the AIDS epidemic, then, is not whether physicians should be required to treat every potential patient who insists upon care, but whether they should be permitted to refuse to treat a class of patients out of fear of contracting a disease, when the empirical evidence demonstrates that their actual risk of infection ranges from low to negligible.

Many states have enacted legislation to address the problem of testing and informed consent. Physicians in New York State, for example, are subject to a statute and regulations concerning this aspect. The law defines the obligations and responsibilities of physicians and other health care providers with respect to informed consent and the confidentiality of HIV-related information. An informed consent form developed by the State Department of Health must be used every time an HIV test is performed. The regulations also require that counseling be provided before and after all HIV tests, and they spell out in detail the circumstances in which HIV-related information can be released without patient consent.

When to withhold or release information that a patient is HIV-positive is a pivotal issue. Such disclosure may cause patients to be denied insurance and to lose their jobs, and it may have other significant consequences. Under the new law, the physician is allowed to release this information in specific circumstances, e.g., to a health care provider if necessary for the patient's care and treatment. However, the law specifically prohibits disclosure solely for infection control purposes. This has outraged certain physicians, especially surgeons and anesthesiologists. One solution would allow primary care physicians to use their judgment in revealing this information, when appropriate, within the institution.

The New York law and the laws of several other jurisdictions create serious problems for health care providers, which it is believed could be avoided. For example, a house staff officer is stuck with a needle after drawing blood. The patient refuses to have an HIV test, and according to the law, the refusal is honored. The recipient of the needlestick has no way of knowing whether he or she has been exposed to a patient who is antibody-positive. Because there is a discrepancy between infection and antibody positivity, the house staff officer's own HIV test would not be conclusive for a period of six weeks to a year or more. The rules, intended to protect the patient's privacy, have made it impossible for a health care worker in a very real high-risk situation to determine whether infection by a patient has occurred. If hepatitis B were the concern, in appropriate circumstances, the resident could draw a sample without permission.

Although the public policy underlying this law may be well meant, a compromise is possible. The person who has sustained an accidental needlestick in a health care institution should be able to have a sample of the patient's blood drawn and arrange for an anonymous test of that blood. The house staff officer or technician who was the victim of the accident need not inform the patient, the patient's physician, or anyone else of the finding, but would have the right to know the results of the test so that appropriate steps to protect self and family could be taken.

Many controversial issues related to morals, ethics, and medical practice have been settled over time. HIV infection and AIDS, however, have become such a major political and emotional issue that the evolution of appropriate solutions has not taken place.

No Need to Tell Their Patients

Physicians who are seropositive for HIV should be extended at least the simplest of civil liberties that are extended to all other citizens, the right to privacy and the right to work so long as others are not at risk. This, despite a recent report which showed that 33% of the public believed that an infected physician could transmit AIDS to them.

The AMA has stated that if risk does not exist, disclosure of the physician's medical condition to his or her patients will serve no rational purpose. Thus, there is no ethical obligation for the physician to volunteer the information. If a patient should ask, the physician has the right to decline to answer the question based on the same arguments. Physicians should not disclose to their own patients whether or not they treat other patients who are HIV-positive.

Seropositive physicians must establish limits to their practices, so that there will not be a risk of transmission of disease to their patients. However, they do not have to tell their patients that they have the disease. Physicians have a right to confidentiality in matters that are not pertinent to their practice. The laws and ethical principles should discipline a physician who does not abide by the guidelines provided for the good of the patients.

Counseling Patients About Prevention

The Food and Drug Administration (FDA) is urging that physicians and other health professionals help educate patients about ways to prevent the spread of HIV. It should be stressed to patients that because AIDS is a sexually transmitted disease (STD), sexual abstinence or a mutually monogamous relationship with an uninfected partner is the best insurance against acquiring the disease, except when one partner is an intravenous drug abuser, in which case, mutual monogamy offers no protection.

Condoms

For sexually active persons, the only instance when condoms are unnecessary for reduction of infection risk is within a long-standing, mutually monogamous relationship in which neither partner uses IV drugs, and neither partner is infected with HIV. This applies to any sexual activity where the exchange of semen and/or blood is possible, including vaginal, anal, and oral sex.

Recent studies have indicated that natural membrane condoms are not able to contain and, therefore, are unable to protect against infection from the HIV virus. Therefore, the FDA allows only latex condoms to be labeled for the prevention of STDs, including AIDS.

Because the diameter of the HIV virus is about 1/25th that of spermatozoa, there was initially some question about whether condoms could contain the virus. Subsequently, however, in vitro tests of latex condoms and epidemiologic data confirmed that the HIV virus does not pass through an intact latex condom.

To maximize protection against STDs, it is important that condoms be used properly. The FDA has sent a letter to all U.S. condom manufacturers, importers, and repackagers regarding the labeling of condoms for prevention of STDs. The letter stated that only latex condoms could be labeled for the prevention of STDs, including AIDS. The FDA does not allow natural membrane condoms to be so labeled because they have a different permeability than latex, and may not lend themselves to the same degree of uniformity. However, regardless of the product's labeling and composition, the FDA requested that all condoms contain adequate instructions for use to maximize the degree of protection they afford.

The FDA suggested the following as an acceptable labeling statement for latex condoms:

• When used properly, the latex condom may prevent the transmission of many sexually transmitted diseases (STDs) such as syphilis, gonorrhea, chlamydial infections, genital herpes, and AIDS. It cannot eliminate the risk. *For maximum protection, it is important to follow the accompanying instructions.* Failure to do so may result in loss of protection. During intimate contact, lesions and various body fluids can transmit STDs. Therefore, the condom should be applied before any such contact.

Risk of Malpractice

There is nothing speculative about the risks of malpractice liability involved in the care and management of patients with HIV infections. One recent verdict against a physician was $28.7 million. Such risks are borne not merely by those who specialize in the treatment of AIDS and ARC, such as infectious disease specialists and oncologists, but by all clinicians. It behooves the practitioner, therefore, to be aware of potential pitfalls that could serve as grounds for a lawsuit, so that with foresight, such pitfalls may be avoided.

The avoidance of potential perils will have an even more important reward: an increase in the quality of care for patients.

Failure to Diagnose HIV Infection

In 1988, a million dollar judgment was entered against a Massachusetts physician who failed to diagnose *Pneumocystis carinii* pneumonia in a 32 year old woman, the result of taking an inadequate history and the failure to identify her as a high-risk patient. More such actions will undoubtedly be brought in the future.

HIV infection in its early stages usually is asymptomatic. Legally, there is no requirement to test an otherwise healthy patient for HIV. Unless such testing becomes customary in medical practice, lawsuits by low-risk individuals who were asymptomatic but seropositive at the time of examination, claiming that they should have been tested, are unlikely to succeed. However, the presentation of AIDS and ARC syndromes varies widely, and may have a lengthy and plausible differential diagnosis. A high index of suspicion, therefore, must be maintained, and if HIV is even remotely considered as an underlying etiology, an antibody test should be performed.

The importance of a complete history cannot be overstated. In the Massachusetts case cited above, the patient was female and did not abuse intravenous drugs, but her husband *was* an IV drug abuser. Hence, the physician might have been well-advised to perform an HIV test, even in the absence of severe pulmonary symptoms.

The physician must consider what tests to perform. In addition to the ELISA and Western Blot tests, there now exists the polymeris chain reaction (PCR), which is quick, inexpensive, and accurate. When a patient is judged to be at risk for HIV infection, the physician may wish to perform the PCR, as well as other tests, in order to be as certain as possible of the results.

In addition, physicians must be aware of the "window" between the time the patient is infected with HIV and the time an HIV test will turn positive. A patient who falls within this "window" is a false-negative. Where suspicion of HIV is high enough, a patient should be considered as having the virus, even when test results are negative, and the tests should be repeated after an appropriate interval.

Failure to make a timely diagnosis of progressive HIV infection can have a significant negative impact on a patient's prognosis. First, there are treatments and prophylactic measures that can prolong the life of an HIV-positive patient and enhance that life's quality. Such measures are known to be most effective in the early stages of the infection. If diagnosis is delayed, the patient will not be given the available prophylaxis and active treatment until the infection is discovered, possibly resulting in an acceleration of the disease process, ineffective treatment of opportunistic diseases, and early death.

Second, until a diagnosis of HIV infection is made, a patient will not be in a position to take steps to avoid exposure to other infections to which he or she would have increased susceptibility. Such avoidable infections might then be contracted, with results that could be devastating. In addition, a patient who is *re*infected with HIV has a worse prognosis than one who has been infected only once, and timely diagnosis is essential to enable the patient to avoid multiple exposures to the virus.

Third, a delay in diagnosis that led to a delay in needed prophylaxis and treatment could lead to emotional distress. Such emotional distress could be grounds for a legal action seeking damages to cover the costs of the resultant loss of income, psychotherapy, or pain and suffering.

Erroneous Diagnosis of HIV

As with many screening tests, the initial test for HIV antibody - the ELISA test - has a high sensitivity, but a relatively low specificity. Thus, this test produces some false-positives. A positive ELISA test must be supplemented with the more specific Western Blot test or the PCR, in order to have any reasonable certainty that the results are accurate. Failure to do so could lead to an incorrect positive diagnosis of HIV infection.

There are several grounds for potential liability if a physician mistakenly tells a patient that he or she is seropositive. A patient in this position may be denied employment or dismissed from employment, or may decline to seek employment. The physician could then be sued for any damages when the error becomes known.

In those jurisdictions that do not require a physical touching in order to establish a case for negligent infliction of emotional distress, an incorrect diagnosis may lead to an action for emotional injury. Another possible ground for liability is the tort of "outrage", where the emotional injury was inflicted intentionally or recklessly. Patients who believe, rightly or wrongly, that they are infected with HIV are apt to feel some distress, and in many cases, will develop full-blown anxiety or depression, leading to a decreased level of social and occupational functioning. Where the diagnosis was erroneous, damages against the physician could include the costs of counseling, lost wages, or pain and suffering.

Patients have committed suicide soon after being told that they had tested positive for HIV. When the decedent in such a case turns out (on autopsy, perhaps) not to have contracted HIV after all, the physician may be the subject of an action for wrongful death.

Failure to Inform Patient of Seropositivity

Occasionally, an institutional physician who examines a patient for an employer, an insurance company, or a prison discovers that a patient is HIV-positive. The physician's duty in these circumstances is not that of the ordinary physician-patient relationship, and some courts have held that the physician has a legal obligation to inform the patient of the test results. Similarly, blood donor screening may uncover seropositive blood, and the legal duty to inform is murky in this instance as well.

Uncertain though the physician's obligations may be, it is clear that the physician takes a considerable risk whenever he or she knows that a patient is infected and does not inform that patient. Such actions have been upheld for other diseases in several jurisdictions; for example, in a 1981 Louisiana Supreme Court case, a hospital hired by an employer to perform a pre-employment examination was found liable for failure to disclose a diagnosis of tuberculosis to the prospective employee. All of the possible grounds for suit that were covered in the discussion of failure to diagnose HIV infection apply here as well.

Where there is a clear physician-patient relationship, the physician may refrain from informing a patient of a positive test because the physician thinks the patient is too unstable to handle the news. There is a doctrine called "therapeutic privilege" that would appear to allow physicians this discretion, although courts have been loath to invoke it. Where there is some question about a patient's capacity to deal with a diagnosis, the physician should tell the patient, and then be responsible for counseling the patient as well.

Inadequate Counseling

A patient usually incurs emotional distress on discovering that he or she is positive for HIV. Such distress may be intensified if the patient is unaware of the significance of the test results. In addition, patients need to know how to modify their personal activities to avoid undue danger to their own health, as well as to avoid transmission of the disease to others. Thus, the physician has a clear obligation to arrange for counseling that effectively teaches the patient the meaning of the diagnosis and the behavioral changes indicated. If this is done and documented adequately, the physician will not be liable for damages to the patient that result from the patient's failure to follow the counselor's advice.

Patients should always be informed that there is a "window" during which a recently infected individual will show a negative HIV titer.

Treatment

The American Medical Association is completing a set of guidelines for early HIV treatment. Areas covered by these recommendations include the medical history, disease staging, and vaccinations to prevent opportunistic infections. When available, the guidelines will indicate what is considered reasonable by the medical profession, and they may be admissible in the examination of an expert witness in a court of law. Of course, a jury may be persuaded by expert testimony on the other side, but it would be advisable for a physician to avoid falling below official AMA standards.

In particular, early prophylaxis with AZT (zidovudine) is now indicated. Where T-4 cell counts have dropped appreciably, AZT will bolster the immune system and help ward off *Pneumocystis carinii* pneumonia. Failure to prescribe AZT when it would be reasonable to do so could accelerate the progress of the disease. Further breakthroughs in treatment may be expected, and physicians are advised to stay current.

Failure to Obtain Consent

Many states have enacted statutes that require written formal consent from a patient before an HIV antibody test is performed. Nowhere has it been held expressly that such consent is dispensable, although some states have deleted such requirements which had previously existed in the law. The best advice for all physicians, therefore, is to obtain written consent whenever possible when an HIV test is done.

But what if a patient suspected of being infected with HIV appears likely to refuse to consent to testing? To test under these circumstances would obviate the requirement of informed consent; to fail to test might not only violate the patient's best interests, but place others at risk as well. A physician's best course in this circumstance is to obtain the advice of counsel.

Some states no longer require by statute that physicians provide counseling to patients prior to conducting an HIV test. However, since informed consent requires that a patient understand the nature and significance of that to which consent is given, it always is important to document that such an explanation has been made.

There may, of course, be instances in which a patient is unable to consent, but is in a known high-risk group. When there are specific reasons for testing, physicians may be protected if they obtain consent from the next-of-kin or another authorized surrogate.

Wrongful Birth

One of the ways in which HIV is contracted is via the placenta during pregnancy. There is a trend in the courts to recognize a cause of action for wrongful birth when a baby is born diseased or injured as a result of medical negligence. Hence, when a physician has failed to diagnose the viral infection in a pregnant woman, or has failed to inform her of positive test results, the physician may be subject to such an action. Liability could include damages for medical expenses, increased childrearing expenses, and pain and suffering of the parents, as well as of the child.

The Centers for Disease Control have recommended that HIV-positive women who are pregnant or of childbearing potential be counseled about the risk to their infant, in order that they may make an informed choice about whether to terminate or to delay pregnancy.

Negligent Transmission of HIV

In June, 1990, an Arizona jury found a neonatologist liable for $28.7 million for infecting a newborn with HIV by negligently transfusing HIV-infected red blood cells and plasma. While blood now is routinely screened for HIV, making this mode of transmission less likely today, a physician may still be liable for failure to take adequate precautions against the spread of the disease. Not only blood transfusions, but transfusions of sperm and organ transplants may be sources of HIV transmission.

The Centers for Disease Control have issued guidelines for prevention of HIV transmission. These guidelines should be followed strictly. Transmission of the virus to a colleague, when such transmission might have been avoided had the guidelines been followed, already has occasioned a major lawsuit in New York.

Breach of Confidentiality/Breach of Duty to Warn

Many states have enacted statutes that prohibit disclosure of HIV test results to anyone other than the patient and specified others. However, such laws vary widely, and may conflict with other laws that place on physicians a duty to warn. A physician with questions about the law in his or her own jurisdiction is best advised to contact local counsel.

Circumstances in which confidentiality of HIV test results may be breached (depending on state law) include the following:

—Where the physician has reason to believe that the patient poses a danger of viral transmission to a third party, such as a spouse or a sexual partner, or an adoptive or foster home parent. In the 1976 *Tarasoff* case in California, a psychiatrist was found to have violated a duty to warn when his patient, after telling the psychiatrist of his intention to kill a particular victim, did so. While this holding has not been applied to the transmission of a communicable disease, a physician who does not warn a spouse may be liable if the spouse does contact HIV.

—In conducting contact tracing, where a physician has reason to believe that a sexual or needle-sharing partner already has contracted the virus. Prophylactic medication may be indicated for such a partner.

—Where a state has a mandatory reporting requirement, such a requirement supersedes any law that would treat such reporting as a breach of confidentiality.

It may be necessary to devise a special medical records system to keep HIV test results confidential from all health professionals, except those who are directly involved in the care of the patient.

Conclusion

The dramatic consequences of HIV infection, and its emotional and political aspects, call for special consideration by physicians who are faced with infected patients. The best rule of thumb in this area, as in others where the threat of malpractice looms, is that the physician's best protection is his or her own competence and dedication. In other words, good medicine makes good law. However, the state of the law remains in flux, and physicians must determine what safeguards are required in their own jurisdictions.

INTERNAL MEDICINE/FAMILY PRACTICE

Introduction

The primary care physician is at the fulcrum of medical practice in this country. The internist/family practice physician is almost always the primary care physician. Although these physicians are not at the top of the malpractice hit parade, it is logical to present the numerous legal doctrines applicable to the various branches of medicine and surgery under this heading. It behooves the various specialists to consult this chapter to obtain an overview of applicable legal principles. Actually, the commonest causes of malpractice for the family practice physician and the internist involve misdiagnosis or late diagnosis, errors in orders and the prescription of medications, and failure to order laboratory tests and to act in timely fashion on the basis of the results of such tests. However, all physicians occasionally "stumble", and suffer the consequences of a malpractice suit based on the various principles described.

The Physician-Patient Relationship

The "life" of medical practice, both generically and specifically, is the physician-patient relationship. Both medically and legally, it is considered a "sacred" or fiduciary relationship. The physician-patient relationship is generally considered to be a contractual one. The physician-patient contract may be entered into with the physician by a third party on behalf of the patient, as in the case of the house officer. The obligations, duties, and responsibilities of the house officer under the contract has limitations. It is different than that of the private physician-patient relationship. This will be discussed below.

Standard of Care

The standard of care to which a health officer may be held will depend on the jurisdiction in which he has his practice, what procedures or treatments may be utilized in the practice, and the nature of the patient's complaints. A single rule establishing the standard of care that is valid for all physicians in all states, and encompassing all specialties and procedures in all clinical circumstances, is impossible to formulate. In general, a house officer is held to a standard of care commensurate with his training. Each physician must make an effort to determine the current standards in his geographical area or in a similar locality, or the national standards for the branch of medicine he practices.

The physician must have adequate knowledge and skill and use it with adequate care in his dealings with a patient. The reasonably pruphysician, acting under the same circumstances, is the standard by which his conduct will be judged. He may also be liable if he knows what to do, but for some reason, does not do it carefully or omits doing it at all.

If another course of treatment would appear to be more beneficial than the one being used, the physician must adopt it. If a patient's condition or the nature of his or her illness or injury is such that the usual and accepted method of treatment would present unusual hazards to him or her, a departure from it is not considered negligence. If established treatment has been less than successful, and the patient's condition is sufficiently serious to necessitate an unproven approach, a physician can justify innovative treatment techniques as being in the best interest of his patient and not as a procedure to elicit research information. This is probably not applicable to house officers.

In the past, courts recognized a standard of care as applying to practices in the same or similar locality or community. However, recently, national standards have been invoked for health professionals and hospitals. Increasingly, internal medicine and family practice house officers are being held to a national standard of care defined as that ordinarily exercised by house officer members of these specialties under similar circumstances. Legally, "doing the best you can" is not a plausible defense.

Where there is more than one recognized method of diagnosis or treatment alternatives and neither is used exclusively and uniformly by other practitioners in good standing, a house officer is not negligent if, in exercising his best judgment, he selects one of the approved methods, and the results turn out poorly. It may have been a wrong selection, or one not favored by certain other physicians, but this is merely a mistake of error in judgment. In other words, human fallibility is not legal liability. However, it is apparent from a review of recent court decisions that the courts are now allowing awards to patients who are the victims of gross errors or mistakes in judgment.

If the patient is properly treated by an accepted method or an allowable deviation from an accepted method and does not recover and dies, or if the treatment causes some other problem, or a worsening of the condition than that from which the patient originally suffered, the house officer is still not liable if he carefully used standard practice and treatment modalities.

All patients do not recover from their problems; physicians are neither guarantors nor insurers of their patient's good health. Some conditions refuse to respond to all known methods of treatment, and some patients exhibit idiosyncratic reactions to established and accepted methods of cure. The legal definitions of due care and negligence are such that no inference of negligence is raised from the fact that a patient's condition did not improve. A poor result is never sufficient in and of itself to establish negligence by a physician. As long as the treatment was proper, there is no malpractice, regardless of the outcome of the patient's illness.

A house officer whose native language is not English would probably be found liable if his difficulties with the language prevent him from reaching any understanding of the patient's complaints and, as a result, he administers the wrong treatment, no matter how skillfully he applies it.

Judicially Imposed Standard of Care

Generally, courts rely on medically established standards of care to determine a health care provider's duty and breach of that duty. Recently, some courts have required a "preferred" rather than the usual, ordinary standard of care. To that end, the courts have rejected the testimony of medical experts as to the accepted medical standard of care when they thought it inappropriate, and decreed their own standard of medical care.

Causation

Although a physician may have negligently acted or failed to act, and thereby has failed to fulfill the standard of care owed the patient, a successful lawsuit cannot be maintained unless the negligence caused some calculable harm to the patient.

Expert Testimony

Since the alleged negligence involves matters outside the general knowledge of the trier of fact, these criteria must generally be established by an acceptable medical expert, such as another internist or physician, even a nurse, who can establish the requisite knowledge and expertise. A patient can only prove a case against one health care provider through the mouth of another. This means that generally, the patient must find an expert. It is rare for a house officer to be called as an expert.

Res Ipsa Loquitur

A long-accepted substitute for the medical expert has been the use of "res ipsa loquitur", or "the thing speaks for itself". It is akin to the common knowledge doctrine. Three conditions are necessary before this rule may be applied: that in the ordinary course of affairs, the accident would not have occurred if reasonable care had been used; that the thing that caused the accident was under the exclusive control of the defendant; and that the plaintiff did not contribute to the occurrence of the accident.

When the plaintiff proves that these conditions exist, it is regarded in some states as circumstantial evidence of negligence, which a judge or jury may accept or reject. In other states, it is held to create a presumption of negligence. It must be remembered that res ipsa loquitur does not have uniform acceptance and implementation in the various states. Under certain conditions, the absence of an expert is not a shield for the defendant-health care provider.

Agency

Liability may also be imposed under the doctrine of agency and "respondeat superior", based on the acts or inactions of others working under the immediate direction, supervision, and control of the physician. This is based on whether the acts or omissions were in the practitioner's presence or absence, and whether or not the physician had the actual ability to control the employee's conduct. A house officer can impose liability on his employer, and possibly the attending physician, by his negligent acts. He must realize that the patient may elect to sue him, and the hospital or insurance carrier can seek indemnification if they are required to pay on behalf of the house officer.

Keeping Abreast — Keeping Up

The law and medicine have imposed a duty on all physicians, including house officers, to be aware of changing concepts and new developments. Keeping up can be accomplished by reading current medical literature and attending scientific meetings and continuing education programs.

It is not the physician's duty to implement new techniques merely because they are new; usefulness, safety, and efficacy must be reasonably established. What may be accepted as the most advanced practice of internal or family practice medicine one time in a physician's career may be swiftly outdated by new discoveries and advances; it is his obligation to render treatment to his patients based on adequate understanding of those new developments. But a physician who is ignorant of recent developments that are known to and accepted by medical practitioners may be liable if the use of an outmoded method results in harm to the patient. While adherence to the usual practice by which the local medical community deals with a problem is ordinarily a good defense to a charge of negligence, i.e., that everybody does it, may not be an excuse if it is, in fact, a sloppy or careless practice, or contrary to national standards.

Diagnosis and Treatment

The failure to properly diagnose and treat are the most common malpractice allegations being made against primary care physicians today. All physicians, regardless of status, have to maintain a high "index of suspicion". They have to constantly think about the diagnostic possibilities to explain any symptoms and findings. The house officer should not be steered into a diagnosis by the patient. Part of maintaining a high level of suspicion is adopting the philosophy that nothing should be treated routinely. When physician and staff reduce patient care to a rigid routine, discontent and non-compliance follow, and malpractice, based on the resultant negligence, frequently ensues.

Misdiagnosis and Delay in Diagnosis

Failure or delay in the diagnosis of a disease is one of the leading allegations in malpractice cases involving internists and family practice physicians. These failures may result in a patient having to undergo more extensive treatment, reduce his or her chances of survival, lead to earlier or unnecessary death, and cause physical and emotional burdens that more timely diagnosis could have avoided. Liability, based on the doctrine of loss of a chance, may arise from a physician's negligent action or inaction, or both.

Loss of a Chance

Loss of a chance caused by the negligence of a physician has been recognized. The question of how to weigh diminished prospects for a plaintiff whose statistical future expectations are already severely impaired has caused many courts to re-examine the issue: should liability be imposed for negligence that merely increased the probability of an already probable negative outcome?

The majority of U.S. jurisdictions retain the "but for" test, i.e., the negligently injured patient must prove that the chance for recovery or survival was probable, was more likely than not, or was better than even. The rationale for this all-or-nothing approach is that less-than-probable losses are speculative and unfairly impose liability based on unquantified possibilities. The majority position is that what the measure "might have caused" is an insufficient quantum of evidence.

Under the majority theory, a plaintiff with less than a 50-50 chance cannot be harmed to a compensable degree by negligent care.

Wrongful Death

If negligence results in the death of a patient, recovery may be based on the doctrine of wrongful death. A wrongful death is a death that occurs earlier than it would have ordinarily. If negligence is the legal causation of the patient's death, then his or her statutory survivors or personal estate may bring an action in "wrongful death". The action is considered to be a derivative one; it cannot be brought unless the decedent would have had a cause of action had he or she survived.

Its rationale is to benefit the survivors. The action is thus a creature of statute, and allows the decedent's survivors to maintain civil actions. Recovery includes pecuniary damages, or that amount which the decedent could reasonably have been expected to contribute if his or her death had not ensued, plus damages for emotional injury. It is a common source of malpractice lawsuits against family practitioners and internists following alleged failed treatment.

Breach of Warranty — Promises, Promises, Promises

No physician should ever specifically promise anything. That creates a specific contract of warranty. More importantly, the physician must be clear in that his assurances, hopefulness, and positiveness not be confused with a specific promise; otherwise, that may result in a suit for breach of a contract warranty.

Medical History

The medical history is the primary responsibility of the attending physician. It is a critical part of the physician's diagnostic workup. Since attending physicians very frequently rely on the house officer's history, it behooves him to abide by the standard of care. Failure to take an adequate medical history, or an incomplete medical history, may be a significant factor in the failure to make the proper or correct diagnosis. As a result of the failure to obtain an adequate history, a physician may fail to include a disease in the differential diagnosis, or may not give proper weight to a disease when evaluating certain clinical signs and symptoms. This failure to appropriately consider a disease may be negligence, as is the failure to make reasonable inquiries about the circumstances of the illness of the patient.

A physician is also required to ask appropriate questions designed to elicit all necessary and relevant information, but he may not merely rely on information the patient volunteers. The physician is also obligated to pay attention to the patient's complaints. Failure to listen to what a patient is trying to tell him about any symptoms or changes in condition could result in the physician's remaining unaware of earlier indications of serious problems. Furthermore, the physician must follow through until the problem is resolved. Family and racial history, particularly in certain diseases, is an important criterion in evaluating patients for screening.

On the other hand, over-reliance on certain facts obtained in taking the medical history may be just as significant as failure to take an adequate history. Failure to follow the clues of certain symptoms as related by the patient because of a history of certain facts has been a factor in the failure to diagnose cases involving internal and family practice medicine.

Failure to listen to the patient and communicate, which results in adverse consequences, is negligence. It is prudent for the physician to examine earlier records.

If this is not done and causes a misdiagnosis as the result of incomplete data, it may constitute negligence if the result is injury to the patient.

Physical Examination

A patient is entitled to a careful and thorough examination to the extent that the circumstances, the condition of the patient, and the physician's opportunity for examination permit. The same admonitions apply as for history-taking. In other words, a duly careful physician will examine the patient with the necessary thoroughness possible under the circumstances.

Failure to perform a physical examination, performing an inadequate examination, over-reliance on a negative examination, or failure to perform a follow-up examination have contributed to lawsuits for failure to diagnose internal medicine problems. Failure to perform an examination, particularly when a significant symptom has been found, figures prominently in many failures to diagnose internal and family practice medicine problems, as has failure to perform follow-up examinations.

Diagnosis

There usually are serious physical and emotional consequences to the patient after being told incorrectly that a disease is present. While, presumably, it is better to diagnose a disease which does not exist than it is to fail to discover one which actually does exist, in either case, the patient has undoubtedly been harmed by the error.

Testing

A physician has an affirmative duty to obtain or perform appropriate tests in the diagnosis of a suspected disease. A physician who fails to use necessary and appropriate laboratory tests in diagnosing a patient's condition, or fails to act on them properly, may also be liable for negligence. With cost-containment, house officers are frequently precluded from ordering tests without the consent of the attending physician.

An error in the evaluation of a test, which results in an incorrect diagnosis, also virtually guarantees large damages for the plaintiff. Losing track of lab results is a problem that crops up in many hospitals. Reports from a laboratory or a consultant that are lost, ignored, or misunderstood have led to successful malpractice suits for negligence or abandonment.

Invasive tests may be necessary in some cases to make a proper diagnosis. Where the test carries serious inherent risk, it becomes a matter of medical judgment whether or not the patient, whose condition is best known by the attending physician, should be subjected to the procedure. Therefore, the more complicated and dangerous the test may be, the less likely it is that a court will find that a physician was negligent in failing to perform it. If, however, the patient's condition is serious, a physician would be much more likely to be held liable for failing to have ordered a dangerous test than if the condition was no more serious, at worst, than the test itself. In these situations, the house officer is best advised to rely on the attending physician.

Even when a report is negative, over-reliance on that report may be negligence when clinical suspicion should be high. Mere reliance on a test performed by a consultant does not always mean negligence, however. Failure of a physician to read the test report or consultant's recommendation, or communicate the report or recommendation to the patient, may be negligence. Failure to repeat a test or perform additional studies when an initial test is negative may be negligence when clinical suspicion is, or should be, high that a disease may still be present.

Negligence during the performance of a test which damages the patient, apart from the accuracy of the report, may impose liability on the physician. If he recommended an incompetent laboratory, or did not communicate the proper data to direct the laboratory to the target, he may be considered negligent. Also, if the physician fails to communicate the result, particularly if it is abnormal and requires further care and management of the patient, and he or she suffers harm, the physician is legally vulnerable.

Although these activities are not within the province of a house officer, some house officers do have this authority and, therefore, are subject to the same principles.

Duty to Refer and/or Consult

For a practicing physician, there are no absolute rules regarding the seeking of a consultation or making a referral. The house officer is constantly involved in referral and/or consultation. The law puts the responsibility on the physician himself of knowing when these are indicated and whom to call. The physician must be aware of any shortcomings. An essential part of practicing good medicine is knowing when to call for a consultation or refer a patient when there is the need for an appropriate consultation and/or referral. Actually, the physician has the duty to refer a patient to a specialist whenever the physician's equipment or facilities are inadequate, or he does not have the requisite trained assistants if they are needed.

A physician is required to tell a patient (or next-of-kin if necessary) if his treatment is not beneficial. If the physician knows that the treatment is ineffective, he is obligated to adopt one of several alternatives. If a specialist would facilitate the patient's recovery, he must make a referral. This is the responsibility of the attending physician, not that of the house officer.

Failure of a physician, including a house officer, to refer to or consult with another physician or specialist for a suspected, or even known, disease may also be a negligent act of omission. Generally, because of the imposing consequences of treatment — for example, if chemotherapy or radiotherapy is proposed — the patient should be offered the benefit of a consultation to assure adequate exposure to alternative modalities. This is one of the most effective ways to avoid a later allegation of undue influence or pressure. Once the offer of a consultation or second opinion is recorded in the chart, there is significantly less chance for a patient to allege he or she was railroaded into a particular course of treatment without adequate informed consent.

If a house officer encounters a situation that is beyond his knowledge or experience, requesting that a consultation from a specialist colleague be obtained, or referring the patient to a tertiary health care facility, is not only the smart thing to do, it is a duty. For example, a physician, such as a house officer, who does not have the training to perform a given procedure, or who does not ask for the necessary information on which to make a diagnosis or render treatment, may be considered careless as he deals with the patient and, in fact, his care may not meet the highest possible standards. The house officer may be negligent if the patient is injured because he failed to refer the patient to a specialist and lacked the necessary expertise himself to treat the patient properly. Thus, a physician may be liable in negligence if he is remiss in his obligation to realize that he is not capable of treating the patient and should, therefore, have gotten help.

A physician who knows what is wrong with a patient and exactly what treatment is necessary may, however, have an obligation to refer the patient to a hospital elsewhere, which has better facilities or equipment than are locally available. However, before a house officer can be found liable for failure to refer a patient, the circumstances must be such that the duly careful house officer should have known that a problem existed which he was not equipped to solve.

In referral cases, the physician to whom the patient is referred is not ordinarily required to make an independent diagnosis. The requirements of ordinary care are fulfilled by accepting the diagnosis of the referring physician, assuming that there is nothing in the patient's condition to put the consultant on notice that an erroneous diagnosis has been made. If the patient's symptoms indicate that the original diagnosis might be incorrect, the consultant is obliged to make his own evaluation prior to initiating treatment.

In an emergency, of course, a different situation is presented. A physician in a small hospital unit might, in fact, be considered negligent if he sent a patient to a larger hospital, and the patient's condition would be jeopardized by the move. In that situation, good and careful medical practice would require only that the physician do the best he can with whatever equipment he has at his disposal.

In most cases, if a physician refers a patient to a duly qualified consultant of whom there is no reason to suspect negligence and the first physician's involvement with the case terminates at that time, any negligence by the consultant is not imputed to him and he is not liable for it. When the referring physician continues to participate actively in the care of the patient, however, he may be jointly liable with the consultant.

If the house officer's activities are directed entirely by the attending physician or consultant, or if one of these providers assumes all decision-making responsibility, the house officer probably would not be liable, even if he continued to visit the patient in the hospital or involved himself in other cooperative ventures. The controlling factor, therefore, in any question of joint liability in a referral situation is the extent of participation by the house officer in diagnosis and treatment.

Whenever there is a referral or consultation, the physicians between them, with the consent of the patient, must define whether it will be a "one shot" affair, whether the two physicians will continue the care jointly, or the new physician will take over the care of the patient exclusively.

A consulting physician who examines a patient at the request of a house officer on behalf of the primary physician for a "one shot" consultation, but who does not intend to continue to treat the patient, certainly is not legally obligated to do so. This should, however, be made clear to both the patient and the primary physician. If this is not done, it is possible that the consultant may later be sued for abandonment. A physician who refers a patient to a specialist for treatment by means of a transfer of care is held to have relieved himself of any further responsibility to the patient, in the absence of an understanding that he will be associated with the consultant in caring for the patient. Again, this must be explained clearly to the patient and the consultant, in order to avoid any possibility of misunderstanding.

If a consultant writes a note and makes a recommendation, the physician in attendance must either follow that recommendation, or justify in the record why he did not do so. It is difficult later to justify why he asked for the advice of a consultant and then chose to ignore it without any explanation. The attending physician should record all consultations, the results, and his actions based on the consulting physician's recommendations.

In order to get the most out of a consultation or referral, the physician in attendance should:

- Arrange for the consultation/referral to be certain it is accomplished;
- Communicate appropriate information in timely fashion to the consultant;
- Require that the report be returned in timely fashion, and communicate personally with the consultant if necessary, particularly to reconcile any differences; and
- Advise the patient as to the recommendations and decisions. If the physician is the consultant, he has the corresponding responsibility.

Over-Treatment - Unnecessary Treatment

While the physician may be held liable for doing too little too late, there is another aspect to this medicolegal equation. The physician may be held liable for doing too much or allowing the house officer to do so, particularly if it is unnecessary, and liability may be imposed for harm caused by over-reacting. It may appear that the physician is damned if he does and damned if he doesn't; nevertheless, in some instances, he is best advised to do nothing.

Continuity of Care

Due care obligates a physician in attendance to follow up on his patient's progress. He must be sure that his patient understands his instructions pertaining to medication, restrictions on activities, return visits, and the like. Of course, if the patient is a child or young adolescent, the physician should, when appropriate, communicate instructions to the parents, as well as to the child. If the patient is senile or otherwise incompetent, instructions must be given to a family member or other responsible adult. If the patient has difficulty with English, the physician must present the instructions appropriately and be sure that they have been understood. If there is any question of illiteracy, oral instructions corresponding to any written ones, such as those on medication labels, must be given.

The responsibility of any physician is not concluded when the patient's immediate need is met. A house officer assigned to the outpatient department should schedule check-up visits to keep abreast of the patient's progress, if necessary, since these visits are as vital as the need for due care in the performance of the original treatment.

Abandonment

Abandonment, in its classical sense, involves an intentional act on the part of a physician to improperly terminate the physician-patient relationship. Closely related to this is the situation in which there is no such intention by the house officer, but he is so dilatory in his obligation that he does not see the patient as often as due care in treatment would demand, and the patient is thus denied the benefit of the physician-patient relationship.

When a patient in the out-patient clinic is released from direct supervision by a house officer, all responsibility and obligations to him or her do not necessarily cease. If the patient's condition requires continuing care, the house officer who neglects to explain these matters is negligent.

If a house officer talks to an out-patient by telephone, either to receive reports as to his or her condition or to give instructions, he may have a justification for not attending the patient personally. If he elects to make a diagnosis or prescribe treatment by telephone, even if it is later proven incorrect, the patient probably does not have an action for abandonment if a reasonable physician in attendance would conclude that he could make an adequate diagnosis in the case on the basis of a telephone conversation.

Discharging a patient from the hospital is the responsibility of the attending physician. Doing it prior to the time when his or her condition justifies it is abandonment, whether the discharge is because the patient cannot pay the bill, or results from an honest mistake as to his or her condition and need for further medical care. The house officer has a duty to intervene when the discharge is improper.

Failure by an out-patient to return when told to do so by the house officer is, of course, under most circumstances, considered to be contributory negligence if there is a mishap; therefore, the physician whose patient does not follow instructions to report for further treatment is not generally considered guilty of abandonment.

Other actions that may be considered to be constructive abandonment include failure to regularly visit a patient in the hospital, and failure to visit a hospitalized patient adequately or with sufficient frequency to keep aware of his or her problems; a house officer's failure to admit an out-patient to a hospital when it is indicated, particularly in an emergency, or to see him or her after an emergency admission, will undoubtedly be considered to be negligent.

Abandonment may give rise not only to a malpractice action in tort for negligence, but one for breach of contract.

Privacy and Confidentiality

Privacy is a patient's right to have peace of mind regarding the exposure and revelation of his or her body, or depictions thereof, to unauthorized persons; confidentiality is the identical right as to his or her medical information. A patient's right to privacy and confidentiality has one of the highest priorities in our legal system. Statutes and court decisions proclaim the duty to provide, maintain, and enforce a patient's right to privacy and confidentiality, and the perils in failing to do so. The Supreme Court has recognized it as a constitutional right. No longer is privacy and confidentiality merely a moral, ethical, professional obligation; it is now a legal duty. It also applies to house officers. A patient has a right to be advised of the house officer's identity and role in the management of his or her case.

A house officer may be liable for disclosure of confidential information about a patient, even if it is true. Release of information about a patient as a matter of gossip is obviously always unjustified. Social conversation involving a patient invariably is sufficient to give rise to a successful lawsuit against a physician.

Because of the extreme importance of the confidential relationship between any physician and the patient, there are statutes in some states which provide that a physician may lose his license for unjustified dissemination of confidential information. It is also a criminal offense in at least one state.

Publication of information or pictures, or discussion of a patient, without his or her consent, even with obfuscation of the identity, if he or she is or can be identified by name or appearance, may lead to a successful lawsuit for invasion of privacy, even if the pictures or information are published in a medical journal for legitimate educational or scientific purposes. A patient may very well give consent to the taking of photographs to be used in medical journals. However, if the scope of the use of the pictures to which the patient has consented is violated, he or she may have a cause of action. Even if the patient consents to the use of photographs or information, the physician is obliged to protect his or her privacy as much as possible.

It is quite clear that the admission of non-essential or nonauthorized persons during treatment, without the specific consent of the patient, constitutes a violation of his or her right of privacy. The attending physician is obligated to protect the patient's privacy and not cooperate with any adverse interests, unless and until he testifies under a subpoena.

On the other hand, the physician in attendance is protected if the disclosures which he made are required by law. For example, statutes which require reporting of cases of venereal disease, other contagious diseases, injuries sustained in accidents or violence, occupational diseases, or child abuse make it incumbent on the physician to do so. In these cases, he not only has the right to disclose the information to proper authorities, he has the duty to do so, and is immunized against legal liability. Thus, barring statutory obligation to disclose information in a situation in which the welfare of a patient or others demands it, a physician commits a tort when he discusses his patient's business with third parties, without the patient's consent. Discussing a patient's problem with an unauthorized third party is an unlawful disclosure, and breach of confidence is a well-recognized cause of action against physicians. A patient has the absolute right to assume that information he or she has given a physician will not be transmitted without his or her knowledge and consent. This, in truth, applies to all health care providers — nurses and medical or physicians' assistants.

The courts have delineated and circumscribed access to both a patient's body and records in the furnishing of health care services to members of the "health care team". Members of the team include the attending physician, assigned house officers, and all of the nursing personnel, including nursing associates and affiliates (licensed practical nurses and nurses' aides), involved in the care of the patient. Also included are technicians, orderlies, ward clerks, therapists, social service workers, patient advocates, and comparable officer personnel. Why these people? The rationale of the courts is that health care providers are indoctrinated in the obligation of privacy and confidentiality. However, they should be appropriately selected by the authorities. This also includes not permitting one who has limited professional connection with the case to observe a procedure, without the patient's express consent.

What about consultants, students (medical and nursing), and chaplains? They are not automatically members of the health care team; the patient must be informed of their involvement and given the opportunity to agree or reject them. If the attending physician wants to have a consultant accepted by the patient, the consultant must identify himself prior to his involvement. Students should not be identified by the staff as a physician or nurse, but rather as a student physician or nurse. Otherwise, this may result in an erroneous impression or conclusion by the patient, which he or she may later claim to be a breach of confidentiality or invasion of privacy, or even fraud or deceit. The medical practitioner and house officer have a legal obligation to see to it that the patient's rights are enforced. Ward rounds and conferences, even for educational purposes, may be attended only by members of the health care team. Visiting experts, regardless of their background or purpose, may attend or participate only with the the patient's prior consent.

The administration of the health care institution is entitled to review the patient's records for three purposes only — statistical analysis, staffing, and quality of care review. This does not include "doctor" talk!

It is believed by many physicians that they may publish accounts, photographs, or depictions of a patient if they are for educational or public relations purposes, even if they put the patient in an unfavorable light. That may be avoided if the patient (or if incompetent, the next-of-kin) consents prior to publication, and when it is well-intentioned or used to help others.

What if the patient's identity is not revealed, even obfuscated? Non-revelation or obfuscation does not assure the patient's anonymity, and if the patient is recognized, the physician is vulnerable to a lawsuit for breach of confidentiality or invasion of privacy. Problems can be avoided by getting the patient's prior approval.

When a patient is discharged, only the attending physician retains the right to review the records in perpetuity unless the patient's (surrogate's) consent is obtained for others.

The patient should be told of the need to share information with other health care persons and agencies if sharing is required, and he or she should sign the appropriate consent form. The release of confidential information is based on the authorization or consent of the patient, the courts, and any statutes.

Exchange of patient information between health care providers does not diminish any of the requirements of the law to protect the patient's confidentiality. Furthermore, unnecessary revelation regarding the patient's condition without authorization could subject the individual revealing the information to a variety of legal actions, since a physician is charged with the responsibility of providing continuity of health care for his patients. Therefore, no patient should suffer by the failure to transfer adequate information to the succeeding health care provider to ensure continuity of care.

The right to confidentiality is not absolute; it has been abridged by the "law". As to ordinary patients, the physician in attendance may respond to telephone or personal inquiries as to the patient's present status in vague and ambiguous terms only. As to so-called newsworthy patients, the attending physician may respond to telephone or personal inquiries regarding the patient's presence and his or her diagnosis and status in vague and ambiguous terms. Hospitalization may be revealed. The patient (surrogate) may interpose or object to even these disclosures.

In emergencies, reasonable disclosures may be made in the hope of contacting appropriate persons and getting information in turn.

Disclosures must be made on court order and to appropriate persons, such as an insurance carrier or attorney, under the "legitimate interest" doctrine, when a physician is being sued for malpractice.

An attending physician is best advised to secure permission from the patient to discuss his or her medical condition with the spouse, parents, and children, including minors, unless the patient is incompetent.

A house officer should know that access to a patient's records is limited to law enforcement authorities by subpoena only, except for the Criminal Division of the Internal Revenue Service, or in the unlikely event that law enforcement officers are in "hot pursuit". Government agencies charged with providing and receiving reimbursement may have access to a patient's records only when investigating the patient's care (quality of care review), but not when investigating a physician, including a house officer; they need a court order under these circumstances.

The same principles apply to a patient's bodily privacy. Examination or viewing an examination is the absolute prerogative only of members of the health care team; others must be specifically approved by the patient (surrogate), regardless of the virtues of their participation. In any event, the examination, even when approved, must be humane, reasonable, decent, and discreet, exposing only those parts of the body under examination. This applies to both men and women.

Sanctioning of an autopsy is limited to a competent patient before death, and the next-of-kin post-mortem. Viewing and information obtained from the autopsy is limited to the attending physician, the health care team, including the house officer, and the Medical Examiner or Coroner's Office, unless it is an official law enforcement matter.

A patient may seek redress from violation of his or her right of confidentiality and privacy by suing for invasion of privacy, breach of confidentiality, negligence, or battery. Affirmative defenses include consent, waiver, and a release.

Duty to Report

Every jurisdiction has a list of diseases which must be reported to the authorities, in addition to the requirement of warning other proper persons. Laws routinely require physicians to report the diagnosis of certain diseases, such as venereal disease, or the treatment of certain injuries, such as gunshot wounds, or the occurrence of child abuse, to local authorities. Failure to conform to the statutory or administrative requirements not only makes the health care provider liable to criminal penalties, but has been held to constitute negligence per se (not requiring proof of negligence) in civil suits brought by injured third parties.

Brother's Keeper Doctrine

The potential liability of a physician for harm to others caused by his patient because of the physician's negligent care and/or management of his patient is now a well-established judicial concept. An extension of this doctrine to include potential liability to third parties injured not by a physician, but by an incompetent, errant, or "sick" colleague, is demonstrated in recent decisions. If the colleague's incapability is known, or should be known, to another physician, including a house officer, and he fails to intervene against the continued practice of this "bad" physician, he may be sued by the disabled physician's injured patient. The cause of action can be predicated on the failure to intercede and with reasonable foreseeability, prevent the harm.

Privilege

One of the public health responsibilities of any physician is to report "bad" actors, patients, and other health care providers. This is done in order to protect and encourage all physicians to report such individuals to the proper authorities.

In general, there can be no liability for communicating the truth. Since it is often difficult to prove the absolute truth of a statement, the law extends "immunity" or "qualified or absolute privilege", depending on the jurisdiction, to certain communications, predicated on the duty to report, as long as the communication was made without malice. The qualified or absolute privilege applies to communications upon any subject matter in which the party communicating has an interest, or in reference to which he has a duty to a person having a corresponding interest or duty, i.e., to a certain person who has a legitimate interest in the information given, as long as the communication is limited in scope commensurate to one with the legitimate interest, and the communication is made in a proper manner so that others do not learn of it inappropriately.

This privilege also embraces cases where the duty is not a legal one, but where it is of moral or social character. This is particularly important to any physician, who has a duty to report "bad" behavior he observes in his professional role. The best way for a physician to avoid exceeding the absolute or qualified privilege is to limit the communication to factual accounts and avoid personal opinions or statements.

Emergencies — Good Samaritan Statutes

A licensed physician, including a licensed house officer, has no legal or professional duty to treat someone in an emergency situation, which the law generally defines as an immediate threat to health or life. Good Samaritan statutes in every state provide immunity from civil liability for physicians who render aid in a medical emergency, and who are thereafter sued for negligence. The statutes generally vary from state to state. Each physician should consult the applicable state statute to determine the immunity provisions governing medical practice.

Defamation — Libel and Slander

Defamation involves allegations or publication of untrue, defamatory material about a person. It consists of a verbal or written communication to someone other than the person defamed of matters concerning a living individual that injures that person's reputation. Slander is oral defamation; libel is written defamation. Since slander is less weighty than libel, slander is usually not actionable unless actual damage is proved by the plaintiff. However, when slander consists of accusing an individual of a crime or of having a loathsome disease, or imputing ill repute to a woman, no proof of injury is necessary for damages to be recovered. It is also defamatory to cast any reflection on a person's fitness or ability for his or her work. The information must be believed by a third party, who then acts to the detriment of the defamed party. Truth is a defense to an action for defamation.

Physicians have been the objects of defamation suits as a result of their peer review activities in censuring hospital staff members, and offering adverse comments involving former associates or employers. When some proceeding is brought as a result of the adverse remarks, and the subject of those remarks is vindicated, sometimes only because it cannot be absolutely established, a suit for defamation may very well ensue. Therefore, all physicians should communicate only established facts about their patients, colleagues, and associates. The author of the report must have no malice, evil intent, or conflict of interest in making the report. There is no duty to investigate the circumstances, merely that there is a reasonable belief that it is a fact, and made only to the proper parties, under proper circumstances, and in the appropriate fashion or manner.

Outrage

Lately, the courts have been imposing an additional liability for the tort of "outrage". As applied to health care providers, "outrage" is an extension of the doctrine of strict liability, i.e., liability without the proof of negligence. The tort of outrage involves deliberate infliction of mental suffering on another, without physical injury. The aggrieved party may be either the actual victim, or merely a third party affected only indirectly.

There are four elements to outrage:

- The wrongdoer's conduct was intentional or reckless; that is, the wrongdoer deliberately caused emotional distress in a given individual, or the wrongdoer knew — or should have known — that emotional distress would be a likely result of his action.
- The conduct was outrageous and intolerable, offending the generally accepted standards of decency and morality. This requirement serves to limit frivolous "outrage" suits and avoids litigation in situations where only bad manners, unpleasantness, or hurt feelings are involved.
- There was a causal connection between the wrongdoer's action and the emotional distress.
- The emotional distress was severe.

Negligent Infliction of Emotional Distress

Some courts have recognized negligent infliction of emotional distress as an independent cause of action in which a patient's harm was caused or aggravated by the patient's reasonable fear for his or her own physical safety. Now, third parties, such as the next-of-kin or bystanders to someone else's injury, are also regarded as having a cognizable claim.

An action for wrongful infliction of mental distress may be based on either intentional or negligent misconduct. The action will not lie for mere insults, indignities, threats, or annoyances. Internists have been held liable for this tort.

Strict Product Liability

The law has imposed strict product liability on manufacturers of foods, drugs, vaccines, and dangerous instruments for injuries caused, without the need to prove fault. It had not been imposed on physicians because they had been held not to be dealing in products or goods. They had instead been considered to be providing a service only — medical care and management. Any drug or device was merely employed in the course of providing treatment, to the best of their ability and according to accepted standards of care.

This no longer appears to be true; recently, courts have extended this liability to physicians. These cases represent an extension of the strict liability doctrine to health care providers.

Duty to Warn and Duty to Third Parties

A physician's duty of care includes the duty to warn patients of the dangers involved in their care, particularly in the use of a prescribed drug or device. It is increasingly recognized that a physician has the responsibility to identify any reasonably foreseeable harmful situation to a patient (or vulnerable third parties), and attempt to prevent it. Failure to advise the patient of known or reasonably foreseeable dangerous effects of treatment may leave the physician open to liability not only for harm the patient suffers, but also for injuries his patient may cause to third parties.

The courts have recognized a physician's duty to adequately warn regarding the hazard of the communicability of contagious diseases. Depending on the circumstances, the warning should be made known to the patient, and also third parties known to be in proximity to the patient, such as relatives or associates, and/or the proper authorities. This provides an opportunity to prevent the spread of the contagious disease.

The courts have imposed the duty to warn upon a physician when he administers medications with potentially dangerous therapeutic side effects. If a drug is administered that might affect a patient's ability to perform such functions as driving a car, the physician is obliged to explain the hazard to the patient and/or to someone who can control the patient's driving, such as the family, an employer, or the authorities. This duty also applies to patients engaged in any activity which may be hazardous, such as operating machinery or equipment. The administration of antihistamines and psychotropic drugs without adequate warning has been a physician's downfall in several cases.

When a physician identifies a medical condition that may impair a patient's control of his or her activities, the physician has a duty to warn the proper persons — patient, family, employer, and/or the authorities. This is true whether the condition is completely diagnosed or still under study. Epilepsy and other undiagnosed convulsive disorders are medical conditions that physicians have ignored to their legal detriment.

There is the risk that unnecessary warnings may be given; it is a reasonable price to pay to protect the lives of possible victims.

The law is emphasizing the public health responsibilities of the physician, as well as his duties, to individual patients. The duty to third parties is an example of the abandonment of the doctrine of "privity" (individual patient responsibility), and enforcement of the public health responsibilities of physicians.

In certain circumstances, a physician may be liable to third parties he has never seen for an action taken by his patient, arising from his failure to relay necessary information, which resulted in harm to the third person. This is part of the duty to warn. The law recognizes a physician's professional responsibility not to reveal information if, in his judgment, it is undesirable or unnecessary. The physician can protect himself by making an appropriate entry in the patient's record. Even if the failure to disclose is later proven to have been a mistake, this will be considered to be an error in judgment, for which the physician is not legally liable; it is not negligence. The interests of the individual often come into conflict with the rights of the public, and compromise is necessary.

All physicians, including house officers, should consider their obligations to potential third party victims with such conditions as coronary artery disease, cerebral arteriosclerosis, diabetes mellitus, and neuropsychiatric disorders. In practice, physicians can meet their responsibilities by only revealing information that, in their professional opinion, poses a clear and present danger to the public. A physician can be found negligent in failing to notify the local health officer as required by state regulations.

Duty to Control

The physician must be aware of the law regarding the duty to control, including the use of restraints. If a patient becomes disruptive or combative, the nurse must notify the attending physician immediately, or as soon as possible. She may temporarily use restraints only in an emergency, when she concludes that the patient is a danger to himself or others, and in order to avoid potential harm to the patient or to others, until the physician can be summoned to examine the patient and order specific treatment measures. A nurse must realize that she is liable if she fails to act to protect the patient.

Restraints generally require a physician's order, which should include the type of restraints to be used and the reason for the restraints. Restraints should be used reasonably, and care must be used to select an appropriate restraining device and to apply it as safely and comfortably as possible, so as not to impose an additional health hazard on the patient. Chemical restraints may be used only on a physician's order. The patient should be checked often enough to be sure that the restraints are not causing pressure, discomfort, or doing any other harm. Each visit should be documented. The patient should be restrained only for a limited time for the purpose of his or her protection, and the restraints should be removed at the first opportunity. The decision to continue using restraints is equally important and is made by the physician. Restraints are a form of incarceration and should be used only as a last resort after other reasonable means of control have not proven satisfactory. Restraints should not be used for administrative or personnel convenience to the detriment of the patient's freedom of movement.

False Imprisonment

False imprisonment occurs when there is an intentional and unprivileged, nonconsensual confinement of an individual. It is the unlawful restraint of an individual's personal liberty. A reasonable fear of force, rather than confinement itself, is all that is required. The tort of false imprisonment has been found in cases where patients have been detained and/or there has been the use of excessive or unnecessary force in restraining a patient, or where the patient is not a danger to self or others.

Privileged Communication/Testimonial Privilege

Confidential communications between physician and patient have been protected in all but 12 states under statutes entitled "privileged communication" or "testimonial privilege". These laws generally provide that a physician cannot be compelled in civil (not criminal) judicial proceedings to divulge confidential medical information regarding a patient, except when the privilege is waived or released by the patient.

It is a rule established for the protection of the patient, not the physician, so that the patient may feel free to be open and frank about his or her condition. Furthermore, the physician is obligated to protect the patient's confidence and not cooperate with the adverse interests, unless and until he is released by the patient or ordered to testify by the court.

If a patient brings a legal action for personal injury against another person, evaluation of his or her physical and mental condition has been placed into litigation by his or her own acts. Thus, "testimonial privilege" or "privileged communication" is considered to be waived.

The privilege also extends to hospital records, insofar as they tend to disclose what the physician learned in the course of treatment.

The Physician and The Nurse

Nursing has greatly advanced, and has become a primary health care profession; a sophisticated medical specialty with subspecialties about which many physicians have no intimate knowledge. Physicians now must rely on the independent skills and expertise of nurses, just as they depend on members of other allied medical disciplines. While physicians have always recognized the importance of good nursing care, there now are areas of care in which they must defer to nurses.

The courts have also recognized the nurse's specialized knowledge and skills as a health care provider, particularly in areas where physicians have defaulted. Court decisions spelling out the role for the nurse in patient care are astounding in comparison with the earlier, traditional role. The law now asserts that attending physicians share the direct care of the hospitalized patient with the nurses. As in the past, a physician may still be responsible for a nurse's deeds, but now, the law also makes the nurse responsible for the physician's actions, including those of the house officer, including the obligation not only to report, but to actively intervene in, substandard patient management. The hospital administration and staff chiefs must be notified; failure to do so may impose liability on the nurse if the patient is injured.

Admissions, Discharges, and Transfers

The attending physician has primary reponsibility for the admission of a patient. He obviously needs assistance from the appropriate hospital staff members, particularly the house officer. There may be liability in negligence for failure to appropriately accomplish these duties.

A physician is now mandated to have an admission plan and orders concurrent with the admission of the patient. The more urgent the patient's problems, the sooner these documents must be in the hospital record. The house officer and the nurse have a duty to see to it that this is properly accomplished, and must be aware that it is the nurse's duty to evaluate the patient and prepare her own nursing admission plan. This supplements and complements the physician's admission plan. If the house officer or the nurse believes, preferably after consultation, that the plan is inappropriate, he or she must relate this fear to the physician. If they fail to reach an accommodation, they must advise the administration, and then leave it to them to manage the problem.

All discharges must now include a discharge plan, which is a documentation showing that the release is medically appropriate with plans for follow-up care and advice, and instructions for the medical regimen to take place at home. Again, the house officer and/or nurse must concur or intercede as above. These include information that:

- The patient is ready to go; it is not a premature discharge; he or she is properly clothed.
- Appropriate transportation and accompaniment (escort) have been arranged;
- Medication and other forms of therapy are understood by the patient or surrogate, and are available;
- The housing situation and access to it are appropriate;
- Food will be on hand and available; and
- Instructions for future care are communicated, even verified. It is the physician's duty to see to it that this is accomplished.

Transfers to other facilities invoke comparable duties.

Orders

Orders involve the physician, the implementer, and usually, but not exclusively, the nurse. A continuing mainstay of nursing practice is the carrying out of a physician's orders, including those of the house officer. As to orders, all physicians must be cognizant of the fact that nurses are now charged with knowing when an order is incorrect, and she certainly must not implement it, but rather, consult with the physician. The nurse has a duty to follow any order that is not patently erroneous. However, when a nurse encounters an erroneous, illegible, or incomplete order, or it cannot be understood (vague and ambiguous), or is inappropriate, her duty is to contact the physician who wrote the order and obtain clarification. To administer such an order without clarification might result in injury to the patient and legal liability to the nurse. If the order appears erroneous or unsuitable, a reasonably prudent and competent nurse should question the physician. When the nurse is unable to reach the physician, she may not delay clarification of a treatment order, but must contact a "back-up" physician herself or have her supervisor do so, in order that the patient does not suffer for want of attention.

When the nurse is aware that execution of a physician's drug order, or an order involving a device, would be contrary to the manufacturer's recommendation or to medical policy in the institution, she must defer execution of the order until she confers with the physician who wrote the order, or with another physician who is authorized to act for him during his absence. If a particular physician regularly violates manufacturers' recommendations in ordering specific drugs, the nurse should report the problem in writing through her supervisor to the appropriate medical administrator.

The nurse must not blindly follow a physician's order. There is no question as to the legal liability; it involves the physician, the house officer, the nurse, and the health care institution. She has a duty to correctly execute the task she undertakes, and to recognize and report any problem that develops while the order is being carried out.

Verbal or Oral Orders

It has been demonstrated that one of the commonest causes of patient injury and malpractice in health care institutions involves the implementation of oral orders.

A verbal order is a legal order, but is a high risk legally and medically dangerous. The physician who gives a verbal order to a nurse is giving a valid order, and the fact that he opts not to write the order does not change its validity. But if any litigation results, and the physician and the nurse issue contradictory statements, i.e., the physician denies giving the order as such, the issue may come down to the credibility of the physician or the nurse.

Except in an emergency when the physician is concerned primarily with the care and management of a patient, verbal orders are a doubtful convenience to the physician. No matter what the hospital rules allow, a physician would be better protected against malpractice suits.

Telephone orders cannot be disallowed, despite their potential for errors. However, there are ways to minimize their hazards. These orders should be given by the physician in charge, or an authorized health care provider, such as a house officer, nurse, or physician assistant, under the immediate direction, supervision, and control of the physician. No one else is authorized, and the physician or his "mouthpiece" may be administratively and criminally liable under the state Medical Practice Act if an unauthorized person practices medicine without a license.

Medications

A physician, including a house officer, must know that the standard of care requires that he be certain that the medication:
- Is properly indicated, i.e., it is the proper usage;
- Is not contraindicated in the patient;
- With reasonable foreseeability, will not cause complications, adverse, or toxic reactions, or interact with other medications;
- Is ordered with the "proper dosage" schedule; and
- Is ordered to be administered by the proper route, and will not interact adversely with other medications.

To minimize risks in this area, the physician is best advised to do the following. If his instructions deviate from the package inserts or Physicians' Desk Reference (PDR), he must have a good reason for doing so. Drug side effects or undesired results can be caused by administering a medication in a manner contrary to the official product literature.

The physician must be familiar with all the actions of the medications he prescribes. That means consulting with sources other than the manufacturer, if necessary. Ignorance of the composition or the pharmacology of a drug is a weak, if not futile, defense in a malpractice case.

A physician is obligated to give a patient explicit instructions about the possible side effects of any prescribed medication, and to make sure that the patient is aware of any problems which the medication might cause, such as increasing the effects of the patient's ordinary alcohol intake or complications of combining the drug with any other medication.

When the wrong drug is administered by mistake, liability is automatic as a matter of law. Oral administration of medicine intended to be used externally is clearly negligent. So is injection of a drug which should be given orally. However, when the medication given by mistake does not harm the patient in any way, a cause of action is not likely to be successful.

The physician must be careful with abbreviations. Serious errors have occurred with incorrect or misconstrued abbreviations. He should write out the volume or units to be administered. For example, he should always spell out the word "units". The abbreviation "U" can be mistaken for a zero, multiplying the dosage ten times. He should carefully identify the frequency of administration. The physician must be aware of hospital procedures for frequency designations (b.i.d, t.i.d, and so on) to ensure that the medication is administered at the correct times and the correct number of times.

When discharging a patient with medication, the physician must do everything possible to ensure that he or she can take it properly, or make arrangements for someone else to administer it. He should document the instructions he gives to the patient or other person responsible for administering the medication. These are best written out. If they are handwritten, the physician should check the handwriting to be certain it can be read.

Because of his frequent prescriptions for narcotics and other controlled drugs, the physician must be familiar with and conform to the state and federal Controlled Substance Acts, in order to avoid administrative and criminal sanctions, as well as malpractice suits. The same is true for both state and federal Food and Drug Acts.

The physician is best advised to know the laws, rules, and regulations involving "new drugs", which include "investigational drugs", "investigational new drugs", and "experimental drugs". A drug which is already approved by the FDA, but which is used for an unapproved purpose or in an unapproved manner, is a "new drug". These are also referred to as "orphan drugs".

Most of all, the physician must remember that a nurse may not administer a medication which she believes has been prescribed below the standard of care. She has a duty to confer with the physician. If they fail to reach an accommodation, it is the nurse's duty to notify the administration.

Materials, Devices, Equipment, and Facilities

All physicians must exercise reasonably prudent care in selecting materials, devices, and equipment for a specific therapeutic or diagnostic purpose. The physician is responsible for reporting defective equipment, particularly when the defect occurs while he is using it. It goes without saying that he should be vigilant and diligent in using the equipment, and not continue to use defective materials and devices.

Although it is unlikely to involve a house officer, he should be aware that physicians may have a duty to advise former patients of newly discovered dangers associated with the use of medications, devices, materials, and procedures previously performed.

Medical Records — Record Keeping

Medical records are not only important medically, they are frequently legally crucial. Keeping good records is critical both for the prevention of lawsuits, and also for enabling an attorney to defend a physician successfully. Many cases are lost because the records are poorly done. A good record will protect the physician, including the house officer, in two ways. The plaintiff's attorney will submit the record to an outside expert for review before filing suit. If the record is consistent and clear, the expert will probably advise against filing suit, and the odds are that the physician will never hear about that case again. It is critical for the house officer to be in sync with the attending physician.

Even if a suit is filed, a good record will make it much easier for the physician's expert to defend him, and to convince the jury that in spite of the poor outcome, the physician acted consistently as a good physician. Proper record keeping often means the difference between victory and defeat in the courtroom. The courts will allow medical records to be introduced as evidence to impugn a physician's professional activities.

The record should contain a reasonably complete discussion of all the diagnostic and therapeutic events, including the results of same. This establishes the physician's continuity of care, and denotes his vigilance and diligence through constant review and surveillance. Sloppy records are equated with sloppy care; grossly inadequate records are equated with inadequate care.

There are recognized standards for record keeping. The physician must check that on each sheet of the chart, the name of the patient and the date is properly filled in for identification. These details are important and may be critical.

Entries must be made legibly and not be vague or ambiguous. The records must be accurate, adequate, and appropriate. They need to be factual, relevant, pertinent, and material. In order to conform to the standard of care, the physician should record as much as he can, promptly and as often as he can. Certainly, no major or minor event should go unrecorded in the progress notes. If a complication is noted only in the nurses' notes, but does not appear in the physician's progress notes or in the discharge summary, both the expert and the jury will wonder why this patient was not followed more closely by the attending physician.

The record should not only be a trail of diagnostic and therapeutic activity, but should also be evidence of the patient's participation in the decision-making. This means a detailed and signed consent form for *any* intervention, and a written note about the nature of the discussion with the patient and about the patient's comprehension of the discussion.

It is good medical practice for the physician to discreetly document if he suspects a patient is not following the regimen, making sure he notes his observations, as well as patient and family comments generally.

The physician should make a note of every call received. In that way, if he has a regular method of taking notes at home and at the office, he will be able to establish that he has a system. If there is no note of having received a call, he can credibly assert no alleged call was made.

A physician is often asked to countersign entries in patient medical records for house officers, students, and nurses. If the physician's signature appears on the record in a capacity other than having personal knowledge of the particular events, he should explain his capacity and role clearly, and note that he read and approved the entry, so in the event of litigation, his position will not be misconstrued. In addition, there is the requirement that each is under a duty to maintain and complete the records in a timely fashion.

Third party insurance companies, such as Blue Cross/Blue Shield, Medicare, and Medicaid, have been upheld in denying payment for medical services if they were not properly documented and recorded in the patient's record. Health care institutions that tolerate poor record keeping have been held liable for injuries caused by insufficiencies.

Criticisms and indiscreet remarks have no place in the chart. It is not the place for witticisms or derogatory remarks that cast aspersions on the patient, the patient's family, colleagues, an earlier treating physician, or hospital staff. The physician should not include personal observations in the record when they are not factual, are inappropriate, and are not related to patient care.

Because the medical record must be completely accurate if it is to provide a sound basis for care planning and recording, errors in charting must be corrected promptly in a manner that leaves no doubt as to the facts of the case. Every health institution should have a written policy and protocol, well-publicized among all health care providers, that specifies that an erroneous chart entry is to be crossed through, labeled as erroneous, signed by the individual correcting the error with the date and time, and retained in the patient's record. Correct information is then to be entered with that date and time to replace the erroneous data crossed through. Pages of the record that contain erroneous and corrected entries are never to be destroyed. Since erasures in records may create suspicion as to the reason for the change, it is preferable to make none.

Alterations to records can be highly suspect. Records with obvious alterations, particularly any record that can be shown to have been fudged, are absolutely deadly in court. Tampering with medical records may result in large malpractice awards, even when there has been no negligence. Nothing should ever be added, deleted, substituted, or removed.

Nurses and physicians who falsify a patient's record, in order to conceal negligence or a criminal violation (such as infraction of a Medical or Nurse Practice Act), may be found civilly and criminally liable.

Patient Access

The physician must always remember that the record is a legal document, and a patient has a right to view the record and obtain a copy. Every time the physician makes an entry, he must consider that this entry may be seen by the patient, and later by a jury.

The importance of record keeping is accentuated by recent changes in the law regarding a patient's access to records. Court decisions have held that since a patient's medical record is essential to proper administration, the record is the property of the hospital. However, generally, the patient has a right to information contained in the record, and so has a right to inspect it while an in-patient, and inspect and copy the record after being discharged from the facility.

Although a patient's right to see his or her record or secure a copy is absolute, it must be reasonable. When a reasonable request is made, the patient may, at a convenient time, review or even get a copy of the record. If a physician honestly believes that a revelation to the patient may be to the patient's detriment, the provider may exercise professional or therapeutic discretion and withhold the information.

Nurses may explain only their entries in the record. The patient should be encouraged to go over the record with the physician, and the nurse is best advised to make the arrangement. A physician who fails to cooperate should be reported to the administration because of the legal hazards incident to the uncooperativeness.

When a patient is given access to his or her records, it should be supervised and monitored. The physician should make himself available when a patient wants to review the records. Hospitals need only advise the physician when they give a patient access. It should be remembered that patients can always get a court order, i.e., subpoena duces tecum, to get access to their records if they can show the judge adequate cause. A patient may successfully file a lawsuit based on only an iota or scintilla of evidence.

When a patient wants a copy of his record, he or she is entitled to all reproducible items, even if an outside source is needed for the reproduction. The hospital may require the patient to pay the cost of reproduction. The original record should never be given to a patient.

Assumption of Risk

The doctrine of "assumption of risk" means that the patient understands the possibility of all risks of untoward, unpreventable results of either treatment or no treatment, and knowingly consents to the course selected. Where it applies, this is usually a good defense to an action for negligence on the part of a physician. It should be noted that this doctrine is related to the doctrine of informed consent and refusal. If all risks which, in fact, occur have not been carefully explained to the patient, as a matter of law, the doctrine of assumption of risk is not applicable.

MUSCULOSKELETAL SYSTEM

Introduction

Orthopedics involves the examination, evaluation, and treatment of the musculoskeletal system. This includes medical and surgical treatment of injuries, infections, tumors, and systemic problems of the neck, back, arms, and legs.

Only problems of the upper respiratory system are more prevalent than problems of the back. If fractures and dislocations, sprains, strains, contusions, crush injuries, and open wounds of the arms and legs are added to the incidence of back problems, then orthopedic complaints probably cause more people to seek medical attention than problems affecting any other body system.

Too many medical students, primary care physicans, and even orthopedic surgeons consider only the skeleton whenever they think of orthopedics. They fail to realize or to remember that the skeletal system is also the reservoir of calcium, phosphorus, and other minerals. They fail to recall the important role of the skeletal system in the mineral, hematopoietic, and immune systems. They forget that bones articulate through joints whose activity makes possible walking and other movements of the arms and legs.

Surrounding or adjacent to bones and joints of the skeletal frame are skin, fat, fascia, muscles, tendons, ligaments, nerves, and blood vessels. Any externally applied force, which is sufficient to break a bone or cause a fracture, must by necessity cause damage to the soft tissues between the skin and the bone. Such soft tissue damage is often not apparent, but a physician must always consider soft tissue damage whenever he is evaluating a patient with a fracture.

Too many physicians have been ignorant of the soft tissue-skeletal relationship, or they have forgotten this relationship to the misfortune of their patients. Many patients have suffered amputations of arms and legs, even though the fractured bones were healing in a normal fashion. Once a fracture has been reduced and immobilized, there should be no pain. Though x-rays may look good and arteries are bounding, something is wrong. The physician must remove the cast and take a look, and not just order stronger and stronger medication.

The typical medical school graduate has had little exposure to the examination and treatment of a patient with orthopedic problems. The result is that recent graduates and house officers will find themselves ill prepared for participation in this particular area of medicine.

Evaluation

The best defense is a return to basics, though we live in a time of high technology in medicine. While evaluation and treatment of musculoskeletal problems are facilitated by modern high technology, history taking as complete as possible and a complete physical examination remain as basic today as they were in the pre-bionic, pre-computerized era. A physician must be as thorough and comprehensive as professionally possible in taking the history and in performing the physical examination. If the physician should rely upon laboratory studies, x-rays,

CT scans, and other sophisticated procedures without a careful history and physical examination, he will have deviated from the basic duty owed to his patient. It matters not so much which system is used, but each physician must develop his own system and stick with it, even it if makes reading his records dull; risk being repetitious. The physician should not deviate from whatever his system is unless there are bona fide reasons for doing so. A frequent cause of medical malpractice claims against house officers, as well as physicians generally, is failure to diagnose. The physician will protect himself by paying close attention to every complaint of the patient as he takes the history, making the examination correspond to the history, and then ordering the appropriate supportive studies.

Radiography

Following an appropriate history and physical examination, x-rays will generally be required for the evaluation of orthopedic problems. X-rays are often required during this evaluation for differential diagnosis, for determining therapy, and for the protection of the patient and the physician.

When are x-rays appropriate? When a physician is treating a patient who has had an injury, he must obtain radiographic studies. When the history and physical examination lead the physician to suspect a tumor or infection of the bone or joint, x-rays are essential. X-rays are necessary during the evaluation and treatment of patients with congenital and postural problems of the spine and extremities. It would be virtually impossible to treat a patient with arthritis without x-ray studies. Whenever a patient has not had an injury, but he or she does have a musculoskeletal complaint which continues after a reasonably short course of symptomatic treatment, the physician should order x-rays. Whenever the reasonable physician orders x-rays, he will be held to the standard of having found it necessary to do the same.

Roentgenographic examination of the injured body part requires at least two right angle views, the anteroposterior and lateral views. Initial studies of injured joints require at least one oblique view as well. Other views should be requested and obtained as indicated. Children have open epiphyseal lines at the ends of long bones. Therefore, children should always have at least one comparative view of the opposite joint.

When x-rays are ordered, they must be done properly. Many patients may indicate foot when they mean ankle or lower leg. Patients with sciatica or arm pain may have no peripheral problem at all. After the examination, the physician will know that the leg pain is based upon a problem in the lumbosacral spine, or that the arm pain is based upon a problem in the cervical spine. Many children will have knee pain, but the clinical problem will be found to be a slipped epiphysis, Legg-Perthes disease, or sepsis of the hip.

Any x-ray film that cannot be properly interpreted has no value. The physician must demand that the technique of exposing and developing the films should be such that he can see clearly whatever needs to be seen. Each film must be properly identified and marked "right" or "left", with no markers obscuring anatomic structures. The physician is required to review the entire x-ray film. He must not anticipate what the film is going to show, and consequently fail to notice any additional, unexpected information in the film.

When the films are returned to the physician, he must verify that they are properly and correctly identified as to patient and laterality. He should place them on the view box for examination. If the physician holds up the film in order to review it with the ceiling light, his thumb just might obscure the second, more significant fracture in the corner. As the physician reviews the film, it is necessary to examine everything within the four corners of the film. Failing to identify a fracture on an x-ray film often leads to failure to diagnose, one of the most prevalent bases for medical malpractice claims.

X-Ray Views of the Musculoskeletal System

- Cervical spine: AP; lateral, showing 7 vertebrae; open mouth.
- Thoracic spine: AP; lateral, showing 12 vertebrae.
- Lumbar spine: AP; lateral, showing 5 vertebrae; cone-down of L5-S1. Right and left oblique views of cervical or lumbar spine as required.
- Sacrum and coccyx: AP; lateral; lumbar spine views.
- Shoulder: AP in internal rotation and external rotation.
- Elbow: AP; lateral; oblique.
- Wrist: AP; lateral; oblique.
- Carpal scaphoid: scaphoid; wrist views.
- Hand: AP; lateral; oblique.
- Pelvis: AP, showing entire pelvic ring.
- Hip: AP; lateral.
- Knee: AP; lateral, oblique.
- Ankle: AP; lateral; internal rotation.
- Foot: AP; lateral; oblique.
- Long bones: AP; lateral, showing adjacent or nearest joint.

The views indicated above are minimal studies. In every instance, there are specialized views which may be ordered if further study is required. Frequently, initial films of the carpal scaphoid and tarsal navicular will not demonstrate non-displaced fractures. Because these are bones in the wrist and ankle, respectively, which require rigid immobilization, if a fracture is suspected, a rigid cast must be applied. Then the joint should be x-rayed 10 to 14 days later.

Children

Children with skeletal injuries represent special problems. There are open epiphyseal lines at the end of the long bones in children, such lines closing entirely at bone maturity. Fractures which occur within the epiphyses may not be readily apparent, and frequently do not become evident by x-ray until several weeks of healing have passed. It is important to realize that children have weaker epiphyseal lines than joint ligaments. For this reason, the same injury which would result in a sprain in an adult will result in an epiphyseal fracture in a child. Such joint injuries should be treated as fractures in children, even if no obvious fracture is immediately identified.

Whenever any child presents with a joint injury, comparative x-ray views of the opposite joint should be ordered. Only in this manner will the physician be able to avoid confusing a fracture with an open epiphyseal plate. If epiphyseal fractures in children are mishandled, disaster may result with arm or leg deformity, or arm or leg length discrepancy. If the physician has no expertise in properly handling children's fractures, he should refer the child to an orthopedist immediately.

Standard of Care

A house officer, without the training and education required of orthopedic or trauma surgeons, will not be required to render definitive care beyond his expertise. As a physician, however, he will be held to the standard of taking histories and performing evaluations, which will enable him to make a diagnosis and properly assess the gravity of the injury. While the trainee is not required to provide care beyond his expertise, he will be liable for failure to make a diagnosis. The trainee must know and accept his limitations, for he is required to know when he is qualified to provide definitive care, and when he must summon a physician with greater expertise. At every patient contact, the trainee will be held to the standard of care demanded of the reasonable physician under the same or similar circumstances.

Duty to Consent and Refer

The duty of a house officer is to evaluate patients, make correct diagnoses, treat if he has the expertise, and summon a specialist when necessary. If the trainee, or even a generalist, provides care which would normally be provided by a specialist, that physician will be held to the standards of a specialist. If the trainee or generalist summons a specialist, he has the duty of conveying to him an accurate sense of urgency as demanded by the circumstances. The physician must know which problems can wait until the morning, and which problems require immediate or urgent care. This duty is not discharged merely by notifying the specialist that an emergency exists; it is not discharged until and unless the specialist assumes responsibility for the care of the patient. The referring physician must not acquiesce to the specialist's refusal to respond immediately if the referrer considers his attention is urgently required. If the specialist refuses or fails to respond as needed, or if the specialist provides care which the physician knows or should know deviates from the standard, the physician's own liability continues. The referrer must seek alternative expertise. His duty and liability are relieved only when there are no other specialists in the community to whom the patient could reasonably have turned to for assistance.

Any Allergies?

A thousand patients may be given trigger point injections of a steroid or Xylocaine into a spastic or painful muscle mass without any complications. These thousand patients would have had no history of medicinal allergies, and many of them would have reported being anesthetized by their dentists with Novocaine with no ill effects. The next patient is the one who was not questioned concerning his or her allergy history. That is the one patient who had an allergic response to Novocaine the last time he or she received dental therapy. This is the one patient who responds with anaphylactic shock to the same injection that a physician gave to one thousand other patients. To compound the disaster, the physician has no equipment for resuscitation. He has no Epinephrine in the office, has never learned the most elementary CPR, and has absolutely no knowledge of endotracheal or even nasotracheal intubation.

The physician must take an allergy history and be specific concerning what happened whenever the patient was given Novocaine in the past by his or her dentist. If the physician is going to administer injectables, he must have Epinephrine available immediately, and he must be competent in basic CPR. Juries are unforgiving of such oversights or basic inadequacies.

Drug Toxicity

Non-steroidal, anti-inflammatory drugs (NSAID) are wonderful, but they are potentially dangerous. When they are prescribed for patients already taking aspirin, they may cause or exacerbate erosive gastritis, as well as gastric and duodenal ulcers. If they are taken by patients already taking anticoagulants, the result may be potentiation of anticoagulation with ophthalmologic or intra-cranial hemorrhaging. There is no excuse for less than a complete medical history.

Orthopedic Emergencies

Because of pain and disability associated with problems of the musculoskeletal system, particularly fractures, patients will consider that every orthopedic problem is an emergency. In reality, there are only a few bona fide emergencies in orthopedics. Whenever they occur, they must be handled immediately. Failure to treat or failure to treat rapidly may result in death, amputation, or permanent crippling or deformity.

The following are common emergencies:
- Dislocations.
- Displaced fractures near joints.
- Vascular compromise in any injured extremity.
- Neurological compromise in any injured extremity.
- Open (formerly compound) fractures or dislocations.
- Acute bone infection (osteomyelitis).
- Joint infections.

The Telephone!

Too many physicians attempt to treat emergency problems over the telephone, or they will improperly delegate the task of treatment to a nurse, ward clerk, or other person. If the physician is not able to handle the problem himself, he has an obligation to refer the patient to a proper specialist. This is not handled by an order, or by having the ward clerk call the specialist. As the physician on site, the emergency room doctor has the professional duty of conversing with the consulting specialist about the problem that he is unable to treat. In this manner, the urgency of the situation will not be lost during the conversation.

If an orthopedic emergency arises, the non-specialist physician has a duty to recognize it as such. If he is able to treat the emergency situation, then he is required to do so with dispatch. If he does not have the expertise, then he is obligated to summon a medical specialist who does have the expertise, and who will handle the situation.

If the physician learns by telephone that an orthopedic emergency exists, the only advice that should be given to the patient is for him or her to meet the physician at the hospital. If the physician is in the office or clinic when he learns of such an emergency, the duty is to insist that the patient be hospitalized without delay. If the physician is in the hospital, though he may be dreadfully tired or sleepy when the nurse calls, he has the duty of seeing the patient in order to evaluate the problem. He should initiate treatment or contact a specialist. If the physician is working in the emergency room and an orthopedic emergency arises, he should converse with the specialist and insist that he come into the hospital without delay. In any of these circumstances, once the physician has notified the specialist of the emergency situation, his duty is not discharged until and unless the specialist assumes responsibility on site. If the specialist fails to properly take care of the patient, it does not relieve the physician of his duty to the patient. Such duty is relieved only when there does not remain any other specialist in the community to whom the physician could have turned to for assistance.

Displacement Injuries

Dislocations and fractures with gross displacement, especially if they occur close to joints, are dangerous to the nerves and arterial blood supply. These vital structures may be severed, frayed, or compressed by the malpositioned bone or fracture fragments. It is imperative that such dislocations or displaced fractures be reduced as soon as possible.

When such an injury occurs at the elbow, the risk is severe damage to the brachial artery and/or the median, ulnar, or radial nerves. At the knee, the risk is severe damage to the popliteal artery, as well as to branches of the sciatic nerve. At the hip, anterior dislocation of the hip may damage the femoral artery, while posterior dislocation of the hip may damage the sciatic nerve. If such emergencies are not recognized and corrected, the risk to the patient is paralysis of the limb distal to the injury, or necrosis of the target tissues, and eventually amputation. Paralysis and/or limb amputation may be the natural consequence of certain injuries, regardless of the treatment rendered. But paralysis and/or limb amputation should not occur when they can be avoided by non-negligent medical care.

Crush-Soft Tissue Injuries

Every fracture represents a crush injury or contusion of the soft tissues where the bone is also damaged. Frequently, crush injuries of the extremities may result in soft tissue damage far more severe than the obvious fracture. Such soft tissue damage is often not immediately apparent, but it is imperative that the physician always consider soft tissue damage anytime he evaluates a patient with a fracture.

Frequently, the soft tissue injuries are of greater importance than the obvious fracture. Dislocations and displaced fractures are always of significance, and represent emergencies because of the danger to the surrounding or adjacent soft tissues.

Compartment Syndrome

A normal response to injury is the accumulation of extra-vascular tissue fluid within the injured tissues. Because muscles and nerves are soft, the life is virtually squeezed out of these structures. The fascial planes which are fibrous and tough are unrelenting. The muscular walled arteries are the last of the soft tissues to be affected by compression. Consequently, the result is a patient screaming with pain, and the nurse recording excellent circulation because the pulses are bounding and the extremity is warm.

Such is the scenario of vascular compartment syndrome. A physician treats this emergency best when he is aware that it may occur with any type of extremity injury, especially following crush injuries. All circulatory restrictions must be removed, and the extremity must be elevated. If the restrictions are external, such as casts, splints, or bandages, they must be removed. If the problem continues to exist, then the skin and appropriate fascia must be incised. The best way of preventing the complications of vascular compartment syndrome is to be aware of the possibility of compartment syndrome as a complication of any compression injury.

Infections

Bacteria are anathema to bones and joints. Any infection of a bone or joint must be treated vigorously as an emergency. Open fractures (previously known as compound fractures) and open dislocations are contaminated. They must be treated vigorously with at least copious irrigation, debridement of the wound, and prophylactic antibiotic therapy.

If the skin is broken in the vicinity of the fracture, the physician must assume that the fracture is open, and that it is contaminated. This is particularly true if the fracture demonstrates a sharp spike. The bone spike will have perforated the skin and then retracted. If the wound is ignored or treated superficially and inappropriately, the treating physician will be liable for the resulting osteomyelitis. If the wound is not treated according to the standard, the treating physician will be liable for the resulting osteomyelitis or septic joint. The house physician who originally requested the services of the negligent orthopedic surgeon will be held to have known that that physician's treatment of the open fracture or dislocation was a deviation from the standard. This particular scenario generally occurs in the middle of the night, when the orthopedic surgeon prefers to believe that the wound has no communication with the fracture. This is lack of professional honesty, for which he might one day be required to pay. The emergency room physician who summoned this particular orthopedic surgeon may also be liable because he will be held to have known that the orthopedic surgeon's treatment of the open fracture was inappropriate.

It is standard procedure to treat uncomplicated fractures under local anesthesia by infiltrating the fracture hematoma with a local anesthetic agent such as Xylocaine. It is essential that the extremity be scrubbed copiously with alcohol or some similar sterilizing agent. Wiping the area to be injected with a single alcohol swab will not sterilize the area. To inject a fracture hematoma without sterilizing the skin is to risk converting a simple (or closed) fracture into an open (or compound) fracture. The physician must at all times avoid making a patient worse as a result of his treatment.

The Extremities

When a physician evaluates a patient with a fracture or dislocation of the arm or leg, he must examine the neurovascular status of the extremity distal to the injury. If the patient sustains permanent or serious damage as a result of the physician's failure to have properly examined him or her, the physician will have exposed himself to professional liability.

Displaced fractures of the humerus are capable of damaging the radial nerve, resulting in radial nerve palsy. Dislocations about the elbow are capable of damaging the brachial artery, as well as the median, ulnar, and radial nerves. Damage to the brachial artery, if not corrected in a timely manner, may result in ischemia or gangrene of the extremity distal to the elbow. Damage to the nerves may result in paralysis of the extremity. Whether the paralysis is complete or incomplete, or temporary or permanent, may be a factor of the timeliness of diagnosis. Competent evaluation by the house officer or physician may mean the difference between proper care or tragic consequences for the patient.

Similarly, the forearm is a rigid parallelogram comprised of the radius, ulna, and the ligaments of the elbow and wrist. If the ulna fractures proximally with displacement, the radius must dislocate at the elbow. This is the Monteggia fracture-dislocation. If the radius fractures distally with displacement, the ulna must dislocate at the wrist. This is the Galeazzi fracture-dislocation. If the physician identifies only the fracture and does not realize that a dislocation is also present, he will never be able to successfully reduce the fracture. Both injuries must be corrected.

In the leg, a similar parallelogram exists. If a fracture with displacement or diastasis (widening or separation of the ankle joint or distal aspect of the leg) occurs, there is probably also going to be a fracture of the shaft of the fibula. Fortunately, the tibia is so much more substantial than the fibula that little impairment or disability will occur if the fibular fracture is not identified. But the converse is not the case. The physician should never be overly concerned with treating a displaced fibular fracture while overlooking the more significant injury about the ankle or distal tibia. If the physician should make such an error, he will have deviated from the accepted standard of care.

Displaced fractures or dislocations about the knee are emergencies which must be recognized immediately and treated promptly. Failure to diagnose and treat in a timely fashion will result in gangrene of the leg and eventual amputation.

Simple dislocations or fracture-dislocations about the ankle may compromise the circulation to the foot. These are injuries which demand immediate reduction, in order to avoid avascularization of the foot and eventual amputation.

Edema in the Extremities

Fractures and other injuries of the arms and legs frequently result in swelling. This swelling results from the inflammatory response to the injury itself, by the muscles damaged by the force of the injury, or by edema resulting from injury to the veins. The muscles of the extremities are divided into compartments by investing fascial tissue which is tight and unyielding.

Following crush injuries or contusion of the soft tissues of the extremities, extra-vascular tissue fluid may accumulate within the fascial compartments. This is the disastrous compartment syndrome, which is characterized by the virtual squeezing to death of all the tissues within the compartment. As the tension within the fascial compartment increases, the veins, muscles, and nerves are progressively destroyed. The muscular arteries are the last of the soft tissues to be affected by compression. It is for this reason that the compartment syndrome worsens as the nursing staff and house officers record the presence of peripheral pulses.

Indeed, an intact arterial system continues to bring blood into the injured area, increasing the tension within the extra-vascular compartment as the veins become progressively damaged. When any patient with an extremity injury has increasing pain, swelling, and numbness, the physician must consider compartment syndrome. He should not be misled by the presence of a bounding pulse, and not give stronger and stronger medication. Rather, all binding strictures must be removed. These include cast, splint, bandage, and eventually fascia (fasciotomy). The house officer must insist that the treating surgeon respond immediately when there is an indication of compartment syndrome.

The Pelvis

The pelvis is a rigid ring. A solitary fracture of the ring, or a strain of the symphysis pubis or one of the sacroiliac joints, frequently requires only symptomatic care. But if there is any displacement of the ring, caused by a rupture of the symphysis pubis or one of the sacroiliac joints, or a fracture with displacement, there must occur a corresponding displacement on the opposite side of the ring. Failure to identify and treat the instability which results will expose the physician to negligence liability.

The Hips

Patients who fracture their hips are generally elderly and not always in excellent health. For this reason, definitive treatment often must be delayed until their medical status is improved sufficiently to permit their submitting to the risks of anesthesia and surgery. Fortunately, delay in the treatment of such fractures generally will not adversely affect the prognosis. But patients who dislocate their hips are generally young and in improved health. This is fortunate since hip dislocation is an emergency and must be treated without delay. If reduction of the dislocated hip is delayed, the risk of vascular compromise of the femoral head with resulting avascular necrosis increases. If this complication occurs, an injury that would have required a simple, closed reduction will now require prosthetic replacement of the femoral head and neck, with the risks associated with anesthesia and surgery. Posterior dislocation of the hip will damage the sciatic nerve, with permanent paralysis of the leg. The risk of such paralysis increases proportionate to the time the hip remains dislocated. Anterior dislocation of the hip, if not reduced quickly, may result in compromise of the femoral artery, with the danger of avascularization of the leg and subsequent amputation.

The Spine

Fractures of the spine without displacement generally will require only symptomatic care. But if the spine is dislocated or fractured with displacement, the danger exists that the spinal cord distal to the level of injury will be severed or compressed to a degree that death or paralysis results. The house officer must stabilize the injured spine until it is confirmed that no serious problem is present, or until he is relieved by a physician with greater expertise. Failure to recognize an unstable spine, or failure to stabilize such an unstable spine, may result in aggravation of the original injury with grave consequences. It is the house officer who has the duty of preventing such damages, while he protects himself from liability.

Tight Cast

Whenever a fracture has been reduced, there should be no pain. If pain continues or progresses, the physician must consider that the fracture has not been reduced, or that the reduction has been lost. Or he must consider that the cast is too tight or too loose. If the problem involves the fracture itself, then it must be appropriately treated. If the problem is a faulty cast, then it must be adjusted or replaced. The physician has the duty of inspecting the casted extremity, in order to be able to provide the necessary care.

Backaches

Relatively few backaches are caused by direct injuries to the back. Most back complaints, however, are caused by problems with the musculoskeletal system. Nevertheless, physicians should not overlook other systems as the origin of backaches. These include the gastrointestinal, genitourinary, and gynecological systems. If the musculoskeletal system has been definitely eliminated as the origin of the backache, questioning the patient concerning these other systems might prove revealing. Then, if appropriate, refer the patient to the indicated specialist.

Examining the peripheral pulses is part of the orthopedic examination of a patient with a backache. If the patient has decreased or absent pulses, the abdomen must be auscultated. It requires only a second to hear the bruit of an aneurysm of the abdominal aorta. If the aneurysm is dissecting, the renal arteries will have occluded, and the patient, if asked, will inform the physician of recent decreased urination effort. The physician will then make the proper referral of the patient to a vascular surgeon. If the diagnosis is not made, and if the aneurysm ruptures other than intra-luminally, the patient will exsanguinate. The diagnosis will be made at the post-mortem examination. The physician will find it difficult explaining to the widow and to the jury why he treated her late husband with only analgesics and muscle relaxants.

Multiple Injuries

If a patient has multiple injuries, it is important that all of the injuries be treated properly. The physician's liability for failure to diagnose will not be reduced because he treated the most obvious injury.

When a patient has been injured as the result of considerable force, such as a serious automobile accident, an explosion, or a bad fall, the physician must anticipate multiple injuries. He must examine the neck, back, and both arms and legs thoroughly. This is particularly necessary if the patient is in a coma, or for other reasons, unable to provide a history.

Even a patient who falls from a height of several feet might present with multiple injuries. If he or she should land upon the feet and jackknife in such a manner as to land upon the hands, the mechanism of injury is expected to fracture both heels (calcanei), T-12 and L-1 vertebrae, and one or both wrists (radius or carpal scaphoid). Additionally, there may occur dislocation of the elbow or shoulder in the same arm as the wrist fracture. Obviously, each of these fractures and dislocations is important, and it would be malpractice to fail to treat because of failure to diagnose.

Within the same area of the body, there are certain combinations of injuries which are associated. If the proximal ulna fractures with displacement, the proximal radius must dislocate at the elbow. When the distal radius fractures with displacement, the distal ulna must dislocate at the wrist. Failure to diagnose the dislocations associated with these fractures may result in loss of function of the joint and permanent disability.

In the leg, if the fibula fractures with displacement, either the ligaments about the ankle must rupture, or the distal tibia must fracture with displacement at the ankle. While fibular fractures may not require serious consideration, ligamentous ruptures about the ankle and displaced ankle fractures always require intensive treatment, frequently including surgical repair. The longer such appropriate treatment is delayed, the greater the probability of permanent disability.

Surgery

Many musculoskeletal problems require surgical treatment. Not only must the surgeon perform the procedure appropriately for the circumstances, but he must know when to operate, when not to operate, and what to do when an emergency develops during the course of performing the operation. If he proves derelict in either of these obligations, he may be professionally negligent.

The physician who performs musculoskeletal surgery must be very cautious in order to avoid the tragic situation of operating on the wrong extremity. Senile patients whose x-rays are mislabeled may have surgery on the incorrect hip for fracture treatment or for hip replacement surgery. Fortunately, the surgeon discovers the mistake before any irremedial damage is done, but the patient returns from the surgical suite with a difficult to explain surgical scar. When the wrong limb is amputated, the situation is tragic for the patient, the family, and the physician. This situation is compounded by the fact that the surgical indication for the correct amputation continues to exist, and eventually, the patient becomes a double amputee.

A couple of simple procedures work very well in preventing wrong limb amputation. When the patient is admitted into the hospital, the physician might indicate the limb to be amputated with some indelible marking. This should be done with an explanation to the patient, or to the family if necessary. Then, on the day of surgery, before the patient is anesthetized, the physician should ask the patient which limb is to be operated on, and be certain that the response corresponds with the indelible marking, as well as all other clinical parameters. These are two procedures which will prevent the surgeon from ever amputating the wrong limb.

Post-Operative Complications

Post-operative infection is a possible complication following any surgical procedure. It is no less so in orthopedic surgery, but whenever it occurs, it is devastating. For this reason, the patient needs to be informed of the risk, and the pre-operative scrubbing of the patient needs to be more intense than would occur for general surgical patients.

Another usual complication possible following any surgical procedure is bleeding. The patient needs to be informed of the possibility of post-surgical bleeding, as well as the possibility that he or she will need a transfusion of blood or blood products. The blood supply of the nation is safe; but there is still an extremely remote possibility that the transfusion the patient may receive will expose him or her to the HIV virus. Nevertheless, the physician has an obligation to discuss this situation with the patient.

Informed Consent

There is a long-standing controversy concerning informed consent. How much should a patient know? What happens if there develops a complication which was not included in the list of possible complications discussed with the patient? Won't too much information scare the patient away from surgery?

An informed consent for surgery means that permission has been granted by the patient, without duress, for surgical treatment of his or her body, after receiving enough information to make a bona fide assumption of risk. The surgeon must discuss with the patient, in language that he or she will understand, the disease process, the procedure to be done, the indications for the procedure, and the benefits and risks of the surgery. There must also be a discussion of the alternative therapeutic measures, as well as the benefits and risks of such measures. If the patient refuses the proposed procedure, the refusal of treatment must also be informed. The surgeon will be liable if the patient is damaged because he or she refused a proposed therapeutic measure, without having been informed of the consequences of the refusal. The risks that need to be discussed are those material risks usually associated with that particular procedure.

If the physician informs the patient in the manner and to the extent that he would want to be informed if the physician were the patient, he will have properly informed the patient.

Since the surgeon is the one who performs the surgical procedure, it is he who should inform the patient and obtain the consent. Obtaining the informed consent of a patient should be considered a pre-operative condition integral to the physician performing the proposed procedure. The physician must not delegate this task to a nurse, ward clerk, or any other person.

Conclusion

Because of the litigious nature of our society, patients with musculoskeletal injuries will be inordinately interested in the legal process. In automobile accidents, workers' compensation cases, and slip and fall situations, orthopedic patients will be expecting monetary rewards for their injuries, pain and suffering, and real and imaginary disability. The physician will, therefore, be suspect, and more often the object of the disaffection of these patients if a misadventure occurs during the treatment of their injuries and illnesses — or if they suspect that something has gone wrong. Therefore, if a physician intends to treat musculoskeletal injuries, continuing medical education will be an absolute must for him, and he must practice according to the standards of the reasonable physician at all times. Whenever the physician's own expertise is exceeded, he must realize it and refer patients to a specialist whose qualifications are known to him.

NEUROLOGY

Introduction

Neurology remains primarily a consultative medical service. Patients are seen at the request of their attending or primary physician, who is seeking the answer to a particular problem. Occasionally, the neurologist may assume the position of the primary physician for a given problem. This distinction can be important.

Physician-Patient Relationship

An initial area of concern is whether or not contact from another physician geographically distant leads to a physician-patient relationship. The courts often give considerable latitude regarding the evidence necessary to establish the existence of a physician-patient relationship. If the calling physician seeks advice in a general sense, then most likely, a court would not consider this enough contact to constitute a contract. If the physician is calling about a specific patient, even if the neurologist indicates a willingness to accept the care of that patient, still no physician-patient relationship will exist if the patient is competent and refuses to be referred. On the other hand, if the patient desires the consultation, a physician-patient relationship ensues.

Agency

A more difficult area with no clear-cut answer is when the calling physician is dealing with an incompetent patient. Here the specific advice given over the telephone, particularly when acted upon by the calling physician, may face a challenge under the law of agency. Agency is defined as a consensual relationship between two persons. This relationship need not involve compensation, but rather may be gratuitous. The relationship can be formed by an oral agreement. A court may feel that the neurologist is acting as a principal, and the calling physician is now the agent. Even though the neurologist has never seen or talked to the patient, some courts may conclude that the advice was patient specific. If so, the fact that the calling physician acted upon that advice would place the neurologist at risk. A principal may be held liable to a third person for a tort (i.e., negligent medical care) committed by his agent.

Consultant v. Referred Physician

Another area in which courts are divided deals with whether or not there is a clear distinction between the role of the consultant and the role of the physician to whom a patient has been "referred". A consultant is an independent individual actor. When a referring physician receives the advice of a consultant, he need not follow it. Assuming that the consultant has completely carried out the consultation and has made an appropriate recommendation, there should be no liability. Of course, if the consultant has made an error in diagnosis or in the recommended therapy, then both he and the referring physician may be liable.

If the referring physician has clearly requested that the neurologist take over the care of a particular problem, such as a seizure disorder, then all liability for wrongdoing will lie with the neurologist, assuming that the referring physician has transferred the case and has met the duty to chose a competent consultant. Some courts have held the referring physician negligent, too, if he knew the neurologist was negligent.

This scenario must be contrasted with the referral by a neurologist to a neurosurgeon. In such an instance, there is a great division among the courts regarding the responsibility of the referring physician. Some courts have concluded that a neurologist may breach a duty to a patient by failing to discuss and advise the patient vis-a-vis the merits and alternatives of the suggested surgery. Other courts have concluded that such surgery requires significant additional training, and that the various risks and benefits of surgery can only be appropriately told to the patient by the operating surgeon.

Other courts have concluded that a neurologist lacks the training and special expertise necessary to discuss these matters with the patient and advise him or her. Further complicating this issue is the fact that at least one court has based its opinion on the use of the term "consultation", as opposed to the term "referral". The use of the term "consultation" in this court's view leaves an ongoing responsibility with the physician requesting the consultation to both inform and counsel his patient. "Referral" in this court's opinion indicates that the patient has been transferred from the care of the referring physician, and therefore, that physician is no longer under any obligation with regard to the patient, providing the "new" physician is competent.

Control Determines Responsibility

The neurologist should always remember certain salient points governing the degree of legal responsibility for which he may be held accountable. Responsibility is proportionate to the amount of control which the neurologist exercises over the patient.

Standard of Care

The neurologist will be held to a higher standard regarding the diagnosis and treatment of neurologic disease than will the generalist. The neurologist can expect that there will be no modification of the national standard when the legal system looks at a neurologic problem.

Negligence

The neurologist must be aware of the elements necessary to prove negligence. The patient must establish: 1) the appropriate standard of care; 2) the physician's deviation from that recognized standard; and 3) that the deviation from the standard was the proximate cause of the patient's injury.

Examples

1) John Doe is referred to a neurologist for evaluation of a possible seizure disorder. Mr. Doe is a poor historian, and there are no witnesses to the ictus. The entire history is that of Mr. Doe's spouse finding him in a state of altered respon-

sivity on the living room floor.

The neurologic exam is normal, and an MRI and electroencephalogram are ordered. The patient is cautioned regarding driving, but no work history is obtained and no cautionary statements are made regarding work. Mr. Doe rides to work with a neighbor. While operating a wood chipper on the paper mill floor, he has another loss of consciousness, falls into the machine, and is severely injured.

The neurologist can be found liable for negligence in this instance, since he failed to take an adequate history. As a consequence of his failure to elicit that history, he did not warn the patient of the great danger that the sudden loss of consciousness can cause in his work. That failure would thus be directly related to the injury suffered.

The neurologist may find himself liable to a third party when he has failed to warn a patient of dangers regarding certain activities. The most commonly litigated problem in this area involves the operation of an automobile.

2) Mr. John Smith sees a neurologist for a history strongly suggesting a convulsive disorder. The neurologist places Mr. Smith on anticonvulsants, but fails to warn him of their sedating effect. Mr. Smith fails to see a stop sign, hits another vehicle, and causes injury to the driver.

Some courts have maintained that a negligent act cannot be successfully prosecuted absent a direct physician-patient relationship. These courts decline to extend a broad duty to the general public. Unfortunately, there is no clear line, and other courts have reached the opposite conclusion.

3) Ms. Carol Roe is referred by her physician to a neurologist for evaluation of intermittent tingling and weakness on the left side of her body, including her face. The neurologic examination is unremarkable. An electroencephalogram and computerized tomograph are normal. Anticonvulsant medication is prescribed. No follow-up visits are scheduled. No further diagnostic studies, such as MRI or angiography, are performed. Nine months later, Ms. Roe has a definite hemiparesis. She is referred to a different neurologist, who makes the diagnosis of glioma, utilizing an MRI which has been available for use for two years. She dies nine months later, despite appropriate surgical and medical treatment of her tumor. Her family sues the original neurologist for failure to diagnose her tumor, and for "loss of a chance" to survive.

There is sufficient evidence to suggest that further testing during the initial visit should have been carried out. An argument can be made that the risk of angiography at the initial visit outweighs a possible benefit. On the other hand, the MRI scan was available, and the risk of this procedure is minimal. Given the symptom pattern, expert testimony stating that the patient should have been seen at regular intervals in follow-up, thereby allowing for earlier diagnosis, can be anticipated.

Loss Of A Chance

The additional issue in the Roe case is that of a "loss of a chance" to survive, which is a viable basis for a cause of action. Depending on the tumor type, witnesses may testify with a reasonable degree of medical certainty that earlier diagnosis is accompanied by increased survival. Failure to diagnose early, therefore, reduced this patient's chance to survive.

Courts treat the loss of a chance to survive in several ways. The traditional approach would say that if the chance of survival was not at least 50%, then there should be no compensation. This is because it does not appear that the patient would have survived, regardless of the time that diagnosis and treatment were rendered. Recoverable damages might, however, be granted for the extended time of survival that would have occurred with more timely diagnosis and treatment. Some courts allow recovery, even when the loss of a chance of cure is less than 50%. This reduced probability of long-term survival is reflected in the amount rewarded, rather than in an absolute absence of an award.

Informed Consent

Diagnostic studies and treatment involve the doctrine of informed consent, as well as the rules governing liability as discussed above. The informed consent doctrine requires the physician to disclose certain information. He must discuss the proposed procedure with the patient. The risks involved in the procedure must likewise be disclosed. It is not necessary that all risks be disclosed, just "material risks". Those of great severity, regardless of the chance of occurrence, and those of common occurrence, regardless of a minor risk, must be discussed. Alternative methods of diagnosis or treatment and the risks related to these methods must be disclosed. Similarly, the material risks of not going forward with the study or treatment must be disclosed. The above constitutes informed consent.

To establish a lack of informed consent, the patient must show the following. First, that the physician failed to inform the patient of certain material risks. Secondly, that a prudent person similarly situated would have declined the proper study or treatment if he or she had knowledge of the material risk. Finally, that the undisclosed material risk manifested itself, and in fact, is the proximate cause of the injury and damages for which the patient seeks recovery.

Case #4

Joey Jones, age 13, had always been a healthy child. While in class, he is suddenly heard to cry out, lose consciousness, and have generalized tonic-clonic activity. By the time Joey arrives at the emergency room of the local hospital, a documented 30 minutes has passed with no abatement of epileptic activity. The emergency room physician gives Joey diazepam with no apparent effect. The neurologist arrives and appropriately gives parenteral phenytoin. The patient is placed on oral phenytoin during the pendency of his workup. He develops a rash with bullous vesicles and goes on to develop corneal erosions, fever, and cellulitis. A diagnosis of Stevens-Johnson syndrome is made. A suit is instituted by Joey's mother, stating that the neurologist failed to inform her of the risks of administering phenytoin.

The above suit will probably be dismissed on the basis that a case of prolonged convulsive status unresponsive to diazepam created an emergency situation, and a prudent person would submit to the use of phenytoin since such an uncontrolled seizure can lead to permanent and irreversible brain damage, and even death.

This situation should be contrasted with that of an individual being started on phenytoin therapy without any discussion of the material risks attendant to using that drug. The patient then develops Stevens-Johnson syndrome. Here a court could well find that the patient was not informed of the material risks, and alternative treatments were not discussed. A material risk came to pass and was, in fact, the proximate cause of the patient's damage. The patient was denied the right of freedom of choice.

Reportable Diseases

The neurologist must be aware of the laws and regulations governing the reporting of certain conditions. These laws and regulations differ from state to state. Some statutes may require mandatory reporting with appropriate immunity, or they may allow physician discretion. There may or may not be criminal and/or civil penalties for failing to report.

Many neurologic disorders significantly impact on highway safety. Dementias, cerebral vascular disease, Parkinsonism, and episodic alterations in consciousness all have the potential for leading to serious injury to a patient and others, particularly when automobile operation is involved. The common element is the disturbance of sensory, motor, cognitive, or coordinative functions sufficient to affect driving. If stable, these can be compatible with safely operating a motor vehicle. If not stable or progressive, re-evaluation over time may well be necessary. In any event, these diseases must be reported.

Altered states of consciousness require a careful workup to distinguish between epilepsy and other disorders that can affect consciousness or motor control. Such a list would include syncope, cataplexy, narcolepsy, hypoglycemia, and episodic vertigo from a variety of reasons.

Determination of Death

Neurologists frequently find themselves involved in the determination of death when such a determination is made on the basis of irreversible cessation of all functions of the entire brain. Most jurisdictions have adopted the Uniform Determination of Death Act. This Act states "an individual who has sustained either irreversible cessation of circulatory and respiratory functions, or irreversible cessation of all functions of the entire brain, including the brain stem, is dead. A determination of death *must* be made in accordance with accepted medical standards."

It is important that the neurologist keep abreast of what the accepted standards are, both nationally and in the community in which he practices, vis-a-vis the determination of death. In certain circumstances, such as organ donation, the standard may require confirmatory studies utilizing neurophysiologic or imaging techniques. Similarly, individuals who are in this condition as the result of an assault, where criminal prosecution for homicide is probable, may require confirmatory studies to meet the appropriate standard. Violent action as a cause of death may also require notification and involvement of the police, Medical Examiner, and the State's Attorney. Certainly, in the area of organ donation, and to a lesser extent in the criminal setting, the determination of death should be made by a neurologist not directly involved in the patient's care.

Vegetative State

Perhaps the most difficult of the ethical/legal problems confronting the neurologist today is that of the diagnosis of a persistent vegetative state and the decisions regarding treatment for that condition. The Cruzan case recently decided by the United States Supreme Court allows the state to legislate on this issue, i.e., whether the patient previously had indicated a desire not to be healed. It is important that the neurologist be aware of any laws, rules, and regulations in his own particular jurisdiction dealing with what may or may not be life-sustaining treatment, and how the initiation, continuation, or cessation of such treatment is viewed by the state. The neurologist should be certain that the diagnosis of a persistent vegetative state is made in full compliance with recognized national standards, such as those promulgated by the American Academy of Neurology. When cessation of life-sustaining treatment, including nutrition and hydration, is an issue, more than one neurologist should independently examine and diagnose the patient.

Dementia

Failure to diagnose correctly can be particularly troublesome when a patient has a completely treatable, if not curable, entity, but is instead diagnosed as having a disease that cannot be treated or cured. The neurologist will be held to a standard that demands ruling out treatable entities, even when the likelihood of their occurring is small. An example occurs when dealing with dementia. Alzheimer's disease accounts for most of the dementing illnesses seen in a neurologic practice. It is necessary, however, to identify the approximately 10-15% of patients with dementia, in that the disease process may be reversed or halted by appropriate treatment. The differential diagnosis runs through metabolic disorders, vascular disorders, deficiency diseases, toxicity, infection, and several other categories. Additionally, depression, a "functional disorder", can be difficult to differentiate from "organic" dementia.

Expert Testimony

A neurologist may be called upon to give an expert opinion in a legal action. That opinion may play a critical role in the outcome of the case. If the expert's incorrect opinion leads to the plaintiff losing his case or receiving a diminished award, that plaintiff may have a cause of action against the expert. An example is rendering an opinion regarding post-traumatic-seizures too early in the post-injury course.

The increase in head trauma and litigation has conspired to make it well worth the neurologist's time to understand the various sequelae of such trauma, and the pertinent findings and course of such ill-defined entities as the post-concussive syndrome.

OBSTETRICS/GYNECOLOGY

Introduction

A normal pregnancy is not a disease; it is a physiological state in the life of a female! Unfortunately, a pregnancy can produce diseases in the reproductive system inherent in an abnormal pregnancy. There can also be pregnancy-related diseases external to the reproductive system, as well as in the fetus.

Labor and Delivery

Labor and delivery are particularly susceptible to legal complications. The physician's liability is extended for birth trauma for many years by statutes of limitations until the newborn reaches the age of majority, since the full effect of a complication may not be readily assessable, or the parents may not be vigilant or diligent. While the public and their attorneys assume that any irregularity in labor and delivery care is causally related to later untoward sequelae, it has been observed that no more than 15% of cases of severe retardation can be attributed to perinatal events. Most severely depressed babies evidence no detectable neurologic or intellectual damage. At least 50% of all cerebral palsy infants have no documented depression at the time of birth. Since labor and delivery may occur at any time of day or night, the availability of the obstetrician and his ability to be present at delivery, or provide an acceptable substitute based on a "legitimate absence," is important to obviate the risk of a patient claiming abandonment. Finally, while the obstetrician *may* be responsible as "Captain of the Ship" for actions of other professional personnel (nurses, nurse-midwives, anesthetists, etc.), much of the care of the patient during labor and delivery must, of necessity, be provided by these other professionals.

Ultrasonography

Ultrasound poses several areas of potential entrapment of the unwary physician. Misinterpreting ultrasound findings in *dating pregnancy* commonly contributes to litigation. The range varies by several days during the first trimester, and by up to three weeks during the late third trimester. If the patient's dates fall within the range suggested by a sonogram, it is improper to revise the expected date of confinement (EDC). If the gestational age, as determined by ultrasound, encompasses a known date of the last menstrual period (LMP), the information is properly interpreted as consistent with the LMP. It is inappropriate to use ultrasound results as a basis for altering a patient's dates, unless menstrual dates fall outside the limits of uncertainty of the ultrasound examination. A second kind of error commonly occurs in the patient with unknown menstrual dates, who has a late sonogram for dating purposes. The uncertainty of the measurement must be taken into account in the management of the patient. Any ultrasound should routinely be used to measure and report not only biparietal diameters of the fetal head, but also head and abdominal circumferences and femur length. It is important to assess amniotic fluid volume, locate the placenta, and perform an anatomic survey, including at least the cerebral ventricles and fetal kidneys and spine, a four-chamber cardiac view, and visualization of the area of insertion of the umbilical cord.

Intrauterine Growth Retardation (IUGR)

This condition produces several different sonographic patterns. Asymmetric IUGR is the most commmon, showing head and femur size appropriate for the gestational age but abdominal circumference below normal limits. A less common but more severe pattern of IUGR involves femur sparing. Femur length is appropriate for the gestational age, but the head and abdomen are below the 50th percentile for gestational age, the abdomen being more commonly severely affected than the head. The combination of normal abdominal circumference and femur length with a borderline or small fetal head is not a common pattern for IUGR, and usually represents a normal variant, not an anomaly. Only when the head size exhibits severe reduction in size might clinically significant microencephaly be suspected. A relatively short femur, plus abdomen and head measurements consistent with the LMP, tends to represent a genetic variant, although it may be associated with fetal trisomy. Therefore, an ultrasound report relying on average measurements may mask potentially important clinical findings. Calculating such ratios as head circumference to abdominal circumference, or abdominal circumference to femur length, and considering these calculations with regard to the proper range of such ratios, will greatly aid the physician in avoiding misinterpreting sonograms. A pattern of symmetric IUGR is extremely difficult to assess when confirmatory, early clinical findings are absent. The sonogram should be repeated in several weeks to assure that fetal growth is taking place at the expected rate. If subsequent examination reveals an inadequate rate of growth, symmetric IUGR may be present.

Abruptio Placentae

Retroplacental bleeding and abruptio placentae may sometimes be seen on sonography. A negative ultrasound examination, however, does not exclude abruption. If the clinical impression is abruptio, but the sonogram fails to reveal a retroplacental clot, one cannot be assured that the patient does not have abruptio placentae. With proper angling of the ultrasound transducer, an apparent retroplacental clot can often be artificially produced. An ultrasound examination is not helpful in a patient whose clinical course is consistent with abruption. The diagnosis is made or excluded on the basis of clinical examination and electronic fetal heart rate monitoring, rather than on the basis of an ultrasound scan.

Fetal Anomalies

Fetal anomalies are occasionally missed by even the experienced sonographer. An unfavorable fetal position or movement may preclude optimal visualization and diagnosis. For the office-based sonographer, particularly one who lacks extensive experience in diagnosing anomalies, it may be helpful to obtain written informed consent before undertaking any diagnostic ultrasound procedure. Such consent would explain that the examination is expected to provide information about fetal number, position, gestational age, and placental localization, but that the sonographer has no experience, particularly in diagnosing fetal anomalies. This kind of informed consent will provide the patient with realistic expectations that may reduce the likelihood of litigation if an existing anomaly is not detected.

Any patient at significant risk for an anomaly should be referred by the office-based sonographer without significant experience to one with experience in diagnosing congenital malformations. Even the experienced sonographer cannot justifiably be held responsible for failure to detect all congenital defects. The gestational sac or a fetus in a location other than the uterus can at times be identified by high-resolution sonography.

Ectopic Pregnancy (EP)

Ectopic pregnancy is a pregnancy implanted at a site which does not permit development of the conceptus. Most often, it is due to failure of the fertilized egg to pass down the fallopian tube in a timely enough manner that allows proper implantation in the uterus. EP is one of the leading causes of maternal mortality in the United States. One of the most common causes is partial tubal obstruction after tubal infection. In addition, EP may have long-term effects on a patient's reproductive capacity. There is a 50% infertility rate after an EP, and a 10-15% risk of a subsequent EP in women who have had a prior extrauterine pregnancy. The major sources of morbidity and mortality are patient delay in reporting early symptoms, and physician delay in diagnosis and treatment.

Etiologic Factors
Several factors account for the increasing incidence of EP: 1) the greater frequency of pelvic inflammatory disease (PID); 2) the use of a intrauterine device (IUD); and 3) the use of progestin-only oral contraceptives. One of the contraceptive actions of progesterone is its effect on tubal physiology. Proper tubal function is thought to be highly dependent on precise relationships between estrogen and progesterone, and possibly other hormone secretions.

Incidence
EP is more prevalent among blacks than among the white population, due perhaps to a higher incidence of gonorrheal salpingitis in blacks. It is more often seen in lower socioeconomic groups than in private patients. Gonorrheal salpingitis usually involves the endosalpinx and is more likely to precede tubal pregnancy than is post-abortal or postpartum salpingitis, both of which are limited primarily to the peritubal tissue. Endometriosis is considered by most authorities to be an infrequent etiologic factor in EP.

Diagnosis
Known as the "Great Masquerader", EP can mimic many other abdominal and pelvic problems. Early diagnosis depends on several factors — first, "think ectopic"; second, consider the possibility in all women from menarche to menopause who complain of lower abdominal pain. The diagnosis is rarely missed if the patient reports symptoms early, the physician has a high index of suspicion, and modern methods of diagnosis are used.

Differential Diagnosis
Several common conditions can make diagnosis difficult because they may present a clinical picture similar to EP. These include appendicitis, salpingitis,

gastroenteritis, ruptured corpus luteum cyst, and threatened or incomplete abortion.

Diagnostic Tests

Standard pregnancy tests are not reliable in the diagnosis of EP. The placenta secretes less human chorionic gonadotrophin in EP than does the placenta in a normal intrauterine pregnancy.

Radioreceptor assays and radioimmunoassays can detect minute amounts of chorionic gonadotrophin and are almost always positive with EPs, even those aborted from the tube into the abdominal cavity spontaneously. Diagnostic laparoscopy or exploratory laparotomy provide the most specific diagnostic procedures. Sonography, culdocentesis, or colpotomy may be useful adjuncts in diagnosis. While 95% of EP pregnancies occur in some portion of the fallopian tube, cases have been reported occurring in an ovary, in the abdominal cavity, and in the broad ligament.

The principal value of ultrasound in the diagnosis of EP is its ability to help confirm or exclude an intrauterine pregnancy. Failure to identify an EP in a patient who has the clinical signs and symptoms should not lessen clinical suspicion, unless a viable fetus is identified within the uterus. The possibility of a pseudogestational sac is well-described in the literature and should also be kept in mind when pursuing a diagnosis. Not all fluid collections within the uterus represent gestational sacs, nor does the identification of such a sac exclude EP. The only certain way to exclude an ectopic gestation is to identify a fetal heartbeat or definite fetal pole within the uterus.

Treatment

Treatment of EP is surgical intervention in most cases with salpingectomy. Removal of the adjacent ovary at the time of salpingectomy has been recommended as improving fertility by allowing subsequent ovulation to take place from the ovary immediately adjacent to the remaining tube. If there is minimal tubal distortion, and particularly if the other tube has already been removed, an early pregnancy in the tubal isthmus may be removed by linear salpingostomy. The operation, however, increases the risk of another pregnancy in that tube in the future.

Treatment in a few instances may consist of simple milking of a tubal pregnancy past the fimbria into the abdominal cavity for removal. If tubal abortion has occurred without significant tubal damage, no further surgery, except for hemostasis, may be necessary. All blood should be removed from the peritoneal cavity to help prevent future peritoneal adhesions.

There is a positive association between EP and tubal surgery, such as tuboplasty, salpingectomy, and tubal sterilization. Laparoscopic treatment of EP may result in decreased morbidity and costs, ccmpared to traditional management by laparotomy. Fewer medical resources may be required, thereby significantly reducing costs. Laparoscopic linear salpingostomy or salpingectomy may be done with removal of the surgical specimen through an auxiliary puncture site. The pelvis must be thoroughly lavaged to decrease the risk of adhesions. Laparoscopy for treatment of EP is not indicated in the presence of hemodynamic instability, either at presentation or with induction of anesthesia. Where it can be accomplished, there is more rapid recovery and reduction in costs. (Thus, it seems that resident training in the laparoscopic technique of EP management is warranted.)

Informed Consent

The patient should be counseled with respect to her wishes about future pregnancies prior to surgery. A true informed consent must be obtained. Failure to do so, with resulting sterilization, may create liability for the gynecolcgist.

Complications

Complications of EP include the most drastic, i.e., death, when surgery is not timely performed and exsanguination occurs. Chronic salpingitis often follows a neglected, ruptured EP. Infertility develops in about 50% of patients who have undergone surgery for extrauterine pregnancy; approximately 30% of these become sterile. Chronic urinary tract infections and ureteral strictures may occur after infection. Intestinal obstruction and fistulae may develop after hemoperitoneum, peritonitis, or lithopedion formation.

Prevention

To prevent original or repeat EP, the surgeon should avoid unperitonealized areas at surgery, resulting in adhesions that may obstruct the fallopian tubes; treat salpingitis early and vigorously; and perform a D&C promptly for an incomplete abortion.

Legal Implications of EP

If a bad result occurs, negligence may be argued if the physician's care fell below accepted standards. The American College of Obstetricians and Gynecologists has not published guidelines for the diagnosis and treatment of extrauterine pregnancy. While no specific symptoms or signs are indicative of EP, a combination of abormal bleeding with abdominal pain (even without a missed menstrual period) in a woman of child-bearing age should raise an index of suspicion for EP. Radioreceptor assays and radioimmunoassays can detect minute amounts of chorionic gonadotrophin and are almost always positive with EPs, even though aborted from the tube into the abdominal cavity spontaneously.

Failure to diagnose an EP is often associated with certain case characteristics. Often, the physician ignores or misjudges the patient's symptoms, causing a rapid worsening in her overall condition, and leading to a life-endangered situation. Prompt diagnostic laparoscopy when EP is suspected from the patient's symptoms will usually reveal the condition and lead to a satisfactory resolution of the situation.

Failure to use accepted diagnostic tests and procedures when a patient exhibits symptoms compatible with EP may result in legal liability. No matter how many tests or examinations a physician conducts, if EP is not considered in the face of indicated symptoms, or if reasonable skill and care are not used in confirming or excluding the diagnosis, liability may result.

Failure to obtain adequate informed consent, as mentioned earlier, may be the basis for another charge of negligence, or depending on the jurisdiction, a claim of battery or lack of informed consent.

Fetal Heart Rate Monitoring (FHR)

Fetal heart rate monitoring is one of the more prominent subjects in the medicolegal area. The monitor strips often provide important evidence of fetal status in an obstetric malpractice case. Until 1988, continuous electronic FHR monitoring was mandated for all high-risk obstetric patients in labor. In 1988, the American Academy of Pediatrics (AAP) and the American College of Obstetricians and Gynecologists (ACOG) issued guidelines for perinatal care, permitting intermittent auscultation or continuous electronic monitoring for high-risk intrapartum patients. Randomized prospective research has failed to sustain the value of continuous electronic monitoring. Studies in low and high-risk pregnancies have not confirmed the positive predictive value of periodic FHR patterns as they relate to uterine contractions, especially as compared to the accuracy of auscultation. The new guidelines recommend FHR evaluation at least every 15 minutes during the active phase of the first stage of labor. This can be by continuous electronic fetal monitoring (EFM), or by intermittent auscultation. During the second stage of labor, the physician should evaluate the FHR by interpretation of the tracing from continuous EFM or by intermittent auscultation every five minutes. These are for the high-risk patient. For the low-risk patient, it is suggested that FHR evaluation be every 30 minutes during the active phase of the first stage of labor, and every 15 minutes throughout the second stage. Under the new guidelines, both intermittent auscultation and continuous EFM are acceptable.

The application of the guidelines may have to be tempered by the realities of the nursing shortage. Intermittent auscultation more frequently during labor may require more nurses to implement care. While staffing is a nursing issue, when fetal assessment is ordered, the nurse has a legal responsibility to determine if adequate staff are available to implement care and to notify the prescribing physician.

Another problem with intermittent auscultation is the impossibility of interpreting FHR variability. This would preclude assessment of fetal reserve with FHR decelerations. Auscultation alone cannot distinguish the fixed FHR baseline from the FHR lacking decelerations but having minimal or moderate variability. By providing continuous printouts and permitting minute-by-minute fetal assessment, EFM lessens the probability of undiagnosed acute problems. Lack of user knowledge, however, may be a problem. Inadequacies in interpretation and management planning may be apparent in reviewing EFM printouts. Since the interpretation of FHR findings is controversial, it may be hard to defend actions of health care workers relative to monitor interpretation. A normal FHR tracing may be expected to result in a good outcome. FHR abnormalities, however, are not necessarily predictive of a poor outcome or fetal pathology.

How should the guidelines be implemented in order to establish an acceptable standard of care, both medically and legally? 1) New practice policies and protocols should be written in clear, concise form; 2) a general policy as a joint endeavor of the medical and nursing staff of the hospital should identify when and how to perform fetal monitoring; 3) protocols should be defined, specifying the frequency and length of fetal monitoring, distinguishing normal from abnormal findings and outlining appropriate nursing and medical responses; periodic pattern names should be used, such as accelerations and early, late, and variable decelerations, to minimize misunderstanding and intervention; and 5) tracings should be stored permanently by a filing and retrieval system of the actual tracing or microfiche. For large volume facilities, computer disk-stored tracings are best. It is crucial that there be ongoing instructional review of monitor tracings by the obstetrical staff to educate physicians in interpreting tracings. Health care professionals must examine the guidelines, review the literature, and develop practice policies and protocols to meet the goal of optimal patient care, and thus reduce medicolegal risk.

Preeclampsia

Hypertension must be differentiated from preeclampsia. Preeclampsia most commonly occurs in primagravidas. Grand multiparas, in particular, however, can also develop preeclampsia. Hypertension without proteinuria is more suggestive of chronic hypertension, but proteinuria can occur in both conditions. In chronic hypertension of long-standing, physical examination may show retinal vascular changes. The uric acid may rise in preeclampsia. Chronic hypertension is best managed with aggressive therapy, including fetal surveillance with either non-stress or stress testing, or biophysical profile assessment. Severe preeclampsia is best managed by judicious delivery. Milder preeclampsia may respond to bed rest with close surveillance; delivery being indicated for fetal indications of distress or IUGR, or the development of severe preeclampsia.

Cesarean section should be performed in preeclampsia only for obstetric indications or deteriorating maternal condition. The incidence of cesarean sections is increased because of the higher incidence of placental insufficiency and fetal distress. If delivery is operative, the liver should be inspected and palpated, especially when there are abnormal liver enzymes recorded. If general endotracheal anesthesia is used, antihypertensive therapy should be started prior to intubation to prevent further rise in blood pressure during intubation. The use of epidural anesthesia in preeclampsia is controversial because blood pressure can drop if volume contraction is not corrected before placing the epidural. For severe preeclampsia, central hemodynamic monitoring should be used to ensure euvolemia before placing the epidural.

Magnesium sulfate therapy should be continued postpartum for at least 24 hours. The hypertension of preeclampsia may last up to six weeks postpartum and should be treated as indicated. If antihypertensive therapy is required after discharge from the hospital, the patient should be monitored in the office weekly and biweekly. By the six week postpartum checkup, the patient should no longer require antihypertensives.

Preeclampsia may present pitfalls in diagnosis and management. It is important to first make the diagnosis and differentiate it from chronic hypertension. Bed rest and antepartum surveillance are required for mild preeclampsia. Delivery is indicated when fetal lung maturity, fetal distress, or severe preeclampsia occur. Preeclampsia complicates at least 5% of pregnancies. Disastrous maternal and fetal consequences may occur unless a course of aggressive diagnosis and therapy is pursued.

Shoulder Dystocia

Most of the lawsuits arising out of injuries caused by dystocia have been generated by characteristics of the passenger, especially shoulder dystocia. Shoulder dystocia is defined as the arrest of spontaneous delivery of the fetus because of impaction of the anterior shoulder behind the pubic symphysis. It occurs because of a disproportion between fetal and maternal size. There is a substantial increase in the incidence when the fetal weight exceeds 4000 grams. The disproportion between trunk and head size is exaggerated in these large fetuses. Shoulder dystocia is related to fetal weight; thus, clinical factors leading to increased fetal size will also increase the chance of shoulder dystocia. The two most important factors are pregnancy duration of 42 weeks or longer, and maternal diabetes. Labor abnormalities are known to be associated with shoulder dystocia. The most crucial factor in predicting shoulder dystocia is the accurate estimation of fetal weight. Despite advances in ultrasound evaluation, there are no well-documented formulas for estimation of fetal weight with a high enough predictive value that can be used for clinical decision-making in the potentially macrosomic fetus.

There are a number of fetal injuries unrelated to fetal asphyxia that can result from shoulder dystocia, fracture of the fetal clavicle or humerus probably being the most common injury. These rarely result in long-term consequences to the fetus, however. Brachial plexus injury, on the other hand, can cause lifelong disability in the offspring. The obstetrician must, therefore, make a clinical judgment on the weight of the fetus in order to formulate a plan for avoiding brachial plexus injury. The successful management of shoulder dystocia requires critical judgment by the obstetrician. Recognition of the problem before excessive lateral traction is applied to the fetal neck is important.

When a birth is complicated by shoulder dystocia, the following information should be contained in the chart. If the delivery was by forceps or vacuum, there should be a statement of the indication for the instrumental delivery with the approximate time required to deliver the head; a statement should be made on how the diagnosis of shoulder dystocia was arrived at; the approximate time from delivery of the fetal head until delivery of the body should be noted, along with a description of the maneuvers to relieve the dystocia; umbilical cord blood gases of both artery and vein should be measured; there should be an examination of the fetus with particular attention to the movement of the arms; and finally, a full explanation of the problem and of the steps taken to relieve it should be given the patient by the obstetrician. If the infant has suffered an injury, the physician should disclose this to the patient. The best method of avoiding permanent injury is appropriate delivery maneuvers once the problem is identified. Careful chart documentation of the events surrounding the delivery and a fully informed patient are the obstetrician's best allies in this instance.

Breech Presentation

Breech presentations occur in approximately 3-4% of all term deliveries, and in 7-8% of all fetuses at 28 to 34 weeks of gestation. Liability may be imposed on the physician for failure to properly treat and manage injuries to both mother and infant, resulting from breech presentation, and for negligence in failing to perform a cesarean section where indicated.

Fetuses in the breech position are at greater risk than other singleton fetuses for cord prolapse, birth trauma, peripartum asphyxia, and possible neurologic sequelae. Breech presentations are associated with higher perinatal morbidity and mortality than vertexes. The common risks include intrapartum fetal death 16 times the normal risk; intrapartum asphyxia; umbilical cord prolapse; birth trauma; arrest of the aftercoming head; spinal cord injuries; major anomalies; prematurity; and hyperextension of the fetal head. Prematurity has been observed in approximately 25% of all breech deliveries involving such complications of prematurity as intraventricular hemorrhage, respiratory distress syndrome, and hyperbilirubinemia.

The incidence of congenital fetal anomalies has been found to be higher with breech fetuses than with vertex fetuses. These abnormalities include congenital hip dislocation, hydrocephaly, anencephaly, meningomyelocele, and trisomic chromosomal abnormalities.

Birth trauma resulting from difficult breech vaginal delivery has commonly involved brachial plexus injury and bone fractures. Breech fetuses with cephalic hyperextension are at particular risk for complications, including medullar or vertebral injuries, meningeal hemorrhages, and spinal cord transection if the hyperextension exceeds 90°. Umbilical cord prolapse is most common with large fetuses, multiparous women, and non-frank breech presentation. Pre-term breech fetuses are also at higher risk for head entrapment because the head size is relatively large compared with the abdomen until 35 to 36 weeks of gestation. The entrapment occurs from delivery of the fetal body through an incompletely dilated cervix, leading to arrest of the head. Larger fetuses are also at risk for this entrapment problem. There is general agreement that breech fetuses have a higher incidence of birth asphyxia than vertexes. Perinatal asphyxia and the long-term neurologic status of breech fetuses have been widely debated, especially in relation to the route of delivery and degree of fetal prematurity. Profound morbidity from breech deliveries is primarily associated with cerebral hemorrhage, cord prolapse, and head entrapment.

Routine cesarean section for impending pre-term breech delivery appears to improve neonatal outcome and reduce long-term neurologic sequelae. The potential benefit of cesarean delivery for pre-term, nonfootling breech fetuses is less apparent with term gestation. While the liberal use of cesarean section delivery for term breech fetuses does not appear to reduce the incidence of perinatal asphyxia or neurologic sequelae, nonetheless there appears to be a trend toward decreased birth injury and neonatal deaths.

Management strategies in breech presentation include the appropriate use of pelvimetry, Piper forceps, and external cephalic version in carefully selected patients. Successful vaginal delivery may be predicted by clinical and x-ray pelvimetry. Neonatal morbidity in vaginal breech deliveries is less when Piper forceps are applied to the aftercoming head of infants weighing 1000-3000 grams. External version of breech fetuses may be successfully performed at or after 36 weeks, although many will revert to the breech presentation.

Careful selection for vaginal delivery on the basis of x-ray pelvimetry and fetography may be used to rule out head hyperextension. An upper limit of 3500 grams may be used to exclude large fetuses from vaginal delivery. Vaginal delivery in selected cases of frank breech presentation at term can be performed with a minimum of risk for mother and fetus.

Decisions on managing the breech fetus should be based on the facilities available, physician experience, anesthesia needed, type of breech, fetal size, head position and size, pelvimetry, and progress of labor. The ACOG technical bulletin #95 (August, 1986) recognizes that many confounding variables make the assessment of risks difficult. "Either cesarean section or vaginal delivery (in carefully selected cases) may be acceptable for the term frank breech presentation." Further information is needed before specific recommendations can be given for the non-frank breech fetus. The following are offered to reduce risk in the management of term frank breech: 1) identify fetal malpresentation; 2) rule out congenital anomalies; 3) obtain informed consent (risks, benefits, alternatives) for external cephalic version, vaginal versus cesarean delivery, and timing of delivery; and 4) document important decisions into the medical chart. It is currently standard practice to consider vaginal delivery of carefully selected term breech fetuses; however, laboring non-frank or premature breech pregnancies are often better served by operative delivery.

Breech fetuses with distress, cord prolapse, head hyperextension, prematurity, inadequate pelvimetry, and weight greater than 4000 grams should also be delivered by cesarean section. Appropriate surgical, anesthetic, and monitoring facilities can make the physician less vulnerable to legal liability.

Apgar Score

The Apgar score was devised as a quick method of assessing the state of the newborn infant. Its misuse, however, has led to an erroneous definition of asphyxia. Intrapartum asphyxia implies fetal hypercarbia and hypoxemia. Metabolic acidemia will result. Because intrapartum disruption of uterine or fetal blood flow is rarely absolute, "asphyxia" is not a precise term. More precise terms include "hypercarbia", "hypoxia", and "metabolic and respiratory or lactic acidemia". These are more precise for immediate assessment of the newborn, as well as for retrospective assessment of intrapartum management. While the Apgar score is convenient for reporting the state of the baby and the effectiveness of resuscitation, it must be placed in proper perspective for assessing asphyxia and for prognostication of future neurologic deficits.

The five components of the score are heart rate, respiratory effort, tone, reflex irritability, and color. Each is given a score of 0, 1, or 2. Some of the score is partially dependent on the physiologic maturity of the infant, including tone, color, and reflex irritability. Thus, the normal premature infant may be scored low purely due to immaturity, with no evidence of anoxic insult or cerebral depression. Other factors affecting the Apgar score include maternal sedation or analgesia (decreased tone and responsiveness); neurologic conditions such as muscle disease or cerebral malformations (decreased tone and interference with respiration); or cardiorespiratory conditions (interference with heart rate, respiration, and tone). The one minute score may indicate the need for special attention to the infant, although a low score does not necessarily correlate with future outcome. The five minute score is a useful index of the effectivenes of resuscitation efforts, particularly the change between one and five minute scores. Because the scores have poor correlation with either cause or outcome, they should not be considered alone as evidence of or consequent to substantial asphyxia. Later scores correlate with future neurologic outcomes when the score is 0 to 3 at 10, 15, and 20 minutes. Substantial cerebral hypoxia leading to cerebral palsy can be presumed only when three criteria are met: 1) Apgar score is 0-3 at 10 minutes (absent other causes); 2) hypotonicity of the infant for several hours; and 3) the infant has seizures. Confirmation of suspected hypoxia (asphyxia) may be obtained by demonstrating metabolic acidemia in umbilical cord blood.

Cerebral Palsy (CP)

Cerebral palsy is the only neurologic deficit clearly linked to perinatal asphyxia. Mental retardation and epilepsy may accompany CP, but there is no evidence that they are caused by perinatal asphyxia unless CP is also present. The Apgar scores are not evidence alone of sufficient hypoxia to result in neurologic damage. Low scores may be evidence of hypoxia influenced by other factors.

Society refuses to accept the fact that nature and the reproductive process are important. Despite rapidly accumulating information to the contrary, the idea persists that most bad obstetric outcomes result from intrapartum events. A recent study found no factor in labor or delivery that was a major predictor of CP. Despite the improvements in obstetric and neonatal care, there has been no consistent decrease in the frequency of CP in the past two decades. It, therefore, behooves all obstetricians to examine the quality of their care and to document fetal condition at delivery. Fetal acid-base status and cord gases can be easily obtained at delivery. Cord blood will accurately reflect the fetal pH, PO_2, PCO_2, concentration of bicarbonate, and buffer base deficit or excess at the time of birth. Therefore, umbilical pH and blood gas analysis will substantiate that the baby was born in a good metabolic state, and that intrapartum care was appropriate. Once specimens have been collected in heparinized syringes and capped, pH and gas values are stable at room temperature for at least 60 minutes. The specimens do not require immediate analysis, nor must they be placed on ice. Thus, routinely obtaining cord blood for pH and gas analysis at every delivery might be viewed as a good defensive measure and effective risk management.

Pregnancy Termination and Prevention

Claims related to pregnancy termination (abortion) and prevention tort litigation and to the involved informed consent are common. The possibility of recanalization of the tubes after ligation has to be explained to the patient, in advance, as a small but definite possibility. Wrongful birth and wrongful life suits are two additional concerns after a failed ligation. In the former, parents may claim physician negligence in not advising them not to conceive, or in failing to perform necessary tests if the woman was already pregnant (e.g., Tay-Sachs disease), or in failing to advise genetic counseling and denying the parents the option of abortion if the child was defective. In wrongful life suits, a defective child by its parents may claim the physician's negligence denied the parents the choice of not conceiving or of abortion after conception. Recent legal decisions in wrongful birth cases may raise relevant issues in some instances, while those for wrongful life may not be sustained.

Substitute Parenthood

Surrogate motherhood, in vitro fertilization, and genetic engineering permit variations from the usual method of conception. The birth of a child with physical or mental defects following artificial insemination may present major litigation problems. Detailed informed consent is essential prior to insemination. In vitro fertilization has stirred popular interest and concern. There are many ways in which the physician or his associate can be involved in legal complications — if pregnancy does not result, if abortion occurs, or if a defective child is born. In spite of the fact that motivation of most couples seeking in vitro fertilization is very high, and the limited chance of success is well-recognized, there is considerable potential for claims.

Breast Disease

A major cause of legal actions is failure to diagnose breast cancer. Since obstetrican-gynecologists are often the only physicians to examine women regularly, the responsibility for diagnosis often lies with the ob/gyn. Omission of recognized diagnostic procedures, or of recommendations that the patient seek them elsewhere, may lead to claims of malpractice. Recommendations for consultation should be documented. A similar risk occurs if studies, such as cytologic examination of aspirate of a cyst or needle or open biopsy, do not lead to a diagnosis of cancer that is later found, or if such procedures result in an infection or unsightly scars.

Obstetrician/gynecologists, like all physicians who care for women, should instruct or refer the patient to learn about self-examination. The physician should be familiar with the recommendations of the American College of Obstetrics and Gynecology and the National Institutes of Health vis-a-vis mammography, and implement them.

Prolongation of Life and Resuscitation

Obstetrician-gyencologists have to deal with dying adult patients, although stillbirth and early neonatal death also fall within their province. It is clearly a duty of the physician to do all that he can to preserve life, but when all attempts to cure have been unsuccessful and death is imminent, the question of life-prolonging treatment may raise legal and ethical questions. Cases have generally occurred in other than ob-gyn situations, but there is an occasional case that involves such a specialist.

The initiation or continuation of cardiopulmonary resuscitation (CPR) may be in question. Present day CPR usually means that in a hospital, a special team is summoned to apply resuscitative measures, and these measures are continued until the patient is clearly biologically dead, or at least brain dead. The measures include transfer to and maintenance of the patient in an Intensive Care Unit. It may be difficult to decide whether or not CPR should be started in a patient who has no chance of eventual survival. At the present time, a nurse or other professional cannot make this decision; it is the physician's responsibility. There being no written order on the patient's chart not to continue therapy, as well as evidence of informed consent by a competent patient, or a surrogate for an incompetent patient, the nurse and/or other staff members must institute CPR. The physician is on safe legal ground if his decision follows accepted medical standards and protocols devised by the institution and developed from generally accepted principles. How the physician arrives at the decision to resuscitate or not is based on established medical practice, as well as ethical and legal principles.

Genetics

Increases in knowledge about inherited diseases and development of the fetus in utero have given rise to an entirely new set of possible medicolegal complications. Most of these are failures of omission, e.g., amniocentesis not offered or performed negligently, resulting in the birth of a defective child because chromosome analysis was not done. Informed consent is essential prior to amniooentesis, as the procedure carries risks, although very minimal, for the mother and fetus, such as infection, injury to the fetus, hemorrhage, miscarriage, or premature labor.

New diagnostic techniques have made invasive surgical management of fetal disease possible. Intrauterine repair of congenital cardiac and other congenital disorders is now possible. Intrauterine transfusion in severe erythroblastosis fetalis and surgical management of hydrocephalus and urinary tract obstruction are but a few of the areas to be considered. Legal and ethical issues raised by fetal surgery make safeguards important. These include detailed review and consent by all involved.

Gynecologic Surgery

Most lawsuits against gynecologists relate to the surgical aspects of the practice, and are likely to include claims against the hospital and other involved hospital staff members. The difficulty from the defendant-physician's point of view is that lawyers for other parties may defend their clients' rights with little or no regard for the effect of their efforts on other defendants. For example, when a sponge or instrument is left inside the abdomen, and the circulating nurse reported correct counts, the hospital may try to lay the blame on the physician in order to avoid its responsibility for the negligent acts of its nurse employee (vicarious liability and respondeat superior). Problems with anesthesia, blood transfusions, and recovery room mishaps are other acts that may give rise to claims in gynecology. Hysterectomies have been of special concern, fostered by reports of unnecessary surgery. While the rate of hysterectomy is declining in the United States in recent years, the effect of careful monitoring and introduction of second opinion programs have created an uncertain legal impact. Patients have become more aware of the effects and complications of a hysterectomy. The most common include infection, hemorrhage, fistula formation, and emotional and menopausal changes. It is, therefore, especially important to obtain truly informed consent from a patient for a hysterectomy, in order to avoid a charge of unnecessary surgery.

Since the gynecologic surgeon is at extremely high risk of being the defendant in a medicolegal battle, several courses of action are in order. First, he should take an adequate history, looking for past episodes of pelvic inflammatory disease, endometriosis, or diverticulitis. A history of infertility may suggest previous infection or endometriosis. These may be a factor in operative success and should be part of the informed consent.

Smokers should be encouraged to curtail smoking at least three weeks before surgery. Pre-operative pulmonary function tests may be useful if there is a long history of heavy smoking or chronic obstructive pulmonary disease (COPD). A patient with COPD should stop smoking eight weeks before surgery. Pre-operative placement of central circulation monitoring lines may be beneficial in patients with known stenotic valvular lesions or a history of congestive heart failure.

Prophylactic antibiotics should be given to any patient undergoing major surgery who has structural lesions, including mitral valve prolapse and murmur. Detoxification of alcoholic patients before surgery should be accomplished because they are at risk for post-operative withdrawal syndromes, coagulation abnormalities, and metabolism altered by medications or anesthetic agents. Patients with abnormal liver function tests should be evaluated for drug reactions, alcoholic liver disease, and hepatitis, as well as diabetes and renal disease. Other conditions to be studied include evidence of coagulation disorders, history of excessive bleeding from dental extractions, or previous surgery for von Willebrand's disease, which is the most common congenital coagulation abnormality.

Appropriate pre-operative studies are guided by the history and physical examination. Barium enema is indicated for a large posterior mass, history of diverticulitis, recent change in bowel habits or stool caliber, rectal bleeding, hemoccult-positive stools, or a family history of colon carcinoma syndromes. Intraveneous pyelography is indicated for endometriosis with findings on pelvic examination, history of PID, previous pelvic surgery, previous pelvic irradiation, history of diverticulosis, or "frozen pelvis" on pelvic examination.

Hemostatic sutures will minimize blood loss in cold knife conization, and electrocautery is useful to control residual bleeding. Surgical and gauze packing may be placed in the base of the cone and tied in place with lateral sutures. Prophylactic antibiotics counter infection after a vaginal hysterectomy. Proper uterosacral plication will help avoid later prolapse of the vaginal vault. Hysterectomy should be delayed for six weeks after conization to avoid infection, regardless of prophylactic antibiotics.

Common sources of litigation in gynecologic abdominal surgery include wound complications, hemorrhage, and injury to adjacent organs such as the bowel or urinary tract. Basic steps to avoid wound complications include pre-operative showering and cleansing of the umbilicus; clipping rather than shaving the pubic hair; use of Hibiclens or iodoform skin preparations; avoidance of cautery to incise skin or fascia; avoidance of subcutaneous sutures; and use of delayed closure for contaminated wounds.

Marked bleeding usually occurs deep in the pelvis or on the lateral pelvic side-walls. Pressure from a sponge stick or pack should be followed by isolating the bleeding points, and either suturing or clipping them with small vascular clips. Massive hemorrhage should be treated by volume and blood replacement and stabilization of vital signs prior to seeking bleeding points. Hypogastric artery ligation may help decrease oozing from torn veins by lowering pulse pressure distal to the ligation site. A gauze roll pelvic pack may be necessary for persistent oozing and brought out through an open vaginal cuff or abdominal stab wound. It can be removed in two to three days by gently teasing the pack out with saline moistening.

Bowel injuries may be avoided by the following precautions: open cephalad to previous midline incisions; enter peritoneum with a knife, not scissors; use traction and counter-traction when lysing adhesions; lyse bowel loop adhesions one loop at a time; do not lyse adhesions deep in the abdomen until anterior loops are separated; and avoid lap pads in handling previously irradiated bowel.

Untreated intestinal injuries may lead to sepsis or fistula formation. Patients at risk include those with endometriosis, pelvic infection, or granulomatous or inflammatory bowel disease, and those previously subjected to surgery or irradiation. These patients should have a bowel preparation before surgery. Gynecologists may repair most injuries to the small bowel. Minor serosal defects may be safely ignored; full-thickness lacerations should be repaired. A longitudinal defect should be closed transversely to avoid narrowing the lumen. Marked bowel discoloration indicates compromised blood supply or multiple enterotomy sites, and means small bowel resection is necessary. A general surgeon should then be consulted. For serosal oozing or minimal discoloration, simply wrapping the affected bowel in warm lap pads will cause normal color to return. With a large bowel injury, the principal management decision is whether or not to divert the fecal stream. The unprepared bowel may be repaired if the injury is less than 3 cm., especially when the site is below the peritoneal reflection. A diverting colostomy is usually indicated for extensive injury. Since most injuries occur in the sigmoid or rectum, a transverse loop colostomy is appropriate with closure in six to eight weeks. A general surgeon should be consulted for all but the simplest bowel repairs.

Inexperience and technical problems in performing a gynecologic procedure are the major causes of urinary tract injuries. The ureter should be identified and retracted medially. Meticulous dissection of the bladder from the anterior surface of the uterus during a hysterectomy can avoid bladder injuries. Ureteral injuries occur in 0.4-2.5% of all pelvic gynecologic procedures, but only about one-third are recognized at the time. The remainder result in eventual loss of a kidney in about 25% of cases. Injury can be avoided by wide bladder mobilization, avoiding the use of large clamps and massive ligatures near the cardinal ligaments, refraining from indiscriminate cautery to control bleeding, and visualizing or palpating the ureter before clamping the infundibulopelvic ligaments. Intra-operative evaluation is mandatory for a suspected ureteral injury. Injection of dye into the ureter requires distal pressure and is of value in diagnosing crush injuries or transection, but not inadvertent ligation. Crush or ligature injury diagnosed by extravasation of the indigo carmine at the injury site can be managed by resection of the area. If there is no extravasation, a Silastic catheter can be used as a splint, adding a soft retroperitoneal drain. The catheter should be left in place 10 to 14 days. Injuries below the midpelvis, within 4-5 cm. of the ureterovesical junction, can generally be treated by ureteroneocystostomy. For injuries above the pelvic brim, end-to-end ureteroureterostomy is needed. Successful repair requires maintenance of hemostasis, use of a limited number of sutures to avoid necrosis, ureteral catheterization and retroperitoneal drainage, and an absolute lack of tension at the anastomatic site.

Pap Smears

By doing Pap smear tests routinely, it is possible for physicians to find evidence of disease years before any visible symptoms are present and before any damage is done. The sexually transmitted virus known as Human Papillomavirus (HPV) has been proven to be the causative agent for developing cancer of the cervix. HPV is a "silent" infection, usually with no symptoms other than the appearance of a genital wart.

Dysplasia is the term to describe the changes the HPV virus causes in the cell it infects. The normal cells are replaced by the dysplastic cells over a period of several years. The condition can usually be detected by an examination that includes a Pap smear. Proliferation of abnormal cells on the surface of the cervix is superficial and considered pre-cancerous under the rubric Cervical Intraepithelial Neoplasia (CIN). CIN is considered to be the forerunner of cancer. Even though only one in four women with CIN go on to develop cervical cancer, there is no reliable method of predicting which cases will advance to invasive cancer. Treatment should be directed at halting the dysplasia process through destroying the area of precancerous growth by a procedure known as conization.

The physician has a duty to warn a patient of the risks of failing to undergo a Pap smear in the course of his general gynecological care of the patient. A physician may be held liable for failing to inform the patient of the result of a Pap smear when it is abnormal, unless a reasonable effort to do so has been made and documented in the patient's record.

Both the physician and the patient have specific responsibilities in the use of a Pap smear as a diagnostic tool. Since cervical cancer can be managed in different ways, the physician has a duty to disclose and discuss alternatives. Use of the Pap smear permits identification of women who are suffering from cervical dysplasia and carcinoma-in-situ, and who are consequently at risk of progressing to invasive cancer. Identification at the earlier stages permits more effective and simpler treatment. The medical profession has recognized that the Pap smear is a simple and effective way of diagnosing pre-malignant and malignant conditions of the cervix. When a physician has performed a Pap smear and the results indicate that the patient is suffering from an abnormal condition of the cervix, he must take reasonable steps to inform the patient of the results. The patient, however, is responsible for providing the physician with enough information to enable complete communication to take place. This includes disclosing risk factors such as age when sex started, number of different partners, drinking, smoking, use of condoms, internal genital organ infections, venereal disease, and whether partners were circumcised. Inaccuracies in Pap smear testing may soon be almost eliminated by computer-driven scanners in rejecting poor specimens which may be reported as normal, and by picking out slides that are questionable. These will be subject to close attention by human experts. Thus, recent alarms about high rates of inaccuracy in Pap smear test results should be relieved and patient confidence restored.

Contraceptives

Medical, as well as legal, complications may arise from the use of contraceptive devices — IUD, diaphragm, or cervical cap or sponge. The age and status of the woman given contraception advice may also impose legal burdens. The Dalkon Shield story is well-known and has provided the most legal complications, but other IUDs may also be a problem because of the occurrence of perforation, pelvic infection, bleeding, etc. Informed consent and permission to insert IUDs are important. Prevention evaluation and follow-up advice and care are critical. These concerns are less so now that IUDs have been largely withdrawn from the U.S. market.

Recent concern about giving contraceptive advice to minors may also raise legal complications. It is essential that the obstetrician-gynecologist be familiar with state and local laws defining minors and how they may be given contraceptive counseling, i.e., with or without parental consent.

When a patient first requests a physician to prescribe an oral contraceptive, the physician must perform a Pap smear, along with a thorough physical examination, and take a complete medical and family history. Failure to do so breaches an obvious and fundamental duty to the patient. Similarly, when prescribing an IUD, a Pap smear must be included with a complete medical history and thorough physical examination. If indicated, appropriate cultures and other tests for venereal diseases should be done to determine whether it is safe for the patient to use an IUD. An unresolved, abnormal Pap smear is a contraindication to the insertion of an IUD, as well as prescribing oral contraceptives, at least until the infection is cleared.

Hysteroscopy

Hysteroscopy has been proposed as a replacement for Hystero-salpingogram (HSG) in evaluating infertile women. Yet, HSG is the basic outpatient screening measure at most clinics. Hysteroscopy is most useful if any irregularity of the uterine wall or a lesion in the uterine cavity is found at HSG, if cornual blockage is present, or if there is a history of abortion or previous uterine surgery. HSG is less costly, easier to perform, and provides more information than a hysteroscopy does in infertility studies. It is not necessary to perform a hysteroscopy as a screening procedure in infertile women before or at the time of laparoscopy if the HSG is normal. Therefore, it is not the standard to routinely use hysteroscopy in infertility work.

Hysteroscopy in post-menopausal and peri-menopausal bleeding is especially important in detecting pathologic conditions. Intra-uterine abnormalities may be missed with the curette. Information and biopsy yield may be increased when endoscopy is used in addition to curettage. Endometrial polyps may be more readily discovered in the post-menopausal patient by endoscopy than with a curette. Failure to use endoscopy may result in missing pathology, including carcinoma, and inappropriate management. Hysteroscopy is a valuable adjunct to curettage in women with post-menopausal bleeding. The procedure is safe and easy to learn.

The use of hysteroscopy is increasing, and diagnostic assessment of abnormal uterine bleeding is probably one of its main applications. Hysteroscopy has considerable diagnostic accuracy in out-patient evaluation that is directly proportional to the severity of the lesion. Diagnosis cannot rely on endoscopy alone. A biopsy can be done during the examination or immediately after it. Office screening by endoscopy for patients with abnormal bleeding may spare them a D&C. The disadvantages of endoscopy include its potential for pushing cancer fragments out of the tubes or into the vascular channels, its relative expense, and the fact that it does not readily permit directed biopsy. While clinicians have been reluctant to use endoscopy routinely for diagnosis in place of dilatation and curettage (D&C), it is an accurate and cost-effective procedure and well-accepted by patients. Out-patient hysteroscopy with paracervical block, or no anesthesia, may prove to be a reliable means of screening for endcmetrial carcinoma.

Intra-operative hysteroscopy has been used to unify septate uteri to improve reproductive performance. It is effective and safe with low morbidity. It is less costly than transabdominal metroplasty, and the results are at least as good. In addition, pelvic adhesions do not develop and vaginal delivery may be permitted. Conjugated estrogens and medroxyprogesterone are used post-operatively. Patients may be discharged within several hours of the procedure. Post-operative HSG or hysteroscopy should be used to evalute the uterine volume. Hysteroscopy surgery is now the treatment of choice for women who have recurrent abortions due to a septate uterus. The technique is easily learned, and the necessity for laparotomy and transfundal metroplasty is avoided. The use of flexible scissors, instead of a resectoscope, is said to increase the success rate.

If HSG reveals a normal uterine cavity, hysteroscopy is not necessary to diagnose a cause for the infertility. HSG is much less invasive and provides useful information on the uterine cavity and tubes. It is mandated in evaluation of infertility and recurrent pregnancy loss. Direct visualization and operative hysteroscopy are appropriate for intrauterine abnormalities. If the workup reveals normal results, laparoscopy with hysteroscopy seems indicated. HSG is as accurate as hysteroscopy in the diagnosis of normal uteri, double uteri, and diethylstilbestrol (DES).

Colposcopy

Colposcopy has superseded the Schiller test in most centers as the initial step in evaluating abnormal Pap smears. Colposcopy should not be performed and cannot be relied upon without adequate training!! The most important field where colposcopy has increasingly been applied is in the diagnosis and management of early malignant lesions of the cervix. Mass screening programs and routine use of exfoliative cytology in gynecologic practice have revealed a substantial number of young women with suspect or positive smears. The main use of colposcopy in the near future will undoubtedly be in the diagnostic follow-up study of these women.

The low-power magnification of the colposcope reveals not only the neoplastic cervical epithelium, but also alterations of the underlying stromal vasculature resulting from the neoplastic process, which can then be visualized through the thin epithelial layer. The degree of alteration in vascular pattern, in intercapillary distance, and in surface color and texture correlates well with the severity of the neoplastic process. Adequate colposcopic evaluation requires complete visualization of the transformation zone and the lesion in question, as well as correlation between the cytologic and histologic diagnoses and the clinical impression of the colposcopist. Endocervical curettage should be performed as part of every colposcopic examination. An additional criterion of colposcopy adequacy is that the lesion must occupy less than 50% of the exocervix. About 90% of women with abnormal cytologic findings may be adequately evaluated with colposcopy.

The colposcope seems to have its greatest use for two special purposes: 1) in helping to make a precise and accurate diagnosis of lesions of the cervix in patients who are identified as suspect by cytologic or other methods; and 2) in helping to resolve basic scientific problems of the etiology and pathogenesis of cervical neoplasia. In the contemporary, practical application of colposcopy, when first developed, it was directed to the screening of asymptomatic women. This function has now largely been taken over by exfoliative cytology. With cytology, visual examination of the cervix, and biopsy colposcopy is still necessary to void unnecessary radical procedures being applied to a relatively trivial lesion, or inadequate therapy being used for a lesion which may be more extensive than suspected.

A precise and accurate diagnosis of the nature and extent of a malignant lesion of the cervix may be made with the help of the colposcope in approximately 85% of all patients with a cervix suspect by virtue of an abnormal smear or a lesion peculiar to the naked eye. Thus, conization is avoided, and definitive therapy may be immediately instituted with assurance of an accurate diagnosis and substantial savings in hospital time and morbidity. Colposcopy is also useful in the follow-up of cervical lesions and in the diagnosis and follow-up of lesions of the vagina and vulva. Colposcopy is not a difficult procedure, but without further training, maximum benefits are not realized, and serious mistakes can be made. The colposcopist requires a good knowledge of the histopathological changes which take place in the cervix throughout a woman's life span. Although the two basic lesions, dysplasia and carcinoma-insitu, can be fairly well-described in general terms, great variations occur in the cellular picture in both cases. Dysplasia and carcinoma-insitu are frequently found in the same cervix, making it extremely difficult at times to draw the line between marked dysplasia and carcinoma-in-situ. Marked dysplasia should be regarded as a potentially malignant lesion similar to carcinoma-in-situ.

Cytology and colposcopy are complementary methods. The major value of colposcopy is the detection of pre-clinical cancer of the cervix, which would have been missed by cytology. Candidates for colposcopy are: 1) patients with suspect or positive smears; and 2) patients with visible lesions such as erythroplakia or leukoplakia, even if the cytology is negative. If a suspect smear has been reported, the patient is followed up with cytology after treatment for inflammation or hormonal therapy for atrophic changes. Repeatedly suspect cytology necessitates conization, even if repeat colposcopy does not reveal abnormal findings.

Abnormal findings are followed by directed punch biopsies, with or without concomitant cervical scraping, depending on whether the total squamocolumnar junction can be seen or not. The choice of therapy for dysplasia or carcinoma-insitu includes excisional biopsy, electrocautery, cyrosurgery, or conization.

The choice depends more on the distribution of the lesion than on the histopathological diagnosis. Conization is considered definite therapy for carciocma-in-situ if the margins of the cone are completely free. A hysterectomy is performed only for additional indications, such as menorrhagia, myoma, pelvic relaxation, sterilization, etc. If microinvasion is found in a directed biopsy, it is necessary to perform conization for a definite diagnosis. If microinvasion is found in the cone specimen, in carefully selected patients who would like to have more children, conization can be considered definitive if the margins of the cone are completely free. In most cases, a hysterectomy is the treatment of choice.

Colposcopy is only one of many methods with which the gynecologist should be acquainted in the evaluation of benign and malignant lesions of the cervix. It is mandatory that the results of clinical examination, cytology, and histology also be taken into account before treatment is decided upon. A supposedly small, pre-invasive lesion should never be treated only on the basis of the colposcopic patterns. Colposcopy has its pitfalls, as have cytology and histology. This is especially important to remember when destructive methods of treatment are chosen, such as electrocautery, cryosurgery, or laser evaporation. Destructive methods of treatment should never be used if the lesion extends up into the endocervix. In such cases, conization is mandatory. For real screening purposes, the cytologic smear is better; however, if a suspect smear is reported, the use of the colposcope helps tremendously in the decision regarding treatment.

Admonition

Only those medicolegal problems of direct concern to obstetrician-gynecologist providers have been addressed. Of course, the ob/gyn trainee and practitioner are responsible for the proper fulfillment of the general obligations and duties that are normally expected of all physicians.

OCCUPATIONAL MEDICINE

Introduction

Occupational medicine is a discipline of preventive medicine, devoted to the recognition, evaluation, and control of factors associated with the work environment. These factors, if left unchecked, can result in death, injury, and disease to the members of the American working population. The responsibility for identifying and controlling workplace hazards is shared by an occupational health care team, which can include physicians, nurses, psychologists, specialists in industrial hygiene and ergonomics, toxicologists, and epidemiologists. Since occupational medicine is concerned with preventing disease before it results in detectable injury or disease, it is chiefly practiced outside of the acute care hospital setting.

Traditionally, occupational medicine physicians have functioned as employees of large industrial corporations — in a type of practice that is commonly referred to as "industrial medicine". Recently, though, occupational medicine physicians are being increasingly found outside of the corporate setting, in either solo or group private practice arrangements, in free-standing clinics serving small industries, and in specialty referral centers within university medical centers.

Occupational medicine practitioners engage in a broad spectrum of medical activities, beginning with traditional patient care involving the diagnosis and treatment of work-related injury and illness (primary care occupational medicine). In addition, occupational medicine physicians engage in non-traditional types of medical evaluations, which are unique to the specialty of occupational medicine, and which are often the initial component of a larger medical-legal determination.

Work Risk Evaluation

These types of evaluations include determination of a worker's capability to perform specific job tasks (fitness evaluation), and determination of a worker's potential increased risk of injury, based on his or her current health status, past medical history, or genetic makeup, in relation to workplace exposures (risk evaluation).

Medical Surveillance Evaluation

Further, occupational medicine physicians engage in the determination of the health status of workers in particular industries, according to protocols mandated by federal or state occupational health standards (medical surveillance evaluation), and the determination of work-related physical or mental impairment in a worker who is seeking to qualify for benefits under a social compensation system, such as a state workers' compensation system (disability evaluation). Because of this latter involvement in complex social compensation schemes, it is essential that occupational physicians respond expeditiously and truthfully to the myriad of written forms and requests which are part of any medical-legal system.

Legal Issues

It is these non-traditional types of medical activities which create legal issues unique to the practice of occupational medicine. The legal issues involved in occupational medicine can more easily be understood by considering separately two general types of occupational medicine evaluations: (1) fitness, risk, and medical surveillance type; and (2) disability type. Also, unique legal issues arise for occupational physicians in managing the employees' medical information, and in supervising urine testing on workers for the presence of illegal drugs or blood testing for the presence of antibodies to the human immunodeficiency virus (HIV), the causative agent of the acquired immunodeficiency syndrome (AIDS).

Worker Fitness Evaluation

Occupational physicians are often asked to provide an evaluation of an individual's fitness for employment, or increased risks to their health from workplace exposures, based on their current health status, past medical history, or genetic makeup. Even though these evaluations are often legally mandated as part of the regulatory requirements of federal or state governmental health standards, the scientific basis of the determination is not well-established. Moreover, physicians unfamiliar with the legal aspects of such evaluations can easily create the basis for a worker's legal claim of employment discrimination. On the other hand, a physician can be held liable for a worker's fitness evaluation performed negligently which results in harm to the worker.

Occupational and Safety Health Act

The Occupational Safety and Health Act (OSH Act), which is administered by the Occupational Safety and Health Administration (OSHA), a branch of the Department of Labor, is the preeminent federal law designed to protect workers against the impairment of their health from workplace hazards. Under the OSH Act, OSHA has promulgated several hazard-specific health standards which set maximum exposure limits for certain workplace hazards, e.g., asbestos, lead, and cotton dust. As part of the OSHA standard, employers must have their workers evaluated by physicians to detect any impairment from exposure to the particular workplace hazard.

Physicians who perform evaluations mandated by any of these OSHA standards must conform to the requirements of the standards. These requirements stipulate that certain medical procedures must be performed as part of worker fitness evaluations. For instance, physicians who do fitness evaluations for asbestos-exposed workers under the OSHA asbestos standard must order pulmonary function tests, and specific types of chest radiographs at intervals which are spelled out in the standard. Failure to follow the exact requirements of the standard can result in liability for employers.

Other Acts

In addition to the OSH Act, other federal laws are designed to protect occupation-specific workers from health impairments due to workplace exposures. The Mine Safety and Health Act requires that all miners working in a coal mine be given a chest radiograph at specified intervals, and the Superfund legislation mandates medical surveillance procedures for workers in the hazardous waste industry.

Public Protection

Some laws which mandate specific medical procedures for fitness evaluations are designed to protect the public more than the worker. For instance, the Department of Transportation's (DOT) Bureau of Motor Carrier Safety has detailed regulations for the physical examination of drivers operating motor vehicles in interstate commerce, and the Federal Aviation Administration (FAA) has similar regulations for the evaluation of airline flight crews.

Legal Implications

The major legal problem which arises when physicians perform fitness evaluations involves the potential for employment discrimination. Illegal discrimination can arise when physicians base their decision on whether or not a particular worker should be selected for a job based on medical test results which may have no relation to the demands of the job for which the worker is applying. Federal and state laws aimed at preventing discrimination in employment decisions prohibit the use of medical information in such an indiscriminate way.

Employment discrimination on the basis of race, color, religion, sex, or national origin is prohibited by Title VII of the Civil Rights Act of 1964, which applies to state and federal governments and private employers with 15 or more employees. Occupational physicians need to be especially careful when using physical examination or laboratory test results to exclude a worker from a particular job, without being sure that the job requires a particular level of physical or mental capacity which the physical examination or laboratory tests reveals the worker lacks. Workers who fall into one of the legally protected categories of the Civil Rights Act can make a claim that they were denied employment unfairly.

Standards as to Women

Specifically, physicians have gotten into the most legal trouble by using minimum height and weight requirements, as well as strength tests, to decide whether a woman can work in a job traditionally held by a man. Even though such medical test criteria appear to be neutral on their face, such criteria will only be legally permissible if the employer can prove that such criteria are related to the job demands, are essential to the performance of the job, and no other criteria with less discriminatory impact can be used.

Handicapped Persons

Employment discrimination is also prohibited by federal and state laws directed at the protection of individuals with a physical or mental handicap. The important law in this area is the federal Vocational Rehabilitation Act of 1973, which has as its primary purpose to bring handicapped individuals within the mainstream of American life by protecting them against unfair discrimination.

On the state level, 48 states and the District of Columbia have laws prohibiting discrimination in public and private employment based on handicaps, which are similar to the federal rehabilitation law. Basically, federal and state handicap laws prohibit employers from discriminating against "handicapped individuals".

The Rehabilitation Act defines a "handicapped individual" as "any person who (1) has a physical or mental impairment that substantially limits one or more of such person's major life activities; (2) has a record of such an impairment; or (3) is regarded as having such an impairment." Once a worker is found to be handicapped, the employer must make a "reasonable accommodation" to the handicaps of "otherwise qualified" individuals.

Estimates of how many individuals might be covered under the handicapped laws run as high as 40 to 68 million. Accordingly, every physician who performs fitness evaluations and has disqualified a worker from an employment opportunity based on medical criteria, should scrutinize his decision-making to ensure that he is not engaging in discrimination based on a handicap.

Medical Evaluations and Determinations

A good approach to discrimination-proof fitness evaluations requires that physicians first make determinations of fitness based on individualized medical evaluations. Unfounded assumptions about the fitness of a worker for a job based on gender, race, or other stereotypes, or probabilities about the occurrence of disease in the particular group of which the worker is a member, are legally impermissible. A detailed medical examination of each and every individual is necessary. Sound medical information on each worker is essential.

In addition, the medical criteria which the physician uses to determine fitness has to be related to the performance demands of the particular job for which the worker is applying. To make a legally sound fitness determination, physicians need to ascertain the physical and mental performance criteria of the job, and then relate these job requirements to the individual worker's physical and mental capacity to achieve those job demands. Physicians often fail to do this, and their fitness evaluations result in a denial of employment. A lawsuit against the employer for employment discrimination based on a handicap usually follows.

Disability Evaluations
Inability to Work

Patients frequently present to physicians with the chief complaint of "inability to work". The injured person often asserts that his or her injury has resulted from some physical, chemical, biological, or psychological exposure in the workplace. This assertion forms the basis of a claim for benefits under the workers' compensation system of their particular state.

State Disability Systems

Occasionally, patients present to physicians seeking benefits for an inability to perform any gainful activity, either under federal Social Security Disability Insurance (SSDI), or under an insurer's or employer's private disability plan. In these cases, claimants do not have to assert that their injury is related to workplace exposure. This discussion will concentrate on the physician's obligation under state workers' compensation systems, because they are the most common type of disability compensation system under which claimants seek benefits.

Work-Related Injuries

If a worker is to be successful in his or her claim for workers' compensation benefits, he or she needs to demonstrate that the injury, or disease, fulfills the legal definition of a work-related injury, i.e., one "arising out of or in the course of employment". After a worker shows the work-relatedness of the injury, he or she must satisfy a particular legal standard of proof. For work-related injuries, the worker must demonstrate that it is "more likely than not" that the condition would not have been present had the work exposure not been present.

Medicolegal Process

The medicolegal process of determining the work-relatedness of a worker's injury or disease is termed a disability evaluation. Employers, insurance companies, and government agencies refer workers to physicians for the purpose of determining work incapacity, or "certifying" disability. Specifically, occupational physicians are called upon to render their medical opinion about (1) whether an "impairment", or loss of function of an organ or part of the body compared to what previously existed, is present; (2) the extent of any impairment; and (3) whether the impairment can be attributed to the work exposure.

Impairment v. Disability

After the physician supplies the medical evaluation of impairment information, non-medical administrative personnel use this information to determine the "disability" or impact of the impairment on societal or work functions of the claimant, and to determine the specific economic benefits to which the worker is entitled, e.g., medical care, lost wages, rehabilitation services.

Many physicians often find disability evaluations and the entire workers' compensation system to be a morass of legal complexities, and something to be avoided. However, the contribution of physicians to the process of determining impairment and disability is critical to the overall operation of society's compensation systems for injury and disease.

Liability for Negligent Performance

Whether performing fitness, risk, medical surveillance, or disability type evaluations, physicians face legal liability for negligent performance of those evaluations. However, the imposition of legal liability first depends on the nature of the relationship between the physician and the individual being examined. Again, the field of occupational medicine presents some unique legal problems.

It is well-known that when a patient voluntarily presents to a physician for diagnosis or treatment of a particular condition, and the physician examines or begins treating the patient, a physician-patient relationship is formed. The formation of this relationship creates specific legal duties for the physician. If the physician performs those duties in a negligent manner, and the patient is thereby injured, the physician can be held financially liable for the patient's damages.

For physicians who perform fitness or disability evaluations, the imposition of legal liability depends first on the existence of a physician-patient relationship. Without the legal existence of such a relationship, liability is quite limited. For instance, if a patient has not voluntarily sought out the services of the physician, but has been sent to the physician by a third party, such as his or her employer, insurance company, or adversary's attorney, and no treatment is contemplated, or none is given, most courts will hold that the physician is an "independent contractor" of the third party who ordered the examination, and no traditional physician-patient relationship has come into existence. However, if the treating physician undertakes to advise an examinee, thereby causing the latter to rely on the physician's services to his disadvantage, a physician-patient relationship may be formed, and liability may attach.

If no physician-patient relationship exists legally, then the physician incurs only a limited duty to the "patient", i.e., to avoid physically harming the patient during the evaluation itself. However, the issue of what harms are a result of an improper evaluation is far from clear, and much litigation has occurred.

The traditional legal rule imposing only a limited duty on physicians may be changing. Physicians, and those with whom they contract to provide such evaluations, may become liable for (1) improperly returning an employee back to work after an injury; (2) failing to follow-up on laboratory tests drawn during a pre-employment examination; (3) concealment of a worker's medical condition; and (4) failing to provide any medical surveillance programs to monitor the post-exposure health status of employees.

Duty to Divulge Information to the Employee-Patient

A physician-patient relationship is not formed in the usual sense during pre-placement employment physical examinations. Thus, the information obtained during such examinations can be given to the employer, although such information should be limited to those factors necessary to make a job placement decision. But what is the responsibility of the physician to notify the employee of the results of his or her examination?

On the one hand, the Code of Ethical Conduct for Physicians Providing Occupational Medical Services, adopted by the American Occupational Medical Association in 1976, states that physicians should ". . . communicate understandably to those they serve any significant observations about their health, recommending further study, counsel, or treatment when indicated." This view creates an ethical obligation on the part of occupational physicians to inform an employee of any abnormal finding discovered as a result of an examination.

On the other hand, the courts have held that the occupational physician does not have a duty to inform the employee of any specific deviation from health, a conclusion based on the lack of a consensual, voluntary relationship between the physician and employee-patient. But a recent California case clearly indicated that a physician might be held liable for damages resulting from a failure to inform a man who on repeated examinations was found to have radiographic evidence of asbestosis. Even though not legally required, the more prevalent view is that physicians should inform the employee-patient of any known abnormality discovered as a result of an examination.

Compulsory Drug and HIV Antibody Testing in the Workplace

In the last few years, the workplace has become the focus of an important medical-legal policy debate regarding the screening of individuals for the use of illegal drugs and for antibodies to HIV, the causative agent of AIDS. These policy debates have important legal implications for physicians who practice occupational medicine.

Drug and alcohol abuse is a national problem of immense proportions. One of the most controversial methods of identifying individuals who use drugs is urine testing. In the workplace, urine testing is generally used in three ways: (1) for pre-employment screening; (2) for cause, based on a specific incident; and (3) on an unannounced random basis.

If a company decides to test, occupational physicians must become involved in every detail of the program, since a plethora of medical-legal issues can arise from every phase of employee urine screening. Constitutional, statutory, regulatory, and common law principles have been used by employees to legally challenge every aspect of urine drug testing. Although the specific legal criteria vary, depending on which legal principle is involved, the essential issue is whether or not the urine testing program represents a reasonable attempt by the employer to address the drug problem in the workplace.

The answers to four questions determine the legal reasonableness of urine drug testing: Who is being tested? When are they being tested? How is the test being performed? What action is being taken on the basis of test results? Based on attention to these four questions, the occupational physician can play a major role in ensuring that a workplace urine drug testing program is reasonable from a legal standpoint.

First, physicians need to convince employers that to be legally acceptable, urine drug testing should be applied to workers whose drug-related impairment poses a direct threat to fellow employees, or to the public. Second, the timing of the testing can affect its legality. For instance, urine drug testing done at the pre-employment stage, or periodically as part of an overall evaluation of fitness, is legally acceptable. However, urine testing done without an individualized need has been generally viewed by the courts as unnecessary, and therefore, unreasonable. In other words, when no reasonable suspicion exists about the need to test an employee for drugs, employers may face legal challenge.

Third, testing procedures can affect the legality of the testing. The physician needs to ensure the integrity and reliability of test results. A chain of custody must be established to ensure that the sample to be tested did, in fact, come from the employee tested, and all positive urine tests must be confirmed by using a more sensitive testing methodology than the original screening methodology.

Fourth, the action an employer takes after the discovery of an employee with a urine test positive for illegal drugs also determines the legality of the testing. If employees with positive urine tests are given the opportunity to enter rehabilitation programs rather than being summarily discharged, then the drug testing program is more likely to be upheld legally.

Another workplace testing issue which has reached national proportions is testing employees for evidence of antibodies to HIV. However, HIV screening of job applicants and current employees is financially costly, generates inaccurate results, and can lead to legal liability for the employer. Physicians who perform HIV antibody testing for employers need to be aware of the legal implications of such testing.

Employers can be found legally liable under tort doctrines, specific state statutes, and municipal ordinances which prohibit the use of HIV antibody test results in employment decisions, and under federal and state laws which prohibit discrimination on the basis of handicaps.

Tort actions for defamation, invasion of privacy, and negligent (or intentional) infliction of emotional distress can arise from wrongful disclosure of HIV screening results collected by employers and contained in employees' personnel records.

Various states have enacted laws specifically prohibiting employer use of

HIV antibody results to determine employment suitability. Also, several municipalities have enacted ordinances which prohibit employment discrimination based on HIV antibcdy results, unless a legitimate business reason exists. In jurisdictions without specific anti-discrimination statues, violation of the federal Rehabilitation Act may give rise to employer liability.

CONCLUSION

The specialty of occupational medicine is a branch of preventive medicine, the practice of which is permeated by complex federal, state, and local laws. In addition to the standard legal considerations which are arise in all fields of medicine, occupational medicine practitioners must also be aware of legal obligations arising from federal and state laws concerning workplace hazards, evaluations for worker fitness, compensation systems for injured workers, worker screening programs for drug use and HIV antibodies, and many other areas not mentioned in this thumbnail sketch.

ONCOLOGY

Standard of Care

The oncology patient presents particular medical and surgical problems for the physician. There are now recognized specialties in medical and surgical oncology. Consequently, any physician treating a patient with cancer would best be advised to review his care of the patient with someone practicing in the recognized specialty of medical and/or surgical oncology, for the simple reason that once a lawsuit is filed, the treating physician, in most jurisdictions, will be held to the standard of care/standard of practice exercised by reasonably prudent medical oncologists and/or surgical oncologists, depending upon the medical care that is at issue.

In most states, the "locality" rule in determining the standard of care has been abandoned. This is particularly true in areas of medical specialty (cancer, heart disease, etc.), such that a physician's care will not be compared just to other physicians in the immediate community. Rather, the standard of care will be that standard that is practiced by the reasonably prudent majority of physicians practicing in a given area treating a patient of like or similar circumstances.

Physicians should be mindful of the fact that university centers may treat cancer patients as part of a study. Such treatment will not necessarily coincide with that which is recognized and accepted for cancer patients outside of the study basis for standard of care. Rather, standard of care is best defined as that care exercised by the majority of reasonably prudent medical specialists treating cancer patients with the same or similar type of cancer.

There is also greater concern today that corporate medicine, such as health maintenance organizations and preferred provider organizations, may, in fact, impinge on the quality of care given the cancer patient because of an underlying motivation to reduce costs that such organizations accomplish by limiting physicians' fees and hospital fees, thereby prompting the physicians and hospitals to increase their patient volume. In so doing, there is less actual time spent with the patient, and a greater likelihood of medical error. Thus, it is not likely that the standard of care delivered by the health maintenance organization will be held as the applicable standard of reasonably prudent medical care for purposes of a professional negligence or medical malpractice question.

Informed Consent for Oncology Patients

The law in all states requires a physician to obtain the consent of a patient before treating or operating on that patient. In the absence of that consent, the physician may be held liable in a civil lawsuit for battery, assault, and professional negligence or medical malpractice. It has been held that a person of adult years has the right, in the exercise of control over his or her own body, to decide whether or not to submit to lawful medical treatment. The problem arises, however, when the issue is raised as to whether or not that adult person understood to what it was he or she was consenting, because in the absence of a knowing consent, any consent given is deemed vitiated or null and void as a matter of law.

The cancer patient presents a special set of circumstances which, in many states, has prompted the passage of legislation that codifies additional legal obligations for a physician treating a cancer patient, in order to obtain an informed consent to treat. An informed consent to treat is obtained not only to avoid charges of assault and battery, but it is also necessary to avoid malpractice litigation and to ensure that the physician meets the duty of due care in advising the patient of all options available to assure that the consent given is one based on adequate information.

When a knowing and consensual participation in treatment is obtained from a patient, and when there is good communication between physician and patient, there is a much lower incidence of malpractice litigation, even when physician error is present. In order to avoid informed consent problems, a physician should consider and be familiar with the following:

- The controlling state laws of the jurisdiction that may provide specific requirements for a physician to inform the patient of alternative treatment modalities which should be considered.
- Provide information of alternative treatment modalities, and even recommend consultation with a physician who might propose an alternative form of treatment.
- Review the applicable legislation of a given jurisdiction to make certain that, as a physician, any information required by statute is communicated to the patient.

The laws in most states require a physician and/or surgeon to disclose and provide the patient with all the information to which he or she is entitled under a material standard. More simply put, the patient is entitled to be informed of all material facts concerning the risks of the proposed or alternative methods of treatment and their rate of effectiveness, such as would objectively inform a reasonable person of the possible consequences of the proposed course of treatment.

Also, it has been determined that the physician's duty to inform can be measured by a jury's finding as to what a reasonably prudent patient would want to know. Some states require a finding that the physician's failure to obtain an informed consent prior to treatment was conscious or willful before the patient can successfully state an action for battery or assault. In almost all states, however, a failure to obtain the patient's informed consent prior to treatment or surgery constitutes professional negligence or medical malpractice, which can be successfully pled and proven upon showing: 1) that the consent given was insufficient, and thus vitiated; and 2) that the physician's failure to provide the necessary information was a cause of the harm or injury that the patient sustained.

Thus, it is necessary that the injury or damage complained of by the patient be a direct or legal consequence of insufficient information — the lack of informed consent — before the patient will prevail in a medical negligence action premised on a theory of insufficient or nonexistent informed consent.

A significant number of states have statutes that deal directly with informed consent to medical treatment. These states seem to have passed such legislation to control expansion of the doctrine. Consequently, if a physician provides a patient with the type of information which the statute requires and records this fact in the medical records at the time the patient consent is obtained, the physician overcomes any informed consent problem as a matter of law.

When the question is raised as to whether a patient's consent was an informed one, it is generally the testimony from medical practitioners who treat patients of similar circumstances with a similar illness that will determine what information should have been conveyed to the patient, in order to ensure that the patient's consent was informed. In a few states, however, there is also a legislative standard or state statute that articulates what the physician needs to tell his patient.

Unfortunately, most statutes, unlike court decisions, do not emphasize that the patient must comprehend the information conveyed. In brief, the physician and/or surgeon would be most protected if the consent obtained from the patient not only met the statutory requirements, but was also obtained after the patient had an opportunity to overccme the fear and shock initially associated with learning of the cancer.

The physician must determine whether there has been a sufficient lapse of time between telling a patient of his or her cancer and obtaining the consent to treat. Does the patient understand the therapy proposed versus a scenario in which the patient is still in a shock/fear syndrome, and thus agrees to treatment in desperation and confusion?

For oncology patients, informed consent, or informed refusal if care and management are refused, is very important. The physician may choose to use therapeutic professional discretion to keep medical facts from the patient when the physician believes disclosure would be harmful, dangerous, or injurious to the patient.

There are several instances that apply in all states when an informed consent is not necessary: when the patient's life or limb is at serious risk, e.g., emergency, patient is incompetent, or patient wants to remain ignorant. In such situations, the patient's consent is not a necessary prerequisite to treatment. A safeguard would be to discuss the patient's treatment with the next-of-kin and record this fact in the medical record.

Assumption of Risk

The doctrine of "assumption of risk" means that the patient understands the possibility of all risks of untoward, unpreventable results of either treatment or no treatment, and knowingly consents to the course selected. Where it applies, this is usually a good defense to an action for negligence on the part of the physician. It should be noted that this doctrine is related to the doctrine of informed consent and refusal. If all risks which, in fact, occur have not been carefully explained to the patient, as a matter of law, the doctrine of assumption of risk is not applicable.

Misdiagnosis and Delay in Diagnosis of Cancer

Lawsuits by oncology patients primarily involve misdiagnosis or, in reality, late diagnosis. Failure or delay in the diagnosis of cancer is the leading allegation in physician malpractice cases, comprising more than 10% of all these claims.

Lawsuits that allege a failure to diagnose cancer are more than twice as common as cases based on failure to diagnose fractures or dislocations, failure to diagnose pregnancy problems, or failure to diagnose post-operative surgical ccmplications, and are three times more common than cases based on alleged improper treatment or incorrect drug therapy, failure to diagnose infection, improper treatment of a fracture or dislocation, improper treatment for lack of supervision, or improper treatment for an infection.

One of the problems is defining the standard of due care in diagnosing cancer. Many lawsuits now being filed are for failure to diagnose breast cancer. Approximately 50% of suits for failure to diagnose breast cancer named physicians in four areas of medical practice: obstetrics and gynecology, internal medicine, pathology, and general and family practice. Lawsuits against radiologists and other specialists are less common.

Patients alleging misdiagnosis are basically complaining of a "loss of a chance". Almost always, there is the question of whether the misdiagnosis caused the patient's injury to a reasonable medical certainty or probability, or whether the natural course of events were unchanged.

Failure to diagnose cancer or delay in the diagnosis can be devastating to a patient and his or her family. It may result in a patient having to undergo more extensive treatment, reduce his or her chances of survival, lead to unnecessary death, and cause physical and emotional burdens that an earlier diagnosis could have avoided.

Although a physician may have acted negligently and failed to fulfill the standard of care owed the patient, a successful lawsuit cannot be maintained unless the misdiagnosis of cancer caused some calculable harm to the patient.

In failure to diagnose cancer cases, damages are meant to compensate a patient for physical pain and suffering and emotional distress due to the requirement for additional treatment, loss of life, or loss of a chance for survival due to the delay in diagnosis and treatment. Monetary damages may also be awarded to the patient's family for harm done to them.

Delay in diagnosis and treatment of cancer, however, are generally not compensable if the delay did not materially affect the ultimate treatment and outcome of the disease. A long delay in the diagnosis of a uniformly fatal type of cancer, or a very short delay in a potentially curable cancer, may more likely result in a judgment against the physician, especially if the patient presents with a later stage of that cancer at the time of the delayed diagnosis and treatment.

Treatment

Liability may be based on the physician's own negligent action or inaction, or both. There are also legal actions involving proper treatment, and invariably, the question of statute of limitations. The treatment of oncological patients is fraught with perils and pitfalls.

Chemotherapy

Chemotherapy is a treatment used to kill malignant cells. Since cellular destruction occurs by the effect on reproducing cells, those cells dividing frequently are more susceptible. The drugs, however, do not discriminate between normal and malignant tissues, and thus may affect normal organ systems.

Complications

Hypersensitivity reactions may occur and produce edema, rash, bronchospasm, diarrhea, and hypotension. Some drugs, such as Doxorubicin or Mitoxantrone, are cardiotoxic. Bleomycin may cause pulmonary fibrosis. Hair loss (alopecia), leukopenia, and anemia are accepted side effects. An inadvertent overdose has been a source of litigation.

Radiation Therapy

Ionizing radiation may be used in the treatment and palliation of malignant tumors. Radiation sources include the cobalt-60 teletherapy unit, linear accelerator, and radioactive isotopes, such as iridium-192, iodine-125, and phosphorus-32.

The biologic effects of radiation therapy on targeted tissues include cell death from inability to reproduce, metabolic cell failure, or degeneration of the cell structure. These effects are directly proportional to the dose. Because malignancies and normal body organs vary in their sensitivity to radiation, the dosage must be regulated according to the desired results. It is possible to sensitize tissues to increase the response to radiation by the use of oxygen, nitric oxide, metronidazole, or hyperthermia.

The use of radiation therapy is frequently the source of medicolegal problems.

Complications

Even when given in a proper dose, radiation may cause skin burns that are erythematous (red) or desquamated (dry or wet). Ulceration with necrosis may be seen with prolonged healing time and scar deformity, and permanent pulmonary fibrosis has been known to occur in the treatment field for cancer of the breast. Radiation enteritis following treatment of intra-abdominal malignancies is not unknown.

Unorthodox Cancer Treatment

Because patients with cancer are often desperate, a physician must address the legal consequences of administering unorthodox treatment, particularly if the patient insists upon it. Basic to the resolution of these problems are invoking risk benefit judgment, comparing the anticipated benefits from therapy with its risks, and weighing the consequences of no treatment.

Despite persistent efforts to achieve early detection, and exhaustive research aimed at developing effective treatment modalities, cancer continues to be a leading cause of death in the United States. Conventional cancer therapy includes surgery, chemotherapy, and radiation therapy in various combinations, depending upon the nature and extent of disease involved in each particular case. Elaborate treatment protocols have been developed for virtually every stage of every type of cancer which afflicts people. These medical advances have undoubtedly resulted in increased survival or improved quality of life for some cancer patients. However, for many others, conventional cancer therapy has simply come to mean a sequence of painful, even disabling, experiences that do not in any way alter the inexorable course of their disease, and do not make them more comfortable, productive, or fulfilled during the time that remains.

For many years, cancer patients have attempted to seek out whatever ray of hope may be offered, even in the form of treatment that the medical establishment finds to be unproven, ineffective, or even fraudulent. These include metabolic therapy, diet therapy, megavitamins, mental imagery applied for anti-tumor effect, and spiritual or faith healing. Despite recent technologic advances in orthodox medical care, unorthodox cancer treatment is increasing in popularity.

Cancer patients, particularly those who are terminally ill, are vulnerable to exploitation because of their predicament. Desperate for any glimmer of hope, they are easy prey for charlatans intent on financial gain. Traditionally, the law has protected those unable to protect themselves on the basis of parens patriae.

This rationale has most frequently been applied to juveniles and the mentally disabled.

However, the state's interest in protecting its citizens must be balanced against an individual's right to have control over his or her own body and to make decisions regarding his or her own medical care. Most cancer patients are adults in full control of their mental faculties, which distinguishes them from other citizens the state seeks to protect under the parens patriae rationale.

It is this basic conflict between the state's interest in the health and welfare of its citizens and the right of the individual to make decisions affecting his or her own health that has confronted legislatures and courts attempting to deal with the problem of unorthodox cancer treatment.

To date, this conflict has not been resolved uniformly. Considerable variations presently exist among the various states with regard to regulation of unorthodox cancer treatment. Interestingly, where there has been legislative action, most legislatures have granted the individual some measure of freedom in selecting cancer treatment that is unproven. In most states that have acted legislatively, however, this freedom is not unlimited. When courts have considered the subject of unorthodox cancer treatment, they have focused more on the state's right to regulate the lives of its citizens under police power.

Although some states have enacted legislation allowing patients to obtain certain types of alternative cancer therapy, the majority of state legislatures remain silent on this issue. Many of the states that require a licensed physician's prescription for the unorthodox treatment also require that the patient first sign a consent form, indicating that the physician has explained that Laetrile or DMSO has not been proven to be effective in the treatment of cancer or other human disease, and has not been approved by the Food and Drug Administration.

The courts have been reluctant to affirm a cancer patient's right to select his or her own treatment as encompassed by the constitutional right of privacy. There appear to be several reasons for this: 1) an ideal fact situation, clearly defining the issue, has not yet been presented to the courts; 2) because of the rapid progression of many types of cancer, the slow justice often afforded by the court system may not be a practicable forum for terminally ill cancer patients; and 3) the courts seem disposed to defer to the state of orthodox medical knowledge, as set forth in the legislative histories usually quoted in the court opinions.

Certain individual decisions regarding health care have already been recognized as falling within the constitutionally protected right of privacy. Although virtually all cancer patients can be expected, in varying degrees, to be anxious, depressed, or frightened because of their disease, the majority of them are still responsible, mentally sound adults. The parens patriae rationale would not seem to be applicable to such patients, as it would be in cases of juveniles or the mentally disabled. Accordingly, the balance weighs heavily in favor of allowing cancer patients to obtain the treatment of their choice. The state's interest in protecting the health of its citizens can be adequately protected in this context by requiring an informed consent by the patient following disclosure of the nature of the proposed treatment, the fact that it has not been proved by well-controlled scientific studies to be effective, and the availability of conventional treatment.

Privacy and Confidentiality

The patient's right to privacy and confidentiality has one of the highest priorities in our legal system. Several recent court decisions involving these rights bring into focus and highlight the physician's duty to provide, maintain, and enforce the patient's right to privacy and confidentiality, and the perils in failing to do so. No longer is privacy and confidentiality an ethical obligation; it is a legal responsibility and obligation.

The question arises whether, in a particular case, the condition and/or proposed treatment should be discussed with the next-of-kin, not only to answer questions concerning the method of the care and treatment proposed, but particularly when there is any question that the patient is not capable or competent to assure an informed consent. The physician may discuss the proposed treatment with the next-of-kin and record the fact of all discussions with the family, noting the subject matter of the discussion and the family responses, if the patient is incompetent or it is an emergency situation; otherwise, it is a breach of confidentiality or invasion of privacy.

Public Health Duties - Duty to Report

Every jurisdiction has a list of diseases which must be reported to the authorities, in addition to the requirement of warning other proper persons. This includes cancer. In these cases, the physician not only has the right to disclose the information to the proper authorities, he has the duty to do so. The physician should be knowledgeable as to what conditions are required to be reported in his jurisdiction. Failure to appropriately report may lead to civil, criminal, and administrative sanctions.

Duty to Refer and Consult

If a physician encounters a situation that is beyond his knowledge or experience, asking for a consultation from a specialist colleague or referring the patient to a tertiary health care facility is not only the smart thing to do, it is a duty.

The failure of a physician to refer to or consult with another physician or specialist for a suspected cancer may also be a negligent act of omission. The physician should consider the need to offer a patient referral, depending upon the expertise of the treating physician that is, if surgery is the recommended treatment, the patient should be offered a referral to a medical practitioner to review medical management versus surgery, even when there is no legislative requirement for this. Conversely, if chemotherapy or radiotherapy is proposed, the patient should be offered the benefit of a consultation with a surgeon to assure adequate exposure to alternative modalities. This is one of the most effective ways to avoid a later allegation of undue influence or pressure. Once the offer of a consultation or second opinion is recorded in the chart, there is much less chance for a patient to allege that he or she was railroaded into a particular course of treatment without an adequate informed consent.

It is critical that a primary care physician, e.g., family practitioner or internist, be mindful of the need to confer with cancer specialists when taking on the primary care of a cancer patient, in order to assure that the patient receives treatment consistent with the standard of care. This is especially necessary when medical information regarding the cancer patient is evolving at a rapid rate. There are recognized tumor forums/tumor boards associated with hospitals or cancer centers, as well as many teaching institutions, with specialty areas in various aspects of cancer care. These centers will not only be consulted at the time litigation is initiated, but they can well advise the treating physician and safeguard against a medical negligence action based on the allegation that the physician's care fell below the acceptable standard of practice. In the long run, consultation with a physician or surgeon specializing in a given field will be much more cost-effective than defending against a lawsuit for failure to consult. Second opinions are the order of the day in caring for oncology patients.

There are no absolute rules regarding the seeking of a consultation or making a referral. The law puts the responsibility on the physician of knowing when these are indicated and whom to call. The physician must be aware of his shortcomings. An essential part of practicing good medicine is knowing when to call for a consultation or refer a patient, when there is a need for an appropriate consultation and/or referral. Actually, he has a duty to refer the patient to a specialist. Whether the physician's equipment or facilities are adequate or whether he has the requisite trained assistants, if they are needed, are other determinants in referrals or consultations. If either or both of these necessities are not on hand, seeking appropriate medical assistance becomes mandatory.

If a consultant writes a note and makes a recommendation, the physician must either follow that recommendation or justify in the record why he did not do so. It is difficult later to justify why he asked for the advice of a specialist, and then chose to ignore it without any explanation. The physician should record all consultations, the results, and his actions based on the consulting physician's recommendations.

In order to get the most out of a consultation or referral, the physician should:

- Arrange for the consultation/referral to be certain it is accomplished;
- Communicate appropriate information in timely fashion to the consultant;
- Require that the report be returned in timely fashion;
- Communicate personally with the consultant, if necessary, particularly to reconcile any differences; and
- Advise the patient as to the recommendations and decisions.

The physician who is the consultant, has the corresponding responsibility.

Keeping Up-to-Date

The law and medicine have imposed a duty on all physicians to be aware of changing concepts and new developments. This is particularly true in oncology. Keeping up can be accomplished by reading current medical literature and attending scientific meetings and continuing education programs.

It is not the physician's duty to implement new techniques merely because they are new; usefulness, safety, and efficacy must be reasonably established. What may be accepted as the most advanced practice of oncology one time in a physician's career may be swiftly outdated by new discoveries and advances, and it is the physician's obligation to render treatment to patients based on adequate understanding of those new developments. A physician who is ignorant of recent developments that are known to and accepted by other physicians may be liable if the use of an outmoded method results in harm to the patient. While adherence to the usual practice by which the local medical community deals with a problem is ordinarily a good defense to a charge of negligence, that everybody does it is not an excuse if it is, in fact, a sloppy or careless practice, or contrary to national standards.

Failure to properly inform a patient because the physician has not "kept up" may result in a failure to have secured a true informed consent.

Agency

Liability may be imposed on the physician based on the acts or inactions of others, e.g., an employee, under the fundamental principle of agency law. This rule applies whether the acts or omissions were in the physician's presence or absence, and whether or not the physician had the actual ability to control his employee's conduct. This is particularly germane to the oncologist, who frequently requires assistance.

Non-Compliance

There are legal problems involving a patient's failure to comply. Non-compliance is a frequent event in the professional life of the oncologist. It often becomes necessary to invoke as a defense the patient's contributory or comparative negligence.

Contributory Negligence in Cancer Patients

Contributory negligence is conduct on the part of the patient that is a contributory cause to his or her own injuries, which falls below the standard one owes oneself to avoid one's own injury at the hands of another. There is no requirement to act; the duty of self-protection always exists and is violated by unreasonable inaction in the face of danger.

At common law, a plaintiff-patient's contributory negligence is an absolute and complete bar to any recovery for the negligence of the patient, as compared to the negligence of the physician.

Comparative Negligence

Because contributory negligence acts as a complete bar to a plaintiff-patient's recovery, causing many harsh results, the majority of states, by statute or judicially, have adopted the doctrine of comparative negligence.

Under comparative negligence, malpractice recovery places the economic loss on the parties in proportion to their fault. In pure comparative negligence states, the plaintiff-patient can recover a percentage of his or her damages when his or her own negligence exceeds that of the defendant-physician.

Professional Organization Guidelines

The American Cancer Society (ACS) and other similar organizations have issued guidelines for the treatment of various cancers. Although they are not legally binding and do not create a prima facie case, these recommendations are widely disseminated via the mass media and are common public knowledge.

Failure to follow these protocols is not necessarily evidence of negligent failure to diagnose cancer. In fact, many physicians in practice do not follow these guidelines, either due to ignorance or because they disagree with them. However, the success of the ACS's educational program, emphasizing the importance of early cancer detection, may make a delay in diagnosis more difficult to defend.

For example, the ACS recommends a baseline mammogram by age 35 to 40, mammography at one to two year intervals from 40 to 49, and annually after age 50, in all asymptomatic women, based on many studies that show the procedure to be a cost-effective, safe method of detecting breast cancer early. A physician who performs mammography only on palpable masses, when 50% of breast cancers are already metastatic, due to unfounded fears of x-ray exposure or that the test is too costly, may have a hard time explaining this logic when sued for failing to detect a cancer earlier. This may be an even greater problem if the physician belongs to a specialty or society which endorses or has similar recommendations to those of the ACS. The American Medical Association, American College of Radiology, American College of Obstetrics and Gynecology, and the American Academy of Family Practice all have similar recommendations.

Presently, the standard of care owed by a general practitioner in diagnosing cancer is essentially the same as the standard of care owed the same patient by a nationally Board-certified oncologist practicing in the same geographical area in many jurisdictions. The "holding self out" doctrine applies — don't treat if you're not up to snuff. An oncologist is more likely to be successfully sued than is a family practitioner, who has negligently missed a breast cancer in a similar patient under similar circumstances; for example, in those jurisdictions which hold specialists to a higher standard of care than generalists, even though a family practitioner is more likely to be sued to begin with.

For this reason, a rule regarding the standard of care in the diagnosis of cancer valid for all physicians in all states, and encompassing all specialties and procedures in all clinical circumstances, is impossible to formulate. Each physician must make an effort to find out the current standards in his own geographical area or similar locality, and the standards of the national certifying board if he practices a recognized specialty, and he should also be aware of current trends (if his state uses the old locality rule, in particular).

Evaluation

Medical History

The medical history is an important part of the diagnostic workup of cancer, as well as other diseases, and is stressed in the introductory course in physical diagnosis in most medical schools.

Unfortunately, many physicians neglect this important aspect of medical practice once out of medical school, and either take no history at all, or do not go into depth in their patient interviews. Failure to take a medical history, or obtaining an incomplete history, may be a significant factor in failure to diagnose a cancer case.

As a result of failure to obtain an adequate history, a physician may not include the diagnosis of certain cancers in the differential diagnoses, or may not give proper weight to a diagnosis of possible cancer, when evaluating certain clinical signs and symptoms. This inappropriately low suspicion of cancer may at times be negligent.

Family history or racial history of certain cancers is an important factor in evaluating asymptomatic patients for cancer screening, as well as for obtaining the proper, indicated tests in certain symptomatic patients.

Occupational exposure, such as asbestos-related occupations, or social habits, such as alcoholism or smoking, may be important factors in the medical history in evaluating a patient for pulmonary neoplasm, liver cancer, or other malignancies, and if not elicited, could be important in establishing negligence in failure to diagnose certain cancers.

Significant x-ray exposure (e.g., breast neoplasia following tuberculosis, pneumothorax collapse therapy, or thyroid cancer as a sequel to childhood radiation of benign head and neck problems), other radiation exposures (e.g., Thoratrast-induced liver cancer), or chemical exposure (e.g., benzene-induced malignancy) may be significant.

Exposure of a patient's forebears to certain drugs or carcinogens may increase the patient's own cancer risk (e.g., vaginal clear-cell carcinoma in DES daughters). Failure to inquire of this history, warn of dangers, and give guidelines to the patient herself may be negligence.

Over-reliance on certain facts obtained in taking the medical history may be just as significant in certain cases as failure to take an adequate history. Failure to follow the clues of certain symptoms as related by the patient because of a history of cancerophobia has been a factor in certain failures to diagnose cancer cases.

Physical Examination

Failure to perform a physical examination, performing an inadequate examination, over-reliance on a negative examination, or failure to perform a follow-up examination, may contribute to lawsuits for failure to diagnose cancer.

Failure to perform an examination at all, especially after a presenting complaint referable to an organ later found to be cancerous, figures prominently in many failures to diagnose cancer cases, as does failure to perform follow-up examinations.

Ordering a test in lieu of a physical examination will not necessarily protect a physician. Even where a biopsy report is negative, overreliance on one report may be negligent when clinical suspicion should not.

Testing

The physician has an affirmative duty to obtain or perform appropriate tests in the diagnosis of a suspected cancer. Failure of the physician to read the test report or consultant's recommendations, or communicate the report or recommendations to the patient, may be negligent.

A biopsy decision reflects estimates of cancer risk that consider such factors as the size of the abnormality and the presence of calcification. A lesion in a woman at particularly high risk — with a strong family history of breast cancer, for example — might be biopsied when it otherwise would not. The decision to biopsy is also influenced by the physician's experience. A less experienced physician will tend to protect patients by recommending biopsy of lesions that might seem relatively low risk to a more experienced physician. Certainly, it is not necessary to screen women who are at extraordinarily low risk (e.g., a 20 year old woman with no family history of breast cancer). However, three-fourths of women who present with sporadic breast cancer have no previously recognized risk factors.

Recent rulings have made it clear that the consulting oncologist has a legal responsibility to personally notify the physician and/or patient in the event of a positive finding on mammogram. Merely sending a positive report is insufficient; the oncologist must ascertain that the information has been received. Once the physician obtains screening information concerning his patient, he must make certain that the patient is informed of the findings, and that she seeks additional attention if it is needed. A physician who fails to order or recommend a biopsy of a lesion that turns out to be malignant will be in a difficult situation.

PEDIATRICS

General Practices

The rights of parents, minors, and the state converge in the context of health care for children. Usually, their respective interests and rights are in concert, and care is provided accordingly. When they are in conflict, federal and state statutory law, administrative agency rules, and prior judicial decisions are looked to for guidance.

The Rights of Parents

The Federal Constitution recognizes family privacy, including the rights of parents to establish family values and determine medical care for their children. The law presumes that parents can best weigh the benefits and risks of proposed treatment and select options that will serve the best interests of their children. This forms the basis for the legal requirement that, except for emergencies and the care of older children, parental consent is required before treatment can be initiated.

The Rights of Children

The rights of children as individuals emerge progressively along a developmental scheme marked by a growing capacity to comprehend issues in health care decision-making. This maturational process supports the legal precepts that permit older children to seek or refuse treatment, and expect confidentiality in an increasingly personalized and differentiated relationship with physicians.

The State's Interests

Notwithstanding the basic rights of family and child, the state is empowered to override individual rights when necessary. This authority includes the "police power", under which the state may implement health regulations that require, for example, compulsory immunization, newborn screening, and prophylactic ophthalmic treatment for neonates. The state is also authorized to asssume the role of *parens patriae,* under which it may intervene in the private lives of families in order to protect children from abuse and neglect.

Forming the Physician-Child-Patient Relationship

As a corollary to the absence of a legally recognized right to health care in this country, physicians are not required to provide care under any and all circumstances. However, once established, the physician's interrelationship with the child and parents confers important legal duties to provide care which, if not respected, may lead to charges of abandonment. It is important, therefore, for physicians to be aware of actions that may be construed as creating a physician-patient relationship.

With the exception of physicians employed in emergency rooms, public or quasi-public institutions, or in health care organizations in which a patient is a subscriber, physicians are free to refuse to see previously unknown persons who request appointments. However, any response by the physician, possibly including telephone communications, that can be construed as initiating care or giving advice, will establish a physician-patient relationship with an attendant duty to provide continuing care.

The consensual character of the relationship between the physician and the child's parents, however, implies the right for either party to withdraw from that relationship under certain circumstances. The physician may legally terminate his relationship with a patient without fear of charges of abandonment, if the patient or the surrogate is provided with written notice of the termination and given sufficient time to obtain care from an alternate source of equal competence. It is recommended that notification of termination of the relationship be transmitted in written form, preferably by certified mail.

Informed Consent for Infants and Children

During the course of the many health care encounters with children each day, physicians must be cognizant of the source of their authority to treat a minor patient. In situations involving young infants accompanied by a parent, the role of the parent as a responsible surrogate decision-maker is usually straightforward. However, clinical and social situations often occur that affect the source and scope of the physician's authority to treat the child. For example, while it is generally understood that physicians are free to provide emergency care to minors under the presumption of implied parental consent, variations among states exist with respect to the legal definition of "emergency". In most states, "emergency" is defined broadly to include not only situations that may be life-threatening to the minor, but also where delay in treatment may increase the risk to health or prolong physical pain, discomfort, or fear.

Courts will rarely second-guess a physician's determination that an emergency existed as a justification for initiating treatment of a minor. It is not necessary for the physician to obtain a second opinion that an emergency exists before providing treatment. It is advisable, and in some states required, that physicians document the nature of the emergency, the attempts made to contact the parents, or the reasons for having made no attempt prior to initiating treatment. In any case, parents should routinely be notified after emergency treatment of young minors.

Children may be brought for medical attention by adults other than their parents, or by a separated or divorced parent without legal custody. It is generally recognized that a parent can consent to treatment of a child in his or her physical custody, even if not the legal custodian, if the need should arise. Typically, this occurs when a child beccmes ill during visitation with the non-custodian parent. That consent may not be valid, however, in non-emergency situations where the physician has reason to know that the legal custodian would object. When minors are brought in by adult caretakers other than the parents, the legal authority for the physician to provide treatment will depend upon whether an emergency existed, the age and maturity of the child, the severity of the treatment procedure, and the attempts made to reach the parents.

Foster parents may grant consent for emergency, routine, or low risk care. Where placement was voluntary, the natural parents should be consulted before major or risky treatment is provided. Where parental rights have been legally terminated, the responsible foster agency should be contacted before serious procedures are performed.

Recreational camps and schools usually require parents to sign blanket consent forms authorizing a physician to provide treatment. Such blanket consent is valid for minor, low risk, non-invasive care. Except for emergency situations, physicians should obtain specific consent from the parents for more serious or complex procedures. Emergency treatment should be provided without hesitation in all circumstances.

Childhood Immunization Practices and Legal Liability

Primary care physicians play a vital role in preventing the spread of contagious disease by ensuring that children receive routine immunizations according to recommended schedules, that children with certain immunologic deficiencies receive special attention with respect to immunization status, and that appropriate precautions are taken to prevent foreseeable side effects. A variety of new vaccines have become available recently, as have specific recommendations for their use published by authoritative groups. Physicians providing continuing care for children, especially those with compromised immune systems, should consult these sources or their local health departments for current recommendations, in order to avoid potential legal liability for injury resulting from failure to immunize properly.

Following a spate of lawsuits alleging a causal relationship between pertussis vaccine and serious neurologic sequelae, which ultimately threatened the continued availability of vaccine in this country, the Federal Government passed the National Childhood Vaccine Injury Act in 1987. This Act provides greater protection from liability for vaccine administrators and manufacturers through a "no-fault" approach to compensation for injury. Several states, e.g., Florida and Virginia, have passed similar statutes.

Parents should be informed about the benefits and risks of immunizations, and their consent should be recorded in the medical record.

Legal Issues in the Care of Adolescents

Physicians involved in the care of adolescents must be conversant with the medicolegal issues surrounding their rights to grant consent and maintain confidentiality. Although the legal age for maturity in all states is 18 years, minors may legally consent to medical treatment in many circumstances.

The Emancipated Minor

Minors who live independently away from home and make their own day-to-day decisions may be considered legally emancipated with respect to their ability to grant consent for medical treatment. This definition generally includes minors who are married, in the military service, and college students who manage their own affairs (even if supported by their parents). Minors who live at home but contribute to family support and manage their own personal affairs are often considered emancipated as well. A previously married minor will still be considered emancipated, unless the marriage was annulled. Minor parents are considered emancipated and may make medical decisions for themselves and their children in most states.

Mature Minors

Minors who do not meet the criteria for emancipation may nevertheless consent even to non-emergency treatment under certain circumstances. There have been no successful lawsuits against physicians for treating minors over the age of 15 when the following criteria have been met: (1) the minor is capable of understanding the proposed medical treatment and appreciating the risk involved; (2) the proposed treatment is necessary for the benefit of the minor and not a third party; and (3) the proposed treatment is not serious or risky. Except in emergencies or where permitted by statutes, younger minors should not be treated without parental consent; physicians doing so may be held liable, even for non-negligent care.

While mature minors may consent to medical treatment, it is always preferable to seek their agreement to involve their parents in medical decision-making. When minors are treated without their parents' consent, the physician should carefully document in the medical record the circumstances as previously outlined, particularly the minor's capacity to comprehend the nature of the problem, the proposed treatment and risks, and the fact that the minor rejected parental notification. Except for emergency care, where parental consent is presumed, non-consenting parents are not financially responsible for care provided for their minor children.

Minor Treatment Statutes

All states permit treatment of minors for venereal disease without requiring parental consent. Most states permit treatment for drug and alcohol abuse and emotional or psychiatric problems without parental consent. Many states have statutes which allow minors to seek contraceptive advice and care during pregnancy. Some states still allow a pregnant minor to arrange for an abortion on her own; others require either parental or judicial consent. Physicians are admonished to be familiar with the state statutes and case law in their respective jurisdictions.

Treatment of Runaways and Homeless Adolescents

Increasingly, physicians caring for adolescent patients become involved with runaway and homeless minors. Following the general rule, care under emergency circumstances should always be provided under the doctrine of implied consent. In non-emergency situations, minors in need of care who refuse to assist in locating their parents may be presumed to be emancipated and treated with their own consent. Under such circumstances, it is best to document attempts made to locate the parents, and include in the medical record a statement signed by the minor refusing to assist.

Confidentiality

As a general rule, minors who may consent to their own medical treatment have a concomitant right to confidentiality, except where disclosure of medical information is statutorily required. However, in situations where the physician determines that because of the seriousness of the minor's condition or the danger of self-injury or injury to others, and involvement of the parents is important, disclosure would be legally permissible.

In order to maintain the trusting relationship essential for the care of adolescent patients, physicians should discuss in advance the scope of confidentiality that will be respected.

Treatment of Sex-Related Conditions

The right of adolescents to consent on their own behalf is particularly strong for sex-related treatment. The constitutionally protected right of privacy protects young adolescents' rights to make personal decisions concerning their bodies where sex-related conditions are concerned. This includes the use of contraceptives, access to family planning services, care during pregnancy, and the performance of early abortions. Therefore, states are prohibited from enacting legislation containing blanket provisions for parental consent for abortions for mature or emancipated minors. State statutes requiring such consent must include an efficient, non-cumbersome mechanism for a minor to bypass parental involvement through judicial determination of maturity or, if immature, that an abortion would be in her best interests. Whether states can legally require parental notification after the fact is currently an unsettled issue.

Parents may not grant proxy consent compelling an age-appropriate, competent child to have an abortion. The state of the current law of consent and confidentiality concerning pregnant adolescents seeking abortions suggest that the criteria to be applied are the same as for mature minors requesting other forms of non-emergency medical or surgical treatment, i.e., the capacity to understand the nature and consequences of the procedure.

Notwithstanding these freedoms, physicians are advised to encourage teenagers to discuss the problem with their parents and include them in the decision-making process whenever possible. Many of the complex legal issues surrounding pregnancy-related care for adolescents are still under debate within the American judicial system. It is important that physicians be aware of existing state statutes applicable to this area and seek specific legal advice when conflicts arise.

Genetic Counseling

Physicians who care for children occasionally are asked for prenatal advice. During the course of a prenatal visit, prospective parents may request information concerning the risk of recurrence of familial disorders or congenital malformations, usually stimulated by experience with prior children or other family members. Physicians are required to provide accurate information according to acceptable standards of care. Parents who decide to continue or terminate a pregnancy based on erroneous information may bring suit against the physician for negligence in genetic counseling. For example, a physician who reassures a mother of a child with polycystic kidneys that the result of her current pregnancy will almost certainly be a normal child may be subject to such a lawsuit. When patterns of familial disease emerge during routine history taking or questions arise concerning the potential teratogenicity of drugs taken in early pregnancy, referral to a genetic counseling service is advised.

The underlying legal issue in genetic counseling lawsuits involves the loss of parental choice caused by failure to provide accurate information. Typically, such claims are for "wrongful birth", in which parents seek compensation for the incremental costs involved in rearing an abnormal child. A small number of jurisdictions recognize a more controversial claim of "wrongful life", in which the child sues on its own behalf, seeking compensation for having been born with an abnormality as a result of failure to provide the parents with accurate information that would have led to termination of the pregnancy.

Adoption

Pediatricians are often asked to become involved in the complex process of adoption. Typically, requests come from a couple seeking assistance in becoming adoptive parents, or a pregnant woman planning to offer her baby for adoption. These matters are usually governed by state statutes with very specific procedural provisions. It is incumbent upon physicians providing assistance with adoptions to become familiar with the laws of the state in which he or she practices and follow them precisely.

Private adoptions, in which arrangements are made between an unwed mother and prospective adoptive parents through an intermediary broker, are fraught with legal pitfalls. These may occur when the natural mother exercises her legal option to change her mind, or the adoptive parents elect to return the child before a final decree is entered. In either case, the physician involved in a private adoption may become embroiled in a conflict between the parties. In some states, private adoptions, including offering assistance, are outlawed altogether; in other states, they are permitted, but regulated and individually reviewed by state agencies.

The law is generally protective of natural mothers against coercive influences to disrupt their bonds with their offspring. Thus, in many states, statutes hold invalid adoption releases that may be executed prenatally. Similarly, many statutes grant natural mothers the right to revoke their consent for adoption within a reasonable time postnatally.

Consent for adoption placement by an unwed or married natural mother is generally sufficient, overriding objections that may be expressed by the biologic father. However, the biologic father's objection may be held valid if he had been previously married to the mother, or demonstrates continuing interest and acceptance of parental responsibilities.

Physicians are asked to perform pre-adoption physical examinations on newborn infants to certify their eligibility for adoption. Legal liability in negligence may apply for undetected defects that may be material to the prospective parents' decision to adopt. This liability would not extend to defects manifesting later in life, or not detectable at the initial routine examination.

In all states, payment beyond administrative costs of the adoption procedure is considered "baby-selling" and is illegal.

Alternative Procreative Techniques

Infertility among young couples occurs with great frequency. Increasingly, pediatricians may be asked to participate in discussions with prospective parents who plan to obtain a child with the assistance of newer reproductive technology. This may include artificial insemination by donor semen (AID), in vitro fertilization (IVF), embryo transfer, or surrogate motherhood where legally permitted.

Most states have statutes strictly controlling AID procedures. Consent of the husband is usually required for artificial insemination by an anonymous donor. The consenting husband is generally regarded as the legal father by state statute. Legislation specifically governing the more innovative reproductive technologies has not yet been developed in most jurisdictions. Courts tend to apply existing adoption laws in resolving conflicts concerning the respective rights of the particular parents. Therefore, the legal basis for identifying the gestational mother as the natural mother, prohibiting private adoptions, outlawing baby-brokering for money, invalidating prenatal releases for adoption, and rights of revocation by either the gestational mother or adopting couple, will vary by jurisdiction according to existing adoption statutes.

Events in the Delivery Room

All hospitals with obstetrical services must have medical staff policies concerning responsibilities and protocols for the care of high risk neonates. These policies will generally include a definition of the respective responsibilities of the obstetrician and pediatrician during the immediate and transitional postpartum periods, requirements for attendance by a pediatrician at high risk deliveries, responsibilities and guidelines for neonatal resuscitation, requirements for consultation with specialists, and indications for transfer to tertiary care units. These policies may vary among communities, depending upon the resources locally available. Many malpractice claims have been based on injury to the neonate, alleged to have been caused by physician conduct not in compliance with existing hospital policies concerning delivery room care.

Appropriate referral of sick neonates to the care of qualified neonatologists and tertiary care nurseries is another area of potential exposure to medical-legal liability. In many institutions, the process of credentialing physicians for appointment to the medical staff and delineation of privileges includes specific reference to qualifications for the care of sick neonates. Both physicians and hospitals may be held liable for injuries sustained by neonates while under the care of physicians acting beyond the scope of their delineated privileges. As a general rule, physicians providing care in an area customarily within the province of specialists will be held to a concomitant higher standard of care. For example, pediatricians caring for sick, low birth weight neonates will legally be held to a standard at the level of neonatalogists.

Authoritative guidelines for cardiopulmonary resuscitation of neonates, infants, and children have been widely published. While these protocols are not necessarily intended as legal national standards, it is likely that they will be introduced as evidence in malpractice litigation involving claims of negligent resuscitation efforts.

Mandatory Genetic Screening

All states have statutory requirements for neonatal screening of certain hereditary disorders, such as phenylketonuria and hypothyroidism. Technological advances are rapidly expanding the scope of disease and carrier states that can be identified in the early neonatal pericd through mass screening programs.

Occasionally, parents may refuse to permit testing of their newborn infants. Many of the legal issues concerning the constitutionality of compulsory screening programs, use of the information obtained, and the state's obligation to provide treatment and follow-up services are unsettled. While specific, informed consent is not required for the performance of neonatal screening tests, physicians should consult hospital counsel before overriding express parental objections to a screening test.

Decision-Making in the Care of Seriously Ill Newborns — The ''Baby Doe'' Rule

In 1985, Congress passed amendments to the Child Abuse Prevention and Treatment Act, essentially providing that decisions to withhold medically indicated treatment from disabled infants with life-threatening conditions may constitute medical neglect.

The Child Abuse Amendments provide that medically indicated treatment may be withheld only in circumstances where, in the treating physician's reasonable medical judgment, a) the infant is chronically, irreversibly comatose; b) the provision of such treatment would (1) merely prolong dying, (2) not be effective in ameliorating or correcting all of the infant's life-threatening conditions, or (3) otherwise be futile in terms of the survival of the infant; and c) the provision of such treatment would be virtually futile in terms of survival of the infant, and the treatment itself under such circumstances would be inhumane. The statute further provides that under all circumstances, fluids and nutrition must be provided.

The amendments require that state child protection agencies reinforce linkages with area hospitals and develop procedures for reporting, investigating, and, when indicated, intervening in cases alleging this form of medical neglect. Failure by a state agency to comply with the statute jeopardizes continued federal funding.

The regulations also include model guidelines for the recommended (but not mandated) establishment of hospital Infant Care Review Committees to function as review bodies for decisions to withhold treatment from disabled newborns. Appropriate functions suggested for Infant Care Review Committees include education of personnel and families, development of hospital guidelines and policies, and case reviews.

Because legal interpretation of some of the rule's provisions is still unsettled, physicians are encouraged to consult with Infant Care Review Committees where available, when questions concerning withholding treatment from such infants arise. In other settings, well-documented consultation and group discussions with specialists and parents and support of the staff will enhance the legal validity of these difficult decisions.

Child Abuse and Neglect

All states have child abuse statutes requiring physicians and other mandated classes to report cases of suspected physical or emotional abuse, neglect, or sexual abuse to state protection agencies or law enforcement authorities. Typically, child abuse reporting statutes contain the following elements: classes of mandated reporters; the agency receiving the report; provisions for placing children in temporary protective custody without parental consent when necessary; provisions for examination, treatment, and photography of allegedly inflicted injuries; defined responsibility for follow-up investigation; suspension of rules of parent-physician confidentiality in cases of suspected abuse; and guaranteed immunity from civil suit for mandated, good faith reporting of suspected child abuse.

Physicians may be asked to provide affidavits in support of petitions to the court by child protection agencies for protective removal of a child or permanent termination of parental rights. These affidavits are introduced as evidence and, to be effective, must meet a required standard of proof of the etiology of the injury and the risk of further injury to the child before courts will authorize state invasion of parental rights. It is, therefore, important that physicians complete child abuse affidavits in as accurate detail as possible, including estimates of the magnitude and severity of the risk of recurrent injury.

Cases of child sexual abuse usually come to attention shortly after the alleged event, or after disclosure by the child of an alleged abuse occurring at some earlier time. In recent years, there has been a growing trend to bring criminal charges against alleged abusers. In such cases, the child's testimony at the time of trial, as well as earlier statements made by the child to the physician, may be crucial evidence for the prosecution. In order for statements made by the child to the physician about sexually abusive acts to be admissible as evidence, it is important that the physician allow the child to talk freely without introducing leading questions and to record the statements verbatim.

Parental Non-Compliance as a Form of Neglect

Charges of medical neglect may sometimes be brought against parents who fail to comply with a physician's recommendation for treatment of their child. At issue is the legal conflict between the parental duty to provide necessary care, and the parental right to make medical decisions for their children. These cases may take the form of outright refusal by the parents to consent to the recommended treatment, or parental selection of an alternative treatment considered inappropriate by the physician.

Courts have settled the issue of parental religious objections to treatment of their child in favor of mandating treatment on the grounds that parental freedoms of religious beliefs and practices do not extend to placing their minor children at serious risk. Therefore, when such conflicts occur, physicians should immediately seek judicial approval to provide care. In weighing its decision to override parental refusal for treatment for whatever reason, courts will generally consider the severity of the risk to the child, especially if life-threatening or leading to chronic disability, the efficacy and risks of the recommended procedure, the feasibility of deferring the procedure until the child is old enough to decide personally, and the current wishes of an older child. In such cases, physicians are best advised to seek judicial relief.

More difficult are cases in which parents select alternative, often controversial, treatment for their child than that recommended by their physician. When reviewing charges of medical neglect brought against such parents, courts may grant them wide latitude in decision-making if they can show that some qualified medical opinion exists in support of their selection. Again, judicial help should be sought in such cases.

Drugs Not Approved for Use in Children

Many of the drugs prescribed for children will be described in the accompanying package inserts, or in the Physicians' Desk Reference (PDR), as not having been approved for use in that age group. Physicians should be aware of the potential medicolegal implications of utilizing drugs so designated. A physician should note the justification in the medical chart at the time of administration of the drug, and be prepared to defend its use.

Drug testing in children is complex and costly. Drugs designated as "not approved for children", because they were not subjected to testing as they were on adults, are not necessarily contraindicated. While package insert information may be introduced as evidence in malpractice suits, the standard of care will be determined by the manner in which the drug is used in accepted good medical practice.

Special Situations —
Sterilization of Minors

State and federal statutes are very specific about the circumstances in which sterilization of competent or incompetent minors may be permitted and the legal procedures to be followed. In many states, competent minors under 18 may not consent to sterilization. Similarly, in most states, parents may not provide proxy consent for sterilization in their children, except in very specific conditions defined in the statutes. Most common are requests for sterilization of retarded adolescents. Physicians should always seek legal advice and judicial review before responding to such requests. In considering requests for involuntary sterilization of retarded minors, courts will require the petitioners to meet a high standard of proof that the procedure is necessary and offers the least drastic alternative that meets the best interests of the incompetent.

Organ Transplantation and Brain Death Criteria

It is increasingly likely that as organ transplantation technology advances, physicians caring for children will become involved in cases of pediatric cadaver organ donation or living-related organ transplantation. The provisions of the Uniform Anatomical Gift Act may be applied to minor cadaver donors, from which organs may be harvested with the consent of one parent, provided the other does not object. If the minor donor was married, consent should be obtained from the spouse.

A more difficult situation arises when living-related organ transplantation is considered, usually between siblings. Legal advice and judicial review should always be sought in such cases. Courts have permitted organ donations from living-related minors where the risk of the procedure was relatively low and some benefit, usually psychological, to the minor donor, could be postulated. Under any circumstance, a minor's express refusal to serve as an organ donor should not be overridden.

While "brain death" statutes have been enacted widely, it is important for physicians to recognize that the clinical criteria generally applied to adults may not be valid for neonates and very young infants. Consultation with neurologists or neurosurgeons specializing in the care of children is advisable before brain death is declared in that age group.

Legal Aspects of Mental Health for Minors

Important legal issues arise whenever decisions to commit minors with serious mental illness to in-patient units are considered. State laws intended to protect children from malicious commitment vary in their specific provisions for the authority of parents to commit minors, the rights of minors to voluntarily commit themselves, and the rights of minors beyond a certain age to commit themselves, while others require either parental consent or judicial review. In general, children are accorded the same constitutionally protected rights of due process as adults, including, at a minimum, independent psychiatric evaluation to confirm the diagnosis and the need for commitment, as well as periodic follow-up review. Minors' rights to refuse non-emergency treatment with psychotropic drugs are generally considered to be the same as adults. Physicians involved in these situations should be knowledgeable about the state statutes and case law in their respective jurisdictions.

The principles of consent by minors for general medical treatment can be applied to mental health conditions in an ambulatory setting, unless specifically covered by state statutes. Treatment by psychologists or social workers would probably be included in a minor's consent, at least when provided in an established setting such as a mental health center under the supervision of qualified psychiatrists.

The Minor as a Research Subject

Research protocols involving minors as subjects are governed by strict federal and state regulations. Federal regulations provide specific guidelines that must be followed by Institutional Review Boards, subject to state statutory provisions. The major issues to be considered are the level of risk and potential benefit to the subject. Scrutiny by Institutional Review Boards should become increasingly strict as the level of risk to the minor subject increases beyond a minimum, and the potential direct benefit to the subject diminishes. Affirmative agreement, or "assent", should be obtained from children old enough to understand the procedure before a research protocol is approved. Research protocols that expose a minor to more than minimal risk, i.e., beyond those encountered in normal daily life at that age, without the prospect of any direct benefit to the subject, should generally be disapproved, regardless of parental wishes.

Legal Issues Concerning the Care of Children with AIDS

As the number of infants and children with AIDS grows, physicians will become involved in legal, as well as medical and social, issues, especially neonatal testing and, for the older child, educational placement.

Neonatal testing is, in effect, synonymous with maternal testing, with all the attendant social and economic risks of disclosure. Therefore, institutional policies governing consent and confidentiality for HIV testing in adults should apply equally to neonates.

Physicians may be asked to participate in discussions concerning school placement of HIV-positive children. The legal limits of the authority of local school districts to determine the educational disposition of HIV-positive children is still unsettled. It appears that federal laws guaranteeing education for handicapped children and prohibiting discrimination against the handicapped will apply to decisions concerning educational placement of HIV-positive children, requiring school districts to review each case individually to ensure maximum participation in the educational system and appropriate protection of others in the environment.

Conclusion

The legal principles that govern the rights and responsibilities within the physician-patient relationship, standards of care, informed consent and confidentiality, and potential liability in a variety of clinical contexts in adult medicine are the framework within which pediatric medical-legal issues are considered. The practice of pediatrics is distinguished, however, by the triadic relationship among physician-parent-child, and the dynamics of developmental biology that make the pediatric patient an ever-changing subject. These characteristics of pediatric clinical practice create important legal correlates.

While the care of children is necessarily negotiated through their parents, to whom the law accords broad latitude in family decision-making, physicians must recognize the outside perimeters of that authority, beyond which children may be placed at serious risk. Similarly, parental rights as surrogate decision-makers gradually attenuate as the child matures into an increasingly comprehending, independent individual with a justifiable legal claim to self-determination in the health care context.

The key to practicing sound pediatric medicine, unfettered by unreasonable fear of medical-legal litigation, is maintaining a respectful attitude toward the physician-parent-child relationship, recognizing the importance of age and size-relatedness in standards of care, freely utilizing consultation from pediatric specialists and documentation of medical rationale, and communications with decision-makers, as well as other relevant evidence of reasonable medical judgment. Few adverse medical-legal consequences will occur when these principles of practice are followed.

PSYCHIATRY

Introduction

The forensic psychiatrist works in three major areas: regulatory issues, civil cases, and criminal matters. The regulatory issues include legal concepts that affect the physician and his patient: confidentiality; privileged communications; privacy; informed consent; competency; patients' rights, including the right to treatment and the right to refuse treatment; and commitment procedures.

Civil legal matters include such cases as personal injury, e.g., negligence and tort cases; domestic relations matters, such as divorce and child custody; parental rights, and other matters of family law, including juvenile cases; competency matters in medicine and surgery; and malpractice cases.

Criminal matters include the assessment of the defendant at any stage of the criminal process, including competency to make a confession, competency to stand trial, and competency to waive one's rights; criminal responsibility or insanity; and recommendation for disposition, including evaluation of death penalty cases.

Forensic Psychiatry

Forensic psychiatry is that sub-specialty of psychiatry in which the psychiatrist deals with people involved in legal matters, either criminal or civil. His role is more of an investigator than a therapist, and he must have access to all relevant information or data involved in a particular case. Prior medical and psychiatric records, police investigation reports, witness statements, crime scene reports, and autopsy reports are all essential to the investigation by the forensic psychiatrist. Assessment of credibility of the defendant or the plaintiff in civil cases is an important feature of the functions of the forensic psychiatrist.

Standards of Care

All psychiatric patients should, therefore, be medically evaluated, including a complete history and physical examination. Other medical conditions, such as AIDS, subdural hematoma, and encephalitis, sometimes present primarily with psychiatric symptoms. A large number of patients suffer from associated or primary medical conditions, such as diabetes, head injury or hormonal changes. Many have abused or failed to conform to their medications.

Certain treatments should be preceded by the use of laboratory screening units. Liver, thyroid, and renal profiles should be conducted on all patients who are to receive Lithium. Specific tests, such as EEG and CAT scan, should be performed as needed. Psychological testing or neuropsychological testing may also be indicated in the assessment and subsequent treatment of some patients.

Psychiatrists, as do all other professionals, must conform to good, medical (psychiatric) community standards and act like "reasonable individuals" under like circumstances. Traditional concepts of abandonment apply.

Record-Keeping and Documentation

Careful and scrupulous documentation is indicated in the care of all psychiatric patients, but the medical (psychiatric) record should include only clinical data, and never legal opinions or derogatory comments.

Good records are a must. This means not more writing, but better writing. If it is not written, "it probably was not done". Document appropriate care, treatment, opinions, and decisions. A good record is the strongest defense against a lawsuit, or in support of a contention.

State regulations, in most jurisdictions, mandate reporting of sexual abuse and abuse to children. Documentation and recording in the chart is important in such matters, which may reach court proceedings.

Confidentiality

One of the most important ethical issues in medicine is that of confidentiality, which prohibits a physician from disclosing what he or she has learned in the course of treating his or her patient.

When a clinician is requested to perform a psychiatric evaluation by and for the benefit of a court, an employer, an insurance company, an attorney, or a third-party payer, the patient should first be informed by the psychiatrist of the contemplated disclosure and its possible implications; i.e., the patient should know what will be done with the material that is disclosed and how that might affect the patient. A properly executed release form is indicated in such cases.

Duty to Warn

Breach of confidentiality may result in a malpractice case, unless the physician can show that the breach of confidentiality was essential to the protection of the health of the patient or the safety of the community. In emergency situations, the physician may breach confidentiality in order to effect commitment to a hospital when the patient is suicidal or acutely in need of psychiatric treatment to prevent damage to him or herself or others. Based upon judicial reasoning in the *Tarasoff* case and its progeny, the psychiatrist is mandated to breach confidentiality if his or her patient threatens the life or welfare of a third party, or seriously threatens to destroy property, and the psychiatrist believes the threat is sincere and likely to be carried out. In such cases, the courts have decreed that the psychiatrist has a duty to warn or a duty to protect the safety of that particular third party. He or she may carry out his or her duty by breaching confidentiality.

Privilege

The matter of privilege differs from confidentiality in that it relates primarily to the disclosure of information in a court of law. In this case, the patient has the right to seal the lips of his or her psychiatrist, and prevent him or her from testifying in court, unless the patient waives his or her privilege by raising his or her mental state as an issue in either a civil or criminal case.

Psychiatrists must adhere to the principles of "confidentiality", but there are times when privilege does not apply. Disclosure is legally required, for example, when a contagious disease is present, when a crime is contemplated, when a child has been abused, when the evaluation is court-ordered, when the illness becomes an issue in a legal action, and when the patient identifies a specific potential victim who has or can obtain the means to carry out the threat. Jurisdictions vary as to whom and how the notification must be made. States still differ with regard to AIDS notification requirements.

Privacy

The patient's right to privacy is distinguished from both confidentiality and privilege in cases in which lawyers and judges are not allowed to inspect the medical or psychiatric records of an individual who is not a party to the legal proceedings. The patient's right to privacy also extends to prohibiting physicians from intruding upon his or her physical or mental functions.

Patients may keep physicians from conducting various intrusive tests, if they are competent to refuse. In psychiatric cases, the patient may refuse psychiatric treatment, including various types of medication, if the patient is not an emergency, and the patient is competent to refuse. These matters refer to the involuntarily committed patient. Certainly, the voluntary patient has the right to refuse treatment, and may also discontinue treatment or leave the hospital, if he or she chooses. These laws are designed to protect the involuntary patient, who is not free to leave the hospital if he or she chooses. The right to refuse treatment is based on the patient's right to privacy.

Competence

The major difference between the legal aspects of psychiatry and the other fields of medicine reflects the fact that many psychiatric patients are "incompetent". "Competence" is a legal term, the definition of which varies with the specific circumstances. Perhaps, the most important issue for forensic psychiatrists, both in civil and criminal law, is that of competency of the patient, who may be a defendant, a plaintiff, or a witness in either case. It may involve the legally recognized ability to accept or refuse treatment (a valid consent must be "informed, competent, and voluntary"), write a will, contract, testify, stand trial, handle one's estate, and even to be executed. To write a valid will (testamentary capacity), one must recognize that the document and its signing is intended to authorize the transfer of property upon the death of the one who owns the property and signs the document (testator), to comprehend the extent of the property to be transferred, and to whom it will be given. There are always, in addition, certain specific statutory requirements, which must be met before the will will be accepted by the courts as valid (e.g., two witnesses). "Competent to stand trial" requires that the individual understand the charges which have been brought, the consequences of a "guilty verdict", and the ability to cooperate with the defense attorney.

The determination of competency depends upon the nature of the situation which is involved, and the particular questions that need to be addressed. In criminal cases, the psychiatrist must ascertain, by law, whether the defendant knows the nature and consequences of his or her legal situation, and whether he or she can work with his or her attorney in preparing a rational defense. He or she must know, for example, the functions of the judge, the prosecutor, the defense attorney, the jury, and his or her particular role within the court system. In ascertaining the defendant's competency, the forensic psychiatrist must ask these particular questions, and may not presume the answers if the questions are not asked. In civil cases, the psychiatrist must be aware of the legal situation in which the competency is to be assessed. There are different questions for determining whether a person is competent to write a will or to manage his or her own affairs, or to testify in court, or to get married, or to get divorced, or to take care of his or her children, or to enter into a contract. Basically, the patient must know the nature and consequences of the legal situation in which he or she is involved.

Perhaps, the most frequent situation where physicians may require an assessment of competency is in consultation and liaison psychiatry, in which the psychiatrist is asked to determine whether the patient is competent to refuse a particular procedure a surgeon wishes to perform. Patients may refuse surgery and may do so legitimately, even in the case of the possibility of death if they do not have the needed surgery. The psychiatrist may be called to assess the competency of the patient in order to determine whether surgery should proceed, or whether a guardian must be appointed before consent may be given. If the psychiatrist and the surgeon are uncertain about competency, and the procedure is not an emergency, the court should be consulted for determination of legal competency, and the appointment of a guardian when necessary.

Informed Consent

Consent is always an important issue, and it is very important in the treatment of a psychiatric patient, especially when the procedure or the medication has known adverse, as well as beneficial, results. Material and substantial disclosure, properly documented, is essential. This is especially significant with the use of psychotropics, the so-called mind altering drugs, which may cause Parkinsonism, tardive dyskinesia, or other side reactions, that can produce distress to the patient, or even injury to a third person (by causing a vehicular accident, for example).

In medicine, a critical consideration for therapy or treatment is the consent of the patient, although the consent may be presumed or vicarious if the patient is not able to give direct consent. However, in most cases, the patient is required to give an informed consent. This means the physician must give appropriate and complete information to the patient, on which the patient can then make an informed decision about whether to accept or refuse the treatment offered. Courts have determined that the information must not only include what treatment procedure the physician wishes to give, but alternative procedures that may not be as effective, or which may carry a greater risk. The patient is then in the position of choosing the treatment he or she wishes to have, with the consent of the physician. In these cases, there are several elements that need to be observed: 1) The information must be given by the physician and must be complete and appropriate; 2) The information must be given in language that is understandable to the patient; and 3) The patient must be competent to give informed consent. The patient may not make decisions based on a delusional system, or on the basis of a significant mental illness.

Involuntary Commitment — Dangerousness

Involuntary hospitalization, called "commitment", is the result of a judicial determination, often at the recommendation of a physician, that an individual is "dangerous".

During the past 20 years, laws have changed regarding the involuntary commitment of patients for psychiatric hospitalization. Formerly, either one or two physicians could have an individual committed involuntarily for psychiatric treatment if the person was mentally ill and in need of hospitalization. That concept has been found to be "unconstitutionally vague", and since the case of *Lessard v. Schmidt,* courts have ruled that in order for a person to be involuntarily committed to a mental hospital, he or she must be both mentally ill and present "a clear and present danger of harm to self or others". Many states have legislated this dual concept, in order for commitment to be effectuated. Psychiatrists know about mental illness, but do not always know about "dangerousness".

Dangerousness is defined as presenting clear and convincing evidence of a substantial threat of injury to self or others. This concept may include violent acts, destructive behavior, or significant physical and/or mental deterioration. If a patient is violent under certain clinical conditions, or suicidal under certain situations, the clinician may be able to tell the court about the potential for violence under those conditions. However, most laws do not include the conditions, and only ask whether the patient is "dangerous". As a result, many individuals are committed to hospitals as both mentally ill and dangerous. The question that remains is when will the person no longer be dangerous. Does the danger leave when the illness is in remission, or is the potential for violence unrelated to the mental illness? Psychiatrists and hospitals have been sued when patients have been discharged, and then harmed themselves or others shortly after release from the hospital. The presumption is that the patient is no longer dangerous to the community when released from the hospital. These are very difficult decisions for psychiatrists to make, especially when there is no track record of behavior under various conditions. It becomes a matter of guesswork and balancing the rights of the patient to be treated in the least restrictive, alternative manner, consistent with his or her illness, and also protective for the safety of the community. Psychiatrists may be able to predict violent behavior (not dangerousness) when the violence is imminent, or under certain clinical conditions.

General predictions of dangerousness are to be avoided, as they are usually not valid and are not based on scientific determinations. The attending physician is always required to document the basis for a determination of "dangerousness", and may be required to substantiate his or her clinical impression before a judge in an adversary proceeding.

Involuntary Patients' Rights to Treatment and to Refuse Treatment

Some of the major changes that have occurred in the practice of psychiatry over the past two decades include the development of patients' rights within the mental hospital. Involuntarily committed patients have a right to adequate treatment, or their commitment is tantamount to being incarcerated for no good reason. They must receive adequate treatment if the commitment is valid. These same involuntarily committed patients, who have a right to adequate treatment, also have a right to refuse treatment that may be harmful for them. One of the most poorly understood concepts in the development of patients' rights is that of the right to refuse treatment. Traditionally, physicians accepted the responsibility of making the decisions for patients in a paternalistic way. Physicians also understood that patients had a right to receive adequate treatment, but then had difficulty understanding the concept of refusing treatment when they had a right to receive it. Wouldn't granting the right to refuse treatment totally negate a patient's right to receive it? The idea is that involuntarily committed patients have a right to adequate treatment, and it is the physician's duty to make it available to each individual patient, but not to force it upon him or her. Since there are various forms of treatment that may be harmful, the patient should have a right to decide whether he or she wishes to have the treatment or not.

An involuntarily hospitalized individual retains the right to refuse psychotropic or neurotropic medication, unless there is evidence that the individual presents an imminent and significant threat of serious harm to self or others.

The right to refuse treatment began as a religious right in the case of *Winters v. Miller,* and evolved to a right to refuse intrusive treatments, such as electroshock therapy. Currently, patients have a right to refuse a particular type of neuroleptic medication that may have long-term, harmful side effects, such as tardive dyskinesia. In order for a patient to refuse treatment, he or she must not be in an emergency state and must be competent to refuse. Various courts have defined emergency and competency in different ways, but the general concept remains the same.

Tardive dyskinesia is a serious, irreversible side effect of neuroleptic medication. The courts have been seriously concerned about this side effect, and have allowed patients to make decisions about taking medication which may result in tardive dyskinesia or other harmful side effects. Neuroleptic medication is the treatment of choice for schizophrenia, the illness most commonly seen in involuntarily committed patients. Thus, the matter becomes a very serious one, because the physician also has to balance the treatment requirements with the security issues and the least restrictive alternative of treatment for the patient. The physician may often have to decide whether the patient is truly competent to refuse the medication offered. If the refusal is based on a delusional system of the patient's illness, he or she may not be competent to refuse, and the treatment may be given. However, it is advised that before the treatment is given, a second opinion should be obtained from an independent examiner, who records the findings and recommendations in the patient's chart. If the situation becomes an emergency, and medication is required, the physician may administer a temporary dose of medication to handle the emergency, and then reassess the patient's condition and the situation. A physician should not usually give long acting neuroleptic medication in an emergency situation, because the effects of such medication may last for several weeks, long beyond the period of the emergency.

Least Restrictive Alternative

The use of restraints or seclusion techniques is properly regulated by hospital rules and regulations. Patients placed in seclusion and/or restraint should be observed regularly and protected from self-abuse or harm by others. Hospitals, in addition to regulations regarding seclusion and restraint, have specific regulations regarding suicidal patients and elopement precautions. Courts have usually held to the standard developed by hospitals and by national organizations regulating hospital treatment. Psychiatric patients are to be treated in the "least restrictive environment" necessary for the clinical needs of the patients. It would be improper, for example, to place a homicidal or suicidal patient in a situation where he or she may act out his or her destructive behavior on him or herself or others.

Civil Law and Psychiatry

The practicing psychiatrist may become involved in a number of different cases or situations in which the patient has a civil case that affects his treatment.

For example, many patients are involved in domestic relations situations. These may be very complex and difficult to resolve, and take a tremendous toll on the mental state of the patient. The matter may go on for years, and may include the issues of divorce, child custody, visitation procedures, and distribution of property. The litigant must be competent to understand the issues involved at each stage of the proceedings. In many jurisdictions, if the woman is not competent to get divorced, the husband may not become divorced and "dump" the problem on the state. In some cases, individuals may not be competent to get married. The psychiatrist may be called to assess the individual and given an opinion about his or her competency. The determination of custody matters is also very complex and involves the review of records from many sources, including school records, physicians' records, and work records of the parents. Family members and other witnesses may need to be interviewed, in order to determine the fitness or qualifications of each parent. Usually, a child psychiatrist is required for assessment of young children in such situations.

Perhaps the most common area of civil law for the psychiatrist is that of personal injury. A psychiatric patient can be found "not responsible for a crime", but remain liable for a tort (damages in a civil action). There are a number of ways in which a person may be injured, including an auto accident, airplane crash, natural disaster, and toxic or nuclear situations. The psychiatrist may be retained either by the plantiff or the defense in the cases. Irrespective of his or her source of involvement, the forensic psychiatrist must obtain a complete evaluation of the plaintiff, with examination of medical records prior to and subsequent to the accident. A complete and thorough psychiatric examination must be conducted. Psychological testing and other special tests may be necessary in order to determine whether the plaintiff has sustained psychiatric damage and, if so, the origin or etiology of the damage.

Malpractice cases enter the field of personal injury, and may include assessment of psychiatric damages in medical malpractice cases, or evaluation of liability in psychiatric malpractice cases.

Civil Matters

The rules regarding competency often relate to the law of contracts. Does the individual understand the terms of the contract, i.e., the nature and consequences of his or her legal situation? The individual may be unable to understand what he or she is doing for a number of reasons. He or she may be mentally retarded, significantly mentally ill so that he or she is deluded, or in a manic phase without proper judgment. He or she may be an alcoholic, or withdrawing from addictive drugs. He or she may have an organic brain syndrome, or may be easily influenced by designing persons. Assessment of competency includes the determination of whether a person may handle or manage his or her own affairs. In such a case, the patient needs to know the amount of money he or she has, in what form it is, and where it is. He or she must be able to answer simple mathematical questions, and be able to make change in a financial transaction. He or she must be oriented to time, place, and person, and must not be of such weakened intellect that his or her judgment would be overborne by those individuals who wish to deceive or take advantage of him or her.

In order to prepare a will, an individual needs to know about how much money he or she has, and to whom he or she wishes to leave the money; i.e., he or she needs to know the objects of his or her bounty and affection. It may be difficult to determine whether a will is valid on the basis of the testator's competency, because the assessment often occurs after the death of the testator. The assessment of competency is then conducted by evaluating and examining records and witness statements after the fact.

Sometimes, the forensic psychiatrist is asked to examine an individual who is scheduled to be a witness, either in a criminal or a civil trial. The witness may not be competent to testify. Some of the reasons the witness may not be competent is because of mental illness, alcoholism, drug addiction, or mental retardation. He or she may also have a condition known as "pathological liar", in which he or she is unable to tell the truth or distinguish between truth and falsehood. The assessment of competency of children in sexual assault or incest cases is also fraught with the difficulty of the ability of the child to understand the situation and his or her need to be truthful. In those cases, it is strongly recommended that a child psychiatrist be involved because of the complexity of the assessment and determination.

Criminal Matters

"Insanity" is a legal, not a psychiatric, term. Legally, it means "not responsible", i.e., that the defendant was unable to form the legally required intent (mens rea) to commit the crime. It is defined differently in various jurisdictions, and may be defined as "unable to differentiate between right and wrong", "unable to conform to the requirements of the law", or "lack the capacity to comprehend or to control a specific criminal behavior" as a result of mental illness. Alcoholism, intoxication, or drug abuse are not regarded as "mental illness" in this context, and are not accepted as psychiatric defenses to a crime.

Alcoholism is defined by the Veterans Administration as "willful behavior" for the purpose of denying benefits, but as an "illness" for the purpose of providing treatment.

The defendant may be evaluated at any stage of the criminal process, beginning with the early investigative stage, and the determination of the competency of the defendant to have made a confession to the police. Confessions may be determined invalid if the defendant did not understand or could not understand the *Miranda* warnings given by the police. He or she may be mentally retarded and did not understand the words. He or she may be so psychotic that he or she cannot focus on the meaning of the words. He or she may be withdrawing from drugs or under the influence of alcohol, so that he or she is easily influenced by the interrogators and would say whatever was felt they wanted him or her to say, in order to get relief from his or her medical condition. Very few statements are ever thrown out of court, but there are some that are legitimately discarded because the defendant was not competent to give the statement taken by the police.

Perhaps the most important consideration in criminal cases is that of competency to stand trial. In order to be competent to stand trial, a defendant must know the nature and consequences of his or her legal situation and be able to work with his or her attorney in preparing a defense. If the individual cannot work with the attorney in preparing a defense because he or she is excessively paranoid or psychotic and does not trust the attorney, he or she may not be competent. If the individual is so delusional about the charges against him or her that he or she cannot fully appreciate them or discuss them with the attorney in a rational way, he or she may not be competent. Most individuals in these circumstances are sent to forensic psychiatric hospitals where they are treated, and most then become competent. If, after several years of treatment, the defendant does not improve or become competent, the law has declared, in the case of *Jackson v. Indiana* in

1972, that he or she would then be converted to a civil case for treatment in a regular mental hospital until he or she is improved sufficiently to be discharged. The charges against the individual will then be suspended.

Criminal responsibility is one of the major issues in criminal cases where psychiatrists may be involved. The determination of insanity varies from jurisdiction to jurisdiction. In most states, the determination is fairly similiar; i.e., at the time of the commission of the crime, was the defendant suffering from a mental illness so that he or she did not know the nature and quality of the act, or he or she did not know what he or she was doing was wrong. This is the so-called *M'Naghten* test of insanity. Many people are mentally ill or psychotic at the time of the commission of the crime. However, very few are so mentally ill that they do not know what they are doing, or do not know what they have done is wrong. In some jurisdictions, the volitional test of the defendant to control his or her behavior is in effect. That is, if the individual knew what he or she was doing and knew that it was wrong, but could not keep from doing the act because of his or her mental illness, he or she may be found legally insane. It should be noted that the use of the term "insanity" is restricted to legal concepts, rather than medical ones, in this century. Formerly, the mentally ill were called "insane", but currently, the use of the word "insane" refers to a legal finding, rather than a medical condition. This distinction is important. Alcoholism and drug intoxication are not regarded as "mental illnesses" in the context of insanity cases and are not usually accepted as psychiatric defenses to a crime, except to mitigate the level of criminal behavior. This is often known as diminished capacity, but not insanity.

Since the *Hinckley* case, a number of states have adopted a verdict of guilty, but mentally ill. This verdict is designed for those severely mentally ill individuals, who are not found legally insane, and yet, who do have a mental illness that requires treatment. This verdict mandates treatment in a mental hospital until the person is significantly improved, and then able to serve the remainder of his or her sentence in a correctional facility.

The forensic psychiatrist also gives recommendations on the disposition of cases. In juvenile cases, he or she may give an option to the court about whether the juvenile should be waived to adult court or remain in juvenile court. The determination depends upon the nature of the illness of the juvenile and his or her ability to be treated effectively within a particular number of years, or until the age of 19 or 21, depending on the jurisdiction. In adult cases, the psychiatrist may give a recommendation for treatment in a hospital, special treatment for sex offenders, or treatment of alcoholics and drug addicts in special facilities. The psychiatrist may recommend probation under certain circumstances, especially where outpatient treatment is required.

In death penalty cases, psychiatrists have testified regarding the dangerousness of the individual and his or her likelihood of committing further crimes. In some cases, especially in Texas, this testimony has led to the death penalty. In other jurisdictions, psychiatrists may testify to "mitigating circumstances", which may lead to life imprisonment, rather than the death penalty. Finally, psychiatrists have examined individuals on death row, and in some cases, have determined that they were mentally ill and incompetent to be executed. The ethical question has arisen as to whether the psychiatrist should treat a death row inmate who is mentally ill and incompetent so that he may improve and, therefore, become competent and then be executed.

In summary, the forensic psychiatrist deals with individuals who are involved in legal matters, either civil or criminal. Forensic psychiatry is a sub-specialty of psychiatry, with special training programs and Board-certification from the

American Board of Psychiatry. The field has become so complex and sub-specialized that it is recommended that in the cases enumerated above, involving patients' rights, commitment procedures, and civil or criminal cases where mental illness is involved, the psychiatrist have forensic training. The field has grown significantly in the past 20 years, and there are now well over 200 Board-certified forensic psychiatrists, and over 1,200 psychiatrists who belong to the American Academy of Psychiatry and The Law. There are several specialized training programs throughout the country, and increasingly, courses given at the American Psychiatric Association meetings and other national conventions include issues of forensic psychiatry.

Malpractice

Psychiatric patients most commonly become the source of malpractice actions, if and when they injure themselves or others. Psychiatrists may also be found liable for damages if a patient injures him or herself, commits suicide, injures another, elopes, or proves "false imprisonment" (treatment in the absence of an informed consent), or sexual abuse. Clinicians should also take the appropriate steps to avoid such allegations. At all times, they should use good clinical judgment, and always carefully and fully document the risks and the benefits of any order for treatment, a pass, a visit, or a discharge.

In psychiatry, the most common reasons for malpractice include improper diagnosis and treatment, suicide, violence to others, mishandling the transference (sexual exploitation of the patient), and violation of the patient's rights.

PULMONARY MEDICINE

Introduction

The practice of pulmonary medicine, whether invasive or not, is beset with perils and pitfalls that must be guarded against. This discussion will emphasize those situations which are most perilous to the physician from a medicolegal standpoint. Medicolegal problems are more often related to office practice, procedures performed by a pulmonologist, lung cancer, and chest disease.

Diagnostic Errors

Lawsuits that are practice-related involve:
- Incorrect diagnosis.
- Inadequate explanation of reasons for and results of examination.
- Failure to identify and explain any procedures planned or considered and the reasons for doing them (lack of informed consent).
- Medication-related side effects, particularly when not anticipated - usually iatrogenic.
- Adverse outcome, especially in the face of inflated expectations not realistically addressed.
- Failure to perform an adequate, timely evaluation.
- Failure to seek consultation or refer a patient, particularly in light of better results from a second pulmonologist.
- Failure to report to the referring physician concerning the various procedures performed by the pulmonologist.

Thoracentesis and pleural biopsy are particularly perilous. Medicolegal problems arise because of:
- A complicating pneumothorax; unbearable pain; bleeding; "pleural shock"; or failure to obtain fluid or an adequate specimen for laboratory diagnosis.

Arterial puncture and arterial line insertion are a peril when they result in:
- Bleeding; hematoma; pain; or brachial and radial nerve injury.

Swan-Ganz catheter insertion is fraught with medicolegal consequences when there is:
- Perforation of the vessels with mediastinal bleeding or bleeding from the insertion site; occlusion of vessels by catheter curling; or the improper interpretation of pressure and pulse studies, which almost always inevitably result in a medicolegal situation.

The insertion of a chest tube (closed thoracotomy) unfortunately may result in:
- Pneumothorax.
- Bleeding.
- Inexorable pain.

Improper placement of the tube, even without any injury, and certainly if injury results, is followed by legal action.

Bronchoscopy can be beset by medical problems, often followed by legal

concerns. These include:
- Inadequate oxygen supply during the procedure.
- Severe laryngospasm, necessitating intubation or emergency tracheostomy.
- Bleeding from biopsy sites, particularly in transbronchial biopsies.
- Occlusion of left main bronchus by improper placement of the bronchoscope, resulting in atelectasis of the left lung.
- Pneumothorax.
- Bacterial contamination of instruments causing pulmonary disease (infection).
- Transmission of infection from patient to patient, or to other physicians or assistants, following a procedure-induced infection.
- Failure to find a lesion noted on x-ray and biopsying the wrong area.

Although pulmonary function tests may result in a benign diagnosis, legal problems may arise when the studies are not performed when indicated, and/or the results are improperly interpreted. Also, failure to inform the patient, the family, and/or the referring physician of the results, depending on the circumstances, frequently turns out to be a pitfall.

Solitary Pulmonary Nodules

The solitary pulmonary nodule may be a peril for both the patient and the physician. A solitary pulmonary nodule is an intrapulmonary lesion that is spherical in contour and has fairly well-demarcated margins in all projections. Nodules often show up as unexpected findings on a routine chest x-ray. Although nodules less than 8 mm. in diameter are almost always benign, 45% of all nodules are found to be malignant at surgery. Therefore, in the presence of a pulmonary nodule, computed axial tomography and needle aspiration biopsy are critical to the workup of lung nodules. The growth rate is also important in differentiating benign from malignant nodes. Seventeen percent of patients who undergo surgery for a lung carcinoma will later develop a secondary primary lesion.

Patients with suspected lung cancer who have normal chest x-rays and positive sputum cytologies are potential medicolegal problems. They should have a thorough nasopharyngoscopy and bronchoscopy performed. Bronchoscopy has the advantage of visualizing the larynx, vocal cords, and the main stem bronchi. At the same time, a tissue diagnosis is possible. The disadvantage of bronchoscopy is that the yield gets less as the lesion gets smaller and smaller. If the carcinoma is not found in the chest, it is almost always found in the head or neck.

Thin needle biopsy, using either fluoroscopy or computed axial tomography, is very valuable. The procedure is easy to do with the proviso that one knows the segmental anatomy of the lung. The yield is over 90% of positive biopsies, and this is an advantage over bronchoscopy in that even as the lesion gets smaller, a positive biopsy is possible. In some cases, mediastinoscopy will provide a diagnosis and a stage for a lung carcinoma without doing a formal thoracotomy. The final diagnostic modality is a formal thoracotomy.

Informed Consent

Underlying most of the lawsuits involving this specialty is the lack of informed consent, either as the principal cause of action or as a secondary factor. All of the pertinent perils and pitfalls must be made clear to the patient or next-of-kin before the process or procedure is undertaken.

Any unexpected outcome should be fully and frankly explained to the patient and/or next-of-kin.

Competence of Physician

Because of the complex, multifaceted situation involving chest disease, including trauma, one of the first decisions the physician must make is whether he is capable of and competent to treat the patient. This is a judgment each physician must make for himself, although later, this judgment may be called into question. The law does not state that the physician must be a pulmonologist, trauma specialist, chest surgeon, or even have specific qualifications, expertise, and training, except as set up by the medical profession itself. If the physician believes he is competent by training and experience according to these medical standards, the law supports his professional right to proceed.

Often, the critical question is: "Was there a failure to do an act that was necessary for the protection of the patient?" If the physician did not possess the knowledge and skill ordinarily used in like situations, he may be liable. In a thoracic trauma case, the question is: "Does the physician have the expertise to properly manage the patient?"

Consultation and Referral

If the physician has questionable expertise, then he should refer the patient to a physician with the necessary expertise, or seek consultation, depending on the circumstances. This is a duty that may have legal consequences for the physician if he ignores his need for help, and the patient suffers harm. This includes the duty to know when help is needed and who can best supply it.

The failure of a physician to refer to another physician or specialist for a suspected disease, such as cancer, may also be a negligent act of omission. Generally, because of the imposing consequences of treatment, for example, if chemotherapy or radiotherapy is proposed, the patient should be afforded the benefit of a consultation to assure adequate exposure to alternative modalities. This is one of the most effective ways to avoid a later allegation of undue influence or pressure. Once the offer of a consultation or second opinion is recorded in the chart, there is significantly less chance for a patient to allege he or she was railroaded into a particular cause of action.

Keeping Abreast - Keeping Up

The law and medicine have imposed a duty on all physicians to be aware of changing concepts and new developments. It is not the physician's duty to implement new techniques merely because they are new; usefulness must be reasonably established. What may be accepted as the most advanced practice of pulmonary and trauma medicine, as well as surgery, one time in a physician's career may be swiftly outdated by new discoveries and advances, and it is his obligation to render treatment to his patients based on adequate understanding of those new developments. But a specialist who is ignorant of the recent developments that are known to, and accepted by, the profession may be liable if the use of an outmoded method results in harm to the patient. Although adherence to the usual practice by which the local medical community deals with a problem is ordinarily a good defense to a charge of negligence, "everybody does it" is not an excuse if it is, in fact, a sloppy or careless practice, or contrary to national standards.

Protecting The Patient's Legal Status

If the pulmonary disease or thoracic trauma is due to an accident, the physician has the duty to acquire information that will help determine the causal relationship of the event to the trauma or injury to the patient, whether it be a workers' compensation situation, an environmental accident, or personal injury. The physician has the duty to acquire and preserve all the facts to protect the patient's legal status. Documentation and record keeping are necessary to comply with the requirement that the patient be protected in any claim for compensation as a result of chest trauma or pulmonary disease.

Successive Tortfeasor

The physician is also faced with the specter of being a successive tortfeasor. Under the law, the initial wrongdoer is usually responsible for all damages to the victim, including losses due to negligent medical care. However, the original wrongdoer is entitled to seek indemnification from a negligent physician for the amount of damages caused by the negligence, even though the victim selected the physician.

Medicolegal Issues In Lung Cancer

The oncology patient in general, and the lung cancer patient in particular, presents specific medical and surgical, as well as legal problems for the physician. Lawsuits primarily involve misdiagnosis or, more often, late diagnosis. Patient-plaintiffs alleging misdiagnosis are basically complaining of a "loss of a chance". Almost always, there is the question of whether the misdiagnosis caused the patient's injury to a reasonable medical certainty or probability, or whether the natural course of events was unchanged.

Loss Of A Chance

Loss of a chance caused by the negligence of another, a physician, has been recognized in lawsuits. The question of how to weigh diminished prospects for a patient-plaintiff whose statistical future expectations are already severely impaired has caused many courts to re-examine the issue: "Should liability be imposed for negligence that merely increased the probability of an already probable negative outcome?"

The majority of U.S. jurisdictions retain the "but for" test; that is, a negligently injured patient must prove that the chance for recovery or survival was probable, was more likely than not, or was better than even. The rationale for this all-or-nothing approach is that less-than probable losses are speculative and unfairly impose liability based on unquantified possibilities. The majority position is that what the measure "might have caused" is an insufficient quantum of evidence.

Medicolegal issues in lung cancer relate mainly to:
• Failure to diagnose lung cancer.
• Wrongful death during a diagnostic procedure or surgery.
• Pathologic misdiagnosis.

- Fruitless thoracotomy.
- Occupational carcinomas, the latest being radon.
- Unproven and quack therapies for cancer; for example, Laetrile.
- Informed consent issues.

Lung cancer is a complex, multifaceted disease. Liability in treating this disease occurs mainly from a failure to diagnose. Physicians can protect themselves by adhering to strict procedures for diagnosis, referral, and treatment.

Diagnosis

The diagnosis of lung cancer is fairly straightforward. One of the reasons that lung cancers are missed is because of a lack of a strong degree of suspicion, and the lack of periodic x-rays and sputum cytologies, as well as airflow studies. The diagnosis rests upon a complete history, a detailed physical examination, and chest x-rays. These are supplemented by computed axial tomography and bronchoscopy (rigid or flexible).

The medical history is an important part of the diagnostic workup of cancer. The failure to appropriately consider the history may be negligent. Family and racial history, particularly in certain cancers, is an important criterion in evaluating patients for cancer screening, as well as for obtaining the proper, indicated tests in certain symptomatic patients.

Physical Examination

Failure to perform a physical examination, performing an inadequate examination, over-reliance on a negative examination, or failure to perform a follow-up examination may contribute to lawsuits for failure to diagnose cancer. Failure to perform an examination, particularly when there is a significant symptom found, figures prominently in many failures to diagnose cancer cases, as does failure to perform follow-up examinations.

Testing

A physician has an affirmative duty to obtain or perform appropriate tests in the diagnosis of a suspected cancer. Failure to appropriately or properly test, resulting in injury, is very likely to impose liability. However, ordering a test in lieu of a physical examination will not necessarily protect the physician. On the other hand, an error in the evaluation of a test which results in a serious or unnecessary operation, or an incorrect diagnosis that an inoperable malignancy exists, also virtually guarantees large damages for the patient-plaintiff. There usually are serious physical and emotional consequences to the patient after being told incorrectly that a cancer is present. Although presumably it is better to diagnose a malignancy that does not exist than it is to fail to discover one that actually does exist, in either case the patient undoubtedly has been harmed by the error.

A physician may also be likely to be found negligent if he performs radical surgery for a suspected malignancy without ordering appropriate tests first, except in an emergency situation. If his opinion is wrong and the surgery later proves to have been unnecessary, he will undoubtedly be found negligent. In an emergency situation, misdiagnosis that leads to the conclusion that surgery is not required may also result in liability.

Various tests also may be necessary in some cases to make a proper diagnosis, including those that are invasive. Where the test carries a serious inherent risk, it becomes a matter of medical judgment whether or not the patient, whose condition is best known by the physician, should be subjected to the procedure. Therefore, the more complicated and dangerous the test may be, the less likely it is that a court will find that a physician was negligent in failing to perform it. If, however, the patient's condition is serious, a physician would be much more likely be held liable, particularly if the condition was no more serious, at worst, than the test itself.

Even where a report is negative, over-reliance on that report may be negligent when clinical suspicion should be high. Mere reliance on a test performed by a consultant does not always mean negligence, however. Failure of a physician to read the test report or consultant's recommendations, or communicate the report or recommendations to the patient, may be negligent. Failure to repeat a test or perform additional studies when an initial test is negative may be negligent when clinical suspicion is, or should be, high that cancer may still be present. Negligence during the performance of a test that damages the patient, apart from the accuracy of the report, may impose liability.

Standard Of Care

A physician should also be mindful of the fact that university centers may treat cancer patients as part of a study. Such treatment will not necessarily coincide with that which is recognized and accepted as the standard of care for cancer patients outside of the study. Ultimately, the standard of care is best defined as that care exercised by the majority of reasonably prudent medical specialists treating cancer patients with the same or similar type of cancer. Generally, the standard of care will be that standard that is practiced by the reasonably prudent physician practicing nationwide for a patient in like or similar circumstances. The "locality rule" in determining the standard of care has been abandoned. This is particularly true in areas of medical specialty such as cancer; a physician's care will not be compared just with other physicians in the immediate community. The failure to diagnose cancer or a delay in the diagnosis of cancer can be devastating to a patient and the family. It may result in a patient having to undergo more extensive treatment, reduce his or her chances of survival, lead to earlier or unnecessary death, and cause physical and emotional burdens that more timely diagnosis could have avoided. Liability may be based on a physician's own negligent action or inaction, or both.

Failure to follow recommended protocols may be the basis for an allegation of negligence. The American Cancer Society and various professional specialty organizations have for a number of years published guidelines for physicians suggesting schedules or protocols for early cancer detection. Although not legally binding in any way, these recommendations are widely disseminated via the mass media and are common public knowledge.

Failure to follow these protocols is not necessarily evidence of negligent failure to diagnose cancer. In fact, many practicing physicians do not follow these protocols, either due to ignorance or because they disagree with the guidelines. However, the success of the American Cancer Society's educational program emphasizing the importance of early cancer detection may make a delay in diagnosis more difficult to defend.

Treatment

There are also legal actions involving proper treatment. Chemotherapy is fraught with complications. For oncology patients, informed consent, or informed refusal if care and management are refused, are very important. The physician may choose to use therapeutic professional discretion to keep medical facts from the patient when the physician believes disclosure would be harmful, dangerous, or injurious to the patient. The use of radiation therapy is frequently the source of medicolegal problems. Basic to the resolution of these problems are invoking risk-benefit judgment, comparing the anticipated benefits from therapy with its risks, and weighing the consequences of no treatment.

Unorthodox Cancer Treatment

Because patients with cancer are often desperate, a physician must address the legal consequences of administering unorthodox treatment, particularly if the patient insists upon it. Cancer victims, particularly those who are terminally ill, are vulnerable to exploitation because of their predicament. Desperate for any glimmer of hope, they are easy prey for charlatans and their insatiably greedy intent on financial gain. Traditionally, the law has protected those unable to protect themselves, most frequently applied to juveniles and the mentally ill, on the basis of parens patriae.

However, the state's interest in protecting its citizens must be balanced against an individual's right to have control over his or her body and to make decisions regarding his or her medical care. Most cancer patients are adults in full control of their mental faculties, which distinguishes them from other citizens the state seeks to protect under the parens patriae rationale.

It is this basic conflict between the state's interest in the health and welfare of its citizens and the right of individuals to make decisions affecting their health that has confronted legislatures and courts attempting to deal with the problem of unorthodox cancer treatment.

This conflict has not been resolved uniformly; considerable variations presently exist among the various states with regard to unorthodox cancer treatment. Interestingly, where there has been legislative action, most legislatures have granted the individual a measure of freedom in selecting cancer treatment that is unproven. In most states that have acted legislatively, this freedom is not unlimited. When courts have considered the subject of unorthodox cancer treatment, they have focused more on the state's right to regulate the lives of its citizens under police power.

Many of the states that require a licensed physician's prescription for unorthodox treatment also require that the patient first sign a consent form indicating that the physician has explained that the treatment has not been proven to be effective in the treatment of cancer, has not been approved by the Food and Drug Administration for the treatment of cancer, that alternative therapies exist, and that the patient requests treatment with that medication.

Several states have attempted to maintain a precarious balance between its so-called police power and individual rights by reserving the right to prohibit unconventional cancer treatment when it is found to be harmful (as prescribed or administered) in a formal hearing before the appropriate state board.

The most sweeping exercise of police power has been enacted in California, where it is a crime to sell, deliver, prescribe, or administer any drug or device to be used in the diagnosis, treatment, alleviation, or cure of cancer that has not been approved by the designated federal agency or by the state board. The statute has been upheld by the California Supreme Court against a constitutional challenge based upon the right of privacy.

It appears that when a competent cancer patient, or the next-of-kin for an incompetent patient, decides to receive unorthodox treatment, his or her only legal protection is that all information was given, and if it was not, then he or she can sue for lack of informed consent.

The balance weighs heavily in favor of allowing cancer patients to obtain the treatment of their choice. The state's interest in protecting the health of its citizens can be adequately protected in this context by requiring an informed consent by the patient following disclosure of the nature of the proposed treatment.

Non-Compliance

Lesser legal problems involve a patient's failure to comply. It often becomes necessary to invoke as a defense a patient's contributing or comparative negligence; adequate and proper documentation may be the difference between success and failure.

RADIOLOGY

Introduction

Radiology can be considered as a clearing house of diagnosis in the hospital. In this arena, the paths of many clinicians cross; the tests accomplished range from simple chest x-rays to complex interventional techniques involving anesthesia, contrast agents, and instrumentation with various invasive procedures.

The events of medicolegal interest and importance that can happen include:
• Diagnostic error.
• Ordinary falls, inattention to patients, excessive waiting, and other such mundane activities that can occur anywhere in the hospital (particularly at night when transport teams and technicians are short-staffed or at dinner).
• Idiosyncratic reactions to particular pharmaceuticals and chemicals, e.g., various contrast agents used for intravenous and intra-arterial injections, as well as other body cavities such as joint, pleural and peritoneal, and cerebral spinal fluid spaces.
• Complications from specific procedures, e.g., pneumothorax from biopsy with lung needles, hemorrhage from liver aspirations, thrombosis from vessel manipulations, etc. These complications can include those that are largely unavoidable, depending on the inherent hazard or urgency of the procedure, or those due to the negligence of the physicians, nurses, and technicians involved, viz., improper performance of the procedure itself, or inadequate preparation of the patient for the procedure.
• Failure to obtain adequate informed consent from the patient to the procedure; and other forms of poor record-keeping, including, in particular, delayed transmission of important information.

Practice Patterns

The practice patterns of diagnostic radiologists tend to be quite different from those of most other physicians. In general, radiologists spend most of their time studying radiographs of patients with various diseases. They observe abnormalities on the radiograph, place these abnormalities into a framework of disease processes which are known to have similar radiographic changes, and then try to narrow the list down to one or two most likely choices. These choices are then transmitted to the referring physician for application to the patient's disease process. This chain of events contains many possibilities for error, which may lead to medical malpractice litigation.

Missed Diagnoses

According to a published series, 64 to 85% of malpractice actions against radiologists arise because the radiologist has failed to see an abnormality on the radiograph. This is called observer error. Although not generally recognized, observer error is an endemic problem in radiology. Various studies have shown that radiologists, even those who are well-trained and experienced, routinely miss as many as 10 to 20% of radiographic abnormalities. Therefore, a radiologist's conduct does not necessarily fall below the standard of care of the radiological community, simply because he or she fails to observe an abnormality. Whether the alleged missed abnormal finding does, in fact, constitute negligence depends on the nature of the finding and how subtle or obvious it is. For example, there is a major difference between missing a small breast carcinoma in an area of fibrocystic disease and missing a large lytic metastasis to the ilium. As with most instances of alleged negligence, the question of standard of care will be resolved by the jury with the help of expert witnesses. Many times, it will depend on the results of the missed diagnosis, i.e., damage or harm to the patient.

Mistake or Error in Judgment v. Carelessness

At the same time, the question of negligence depends to some degree upon how much the alleged breach of the standard of care was a simple failure to see a lesion, or how much was related to the radiologist's medical judgment. The former type of error is more difficult to defend against because the plaintiff's attorney has the radiograph and can point out the missed abnormality to the jury. If the jury can see a lung nodule, for instance, they have a hard time understanding why a well-trained radiologist should not have seen it as well. On the other hand, the greater the medical judgment involved in the interpretation of an abnormality, the more the error becomes like analogous judgmental errors in other areas of medicine.

Injury Due to Procedure

Most of the remaining 15 to 34% of malpractice actions against radiologists allege that the radiologist negligently injured a patient while performing a special procedure. Such suits frequently involve large claims for damages because the complications, particularly paralysis, have such high medical costs associated with them. Suits which arise from patient injuries frequently allege that the radiologist performed a procedure beyond his or her level of training and expertise, failed to obtain adequate informed consent, inadequately supervised technicians and nurses during the performance of the procedure, failed to anticipate and be prepared for recognized complications, failed to recognize a complication when it occurred, failed to get adequate assistance from anesthesiologists, "Code-Blue" teams, etc., and failed to treat the complication appropriately until help arrived. In fact, most suits arising out of complications of special procedures allege many of these breaches of duty. Therefore, any risk management program in radiology should focus on these areas, and protocols should be prepared to try to prevent them.

Record-Keeping

Poor record-keeping is a problem in many cases alleging inadequate treatment of complications of angiography. Radiologists are not as accustomed to record-keeping as other physicians, and documentation in the patient's chart of what occurred, when it was recognized, and what the radiologist did to help the patient is often inadequate. In fact, inadequate record-keeping is one of the most common reasons an otherwise defensible medical malpractice lawsuit is lost.

Radiologists must become more attuned to making timely, legible, pertinent, and adequate entries in the patient's medical record.

Safety Hazards

Other malpractice problems in diagnostic radiology relate to "slips and falls" in the department and transmission of radiological information. An ongoing program of radiological risk management is important to identify patient safety hazards within the department in a prospective manner and correct them before injuries occur; this is required by the Joint Commission on the Accreditation of Health Care Organizations (JCAHO). Even with such programs, however, it is impressive how many patients fall from stretchers and x-ray tables in radiology departments. Frequently, such problems are corrected by very simple means; for example, using rubber-soled slippers to give patients more traction on the floor as they step off the x-ray table.

Communication

The radiologist has a duty to transmit radiological information to the referring physician in a manner reasonably designed to make the referring physician aware of the patient's radiological diagnosis in a timely manner. Timeliness, of course, varies, depending upon the severity of the abnormality. Too often, however, patients have emergent or urgent conditions, such as bowel perforation, a fracture, or an unsuspected cancer, and the radiologist uses the same means of transmission of the clinical information to the physician as he or she might use to report a finding of minimal significance. Patients have frequently sued a radiologist successfully for failing to make the referring clinician aware that a need exists to act promptly in regard to the patient's care. This is particularly true in the emergency room and during "off" hours.

If the radiologist is not certain that the patient has a treating physician who will be reviewing the X-ray report in timely fashion, and there is a potentially serious or significant disease process demonstrated in the radiology procedure, some courts have recently held that the radiologist may have a duty to alert the patient to those findings.

Non-Radiologists Practicing Radiology

An interesting question that arises about the legal liability of non-radiologists who practice radiology relates to the acceptable standard of care. Is the standard of care expected of such a physician that of a radiologist or that of a non-radiologist? There are many different levels of expertise that physicians can hold themselves out to possess, and they will be held to the standard of care appropriate for the level that they practice. There is only one standard of care for the practice of radiology, whether it be practiced by a radiologist, orthopedist, urologist, or family practitioner. Therefore, at a trial for negligence in interpreting a radiograph, a family practitioner may expect to find the plaintiff's expert witness to be a radiologist, and a radiologist on trial for medical negligence may find the plaintiff's expert to be a family practitioner who has had a great deal of experience in interpreting radiographs. Thus, it is clearly in the best interests of patients that all persons who interpret radiographs have adequate skill, training, and experience to do so safely and competently.

The Future

As radiologists develop new imaging technologies and become more active in intravascular percutaneous therapies, their medical liability exposure will increase. All groups involved in monitoring the care provided by physicians and hospitals will progressively insist on the institution of adequate retrospective and prospective risk management programs. All physicians who practice radiology should eagerly participate with the hospital in trying to find ways to decrease patient injuries.

Admonition

Many malpractice suits are frequently instigated by what the patient perceives to be indecent handling by hospital personnel. Such events seem to serve as a trigger for the lawsuit, which then is pursued based on some alleged negligence. Management of patients is often as important as the radiological procedure.

Radiation Oncology
Determination of Indication for Treatment

Radiation oncology is a method of approach to patients, wherein consultation and treatment of cancer is the main modus operandi. The in-patient visits the department, usually on referral from primary care physicians or from various specialty groups. Many of these patients are either desperately ill, or are in the midst of a staging workup to assess the extent of the cancer, following initial procedures which have led to the diagnosis of neoplasia. The radiotherapist evaluates the patient, determines whether cure or palliation is the goal - or indeed, whether no treatment is to be employed - and sets about arranging for and carrying out further planned diagnostic procedures (such as simulation and computerized treatment planning scans) if irradiation is to be used.

In a Radiation Oncology Department, medicolegal problems can arise from:
• Ordinary errors common to all hospital personnel, e.g., overdosage with appropriate drugs or administration of inapproriate drugs. Patients can be neglected while in the department and suffer injury common to all hospital areas.
• Erroneous prescriptions or delivery of ionizing radiation to the patient. This can be due to human error or to equipment failure, the latter often traceable to human failings of improper calibration or checking of machinery. These problems, however, do not impinge upon the house officer in the ordinary course of events.
• Patient reactions due to the joint use of radiation and other forms of treatment such as chemotherapy too soon after surgery, or an operation too radical for the amount of irradiation needed. In like fashion, chemotherapy concurrent with or following irradiation may lead to complications, unless one or both modalities undergo a modification of dosage.

Radiotherapists often work closely with medical oncologists. The knowledge of which specific chemotherapeutic agents are to be used, their mode of application, and dosages given can be of great importance to the well-being of the cancer patient. The total doses of Adriamycin, for example, that the patient has had in the past may not only determine whether that particular drug can be used again, but may modify the radiation portals, as well as the daily and total doses to be given. A patient who has had moderate to severe chronic obstructive pulmonary disease or Bleomycin or Cytoxan will probably not tolerate doses of irradiation to lung parenchyma which, under other circumstances, would be within acceptable limits.

- Inadequate informed consent is a source of litigation. Radiotherapists may admit patients either on their own service or on those of the other treating physicians. When the cooperating service has the patient in tow, the appropriate resident may be working up and writing orders on patients who are currently receiving therapy, or who have had irradiation given in the past. Such house staff should check closely with their opposite numbers on the Radiation Oncology Service to be certain that the orders are appropriate. Informed consent should be left to the members of the Radiation Oncology Department where brachytherapy (use of radiation sources within the patient's body) is the prime reason for admission. All of the requirements of informed consent must be met.

II.
SURGICAL

ANESTHESIOLOGY

General Considerations

The following are basic concepts that all physicians should keep in mind regarding the practice of anesthesia.

Do not attempt to administer any anesthetic unless you have undergone adequate training in monitoring, resuscitation, and the use of the contemplated agent and technique, or you have continuous, over-the-shoulder supervision by an instructor.

Insist on a thorough equipment check before beginning anesthetic administration, and make certain that all drugs which might be needed are at hand.

Once anesthetic administration has begun, do not leave the patient unless your relief is at least equally competent.

Make an accurate, complete, concurrent record of all activities and observations pertinent to the anesthetic.

Do not, under any circumstances, alter the record. While it is acceptable at a later time to make entries referring back to the anesthetic to attempt to correct errors in the record or to elaborate, it is usually unwise to do so.

Should an untoward complication occur, whether apparent or real, whether major or minor, do not develop an ostrich attitude. Continue to follow the patient closely and frequently. Make appropriate notes in the record. If studies might time the severity or onset of a particular complication, such as sequential electromyography in the case of nerve dysfunction or paralysis, arrange to have appropriate tests performed. If the patient expires, make every effort to obtain a complete autopsy.

Pre-Operative Evaluation, Preparation, and Informed Consent

In the United States, anesthesia is administered by physicians who may be allopathic (M.D.) or osteopathic (D.O.). These physicians may have undergone residency training and have received certification after passing examinations. However, while it is the state that awards a license to practice medicine, it is the responsibility of each institution in which the physician seeks privileges to evaluate the credentials of the anesthesiologist, since the practice of anesthesia is generally hospital-based. Anesthesia may also be administered by dentists. By regulation or statute, except in training, they are usually limited to the administration of anesthesia in connection with dental procedures performed in the office setting. Anesthesia is also administered by nurses who may have undergone training and passed examinations, culminating in the designation of a Certified Registered Nurse Anesthetist (CRNA). Since the administration of anesthesia in all states is considered to be the practice of medicine, nurses may administer anesthesia under the supervision and authority of a physician who may not have had any special training in anesthesia. In some states, such as Ohio and Colorado, anesthesia may also be administered under the supervision of a physician by Physician Assistants (PA).

Responsibilities

Ideally, the functions outlined below should be carried out by the person actually administering the anesthetic.

The three responsibilities of the person administering anesthesia are grouped together, because they are usually carried out at the same time for elective surgery on the night before the scheduled operation.

Pre-operative evaluation as a minimum requires review of the admitting history, physical examination, and pertinent laboratory studies. The anesthetist should also take an independent history. This history must include details of the medical experience of blood relatives, such as an unexplained death after anesthesia, which may be a clue that the patient might be susceptible to malignant hyperthermia. Details of the patient's reactions to all previous anesthetics, whether general, conduction, block, or local, must be elicited. All previous hospitalizations should be considered, since these will be most important in learning the medical conditions from which the patient may be suffering. The patient must be closely questioned regarding medications and drugs, especially over-the-counter drugs such as aspirin. A rapid weight loss regimen may have resulted in electrolyte imbalance, particularly hypokalemia. Although allergy to anesthetic agents, with the exception of the locals, has never been proven, such an inquiry should be made. If the patient claims to be allergic to one agent or another, accept the statement at face value and avoid that agent. Often, the patient will indicate an allergy to procaine or one of the other esters used as local agents, in which case an amide such as lidocaine may be administered.

The anesthesiologist should perform some physical examination. In particular, the teeth should be carefully inspected for chips, and they should be tested for looseness. The ease or difficulty of endotracheal intubation should be determined. If relevant, the heart and lungs should be examined. The skin should be examined for infection, especially if conduction or block anesthesia is contemplated. The anesthetist should verify which side is to be operated on in the case of hernias and extremity surgery.

The goal is to have the patient in the best possible condition before elective surgery. Should more studies be required or more preparation be necessary, the anesthetist, after having gone through the above drill, should know and advise the patient's responsible physician accordingly. It is this function that presumably differentiates the physician from the technician, since endotracheal intubation, insertion of spinal needles, and other technical tasks should be performed equally well by nurses or physicians.

The patient's consent must be obtained. Consent requires that the patient be told in language that he or she can understand what the proposed anesthetic is, the material risks of the proposed anesthetic, what alternative anesthetic agents or techniques are available, what the material risks are of the alternative methods as compared to the contemplated preferred technique, and who is actually going to administer the anesthetic. Not relevant to anesthesia, but required of the surgeon, is a discussion of the possible course if the surgical procedure is not performed. In the case of minors, consent must be obtained from the responsible parent or guardian. In the case of obtunded patients or severe emergencies, consent is usually implied. Special problems such as refusal of blood and blood products by Jehovah's Witnesses must be respected, and may only be overridden by a court order, in non-emergency situations. All of the above must be recorded in the hospital chart.

The Airway and Ventilation

Failure to continuously provide adequate alveolar oxygen is the cause of most major anesthesia-related damage. During administration of anesthesia, the anesthetist must maintain a patent airway into the trachea and provide an adequate inspired oxygen concentration, except, of course, during cardiopulmonary bypass. While in the supine position, as the patient is rendered unconscious by the anesthetic drugs, the tongue will fall back and tend to occlude the upper airway. Some drugs will precipitate laryngospasm. Regurgitation of gastric contents may also cause laryngospasm, as will premature instrumentation of the pharynx and larynx. Patients with a compromised airway due to tumor or infection demand the highest skill when anesthesia is induced.

In order to ensure adequate alveolar oxygenation, not only must the airway be patent, but also adequate concentrations of oxygen must be delivered to the alveoli. The anesthesiologist controls the concentration of oxygen delivered to the patient. While the 20 to 21% present in the atmosphere is more than sufficient for a healthy individual, it is the custom to deliver supplemental oxygen, even to patients under spinal anesthesia. Many anesthetic drugs depress the respiratory drive, while muscle relaxants both paralyze the diaphragm and relax the tongue. Before the administration of any anesthetic drug, all equipment which might be required to establish an airway and to deliver 100% oxygen must be at hand.

In the unconscious, supine patient, the airway can be maintained by holding the mentum forward and cephalad. This maneuver will open the pharyngeal air passage by bringing the tongue forward since it is attached to the mandible. In laryngospasm, the epiglottis closes over the glottis and the mentum forward maneuver will even break laryngospasm if the masseters can be overridden.

An oropharyngeal airway can be inserted to maintain the forward position of the tongue. The airway must be the correct size and properly inserted. If it is too small or if the correct size becomes misplaced anteriorly, then the base of the tongue will be forced back against the pharyngeal wall and the patient's airway will be obstructed. If it is too large, the passage may be into the esophagus.

Improper insertion of an endotracheal tube into the esophagus and failure to correct the position before anoxia develops has resulted in profound brain damage or cardiac arrest. These are the deviations from the standards of care which eventuate in the highest malpractice settlements and verdicts. One way to be certain that the tube is in the trachea after it has been passed is to reoxygenate the patient by face mask. This will assure alveolar oxygenation, even if the tube is in the esophagus. Then, relaryngoscope and visualize the vocal cords alongside the tube. If the anesthetist is working with a student or supervisor, that person should also confirm that the tube is between the vocal cords.

To ensure adequate alveolar oxygenation and carbon dioxide excretion, the anesthetist should assist or control ventilation manually or with a respirator. Assisted ventilation means that the patient is initiating each breath and the anesthetist is increasing the tidal volume. In controlled ventilation, the anesthetist both initiates the breath and determines the tidal volume.

Overdose

All anesthetic agents may be the proximate cause of damage if administered in a relative or absolute overdosage. There are anesthetic agents, such as the narcotics and the non-depolarizing muscle relaxants, for which there are available pharmcologic antagonists, although generally speaking, the duration of action of the antagonists is shorter than that of the narcotic or relaxant. Other anesthetic agents can only be removed, and then not completely, by mechanical means, such as ventilation for an inhalation agent. Most anesthetic agents such as sodium thiopental and locals, once in the body, can only be metabolized and excreted.

Even pre-operative medications can produce an overdose state. These compounds are administered to allay pre-operative anxiety, sedate, produce some degree of analgesia, decrease salivary secretions, and for other purposes. They are usually ordered to be administered parenterally about an hour before anesthetic induction is scheduled to begin. Patients are often not closely observed between the time of administration and when they are brought to the operating suite. If a complication develops during this period, the patient may suffer major damage, and even death.

If a general anesthetic is planned, practically all anesthesiologists will begin by administering sodium thiopental intravenously in order to establish amnesia rapidly. In the weak or debilitated patient, even a very small dose may produce cardiovascular collapse. The solution is highly alkaline; extravasation, or even worse, an intra-arterial injection, will result in necrosis and gangrene. The greatest danger, however, is not to realize that thiopental is only a soporific and not an analgesic. Should surgery be attempted with thiopental as the principal agent, such a large dose is required to keep the patient from responding to pain that an overdose is inevitable.

Diethyl ether is no longer administered to produce general anesthesia, because it is flammable, explosive, and generally speaking, an unpleasant experience for the patient. But it had one great attribute; that is, if the patient was kept breathing while it was being administered, an overdose could not occur. Unfortunately, today's general anesthetic techniques, possibly to achieve maximum muscle relaxation, are based on producing apnea as rapidly as possible. During apnea, the anesthetist has no reliable guide to the depth of anesthesia, because electrocardiographic changes and decreases in blood presssure do not occur until an overdosage has been administered. Furthermore, the non-flammable, halogenated general anesthetics currently in vogue will produce a very relaxed, non-elastic myocardium which cannot respond to closed chest massage when the patient is overdosed.

Overdosage with striated muscle relaxants should be managed with pharmacologic antagonists, if possible, and with prolonged airway maintenance and artificial ventilation. The danger is premature extubation while the patient is unable to maintain and protect his or her own airway and is ventilating inadequately. Extubation should not be done until the vital capacity is at least three times the required tidal volume. Amnesia can be achieved with agents such as diazepam and scopolamine.

While local anesthetic agents such as procaine and lidocaine are, generally speaking, often preferred because they are felt to be quite safe, an overdose remains a risk. Infants and children will suffer an overdose if adult dosages and concentrations are administered. Inadvertent intramuscular injection, particularly in the head and neck, may produce convulsions and cardiovascular collapse. Premature release or leakage of the tourniquets in a Bier block may also result in cardiac arrest. One of the dangers of an epidural block is intravascular injection. Should the epidural dose enter the subarachnoid space, a high spinal will result. Prompt recognition of the high spinal and appropriate support of ventilation and circulation should result in no damage. Another frequent cause of damage to the fetus is a paracervical block for delivery.

Equipment

The anesthesiologist must be familiar with and throughly check all equipment before administering any anesthetic agent. No matter what the proposed technique - local, block, conduction, basal narcosis, or general - the equipment at hand must be such that the airway can be secured and artificial ventilation accomplished.

Unappreciated disconnect of the ventilator in an apneic, unconscious patient was the most frequent cause of anesthetic-associated damage in Great Britain for some years. Although disconnect alarms have been marketed for some time, disconnect is still a hazard.

Today, disposable anesthesia hoses bridge the anesthesia machine and patient, and scavenger systems exhaust the excess agents outside the operating room. One way exhaust (pop-off) valves may be inadvertently shut tight. Improper connection of the systems can result in the inability of the patient to exhale, build up of pressure in the lungs, failure of venous return, and cardiac arrest.

Monitoring and Charting

The true purposes of monitoring are to detect deleterious trends in the patient's condition and to institute corrective measures before preventable permanent, significant damage has occurred. Unfortunately, many anesthesiologists believe that monitoring is primarily a means of recognizing cardiac arrest in a timely fashion. In many litigated cases, the surgeon is the one who brings to the attention of the anesthetist the presence of very purple unoxygenated blood as the incision is made and there is only an ooze with no active arteriolar spurting.

The true purpose of charting is to assist in the recognition of deleterious trends in the patient's condition. A second purpose is to enable review and study in an attempt to discover the cause of major anesthesia-related damage, an exercise which 99 out of 100 defendants testify was never performed, so nothing was ever learned to prevent similar accidents in the future. During induction, termination of anesthesia, and crises, the anesthesiologist is so busy "taking care of the patient instead of the paperwork", the charting for these crucial times is almost always done sometime after the episode and is usually based on memory. Complete, meticulous charting may be considered evidence that the anesthesiologist is knowledgeable, or it may indicate that the chart was prepared at a later date. In any event, charts seldom reveal the deviation from the standard of care.

It is important to appreciate that not every anesthesia-associated death is necessarily due to a deviation from the standard of care. In approximately 10% of autopsies of deaths associated with anesthetic administration, a fortuitous cause is discovered. The cause of the death may be massive pulmonary embolus, massive myocardial infarction, uncal herniation from asymptomatic brain tumor, or fibroelastosis of the heart. Not every death can be explained, even after autopsy, in the current state of knowledge.

The organ most susceptible to oxygen lack is the brain. Within 17 seconds of deprivation of oxygen, whether due to lack of blood flow (ischemia), or to lack of oxygen in the blood (anoxia), humans become unconscious and stop breathing (apneic).

The body continuously monitors, through the carotid body and the carotid sinus, derivatives associated with blood flow and oxygenation of the brain; these structures initiate appropriate reflexes when indicated. The anesthesiologist can monitor the blood flow by keeping a finger on the carotid artery just above the clavicle, and the state of oxygenation by observing the color of the blood in the surgical field. Attempting to detect cyanosis or blue blood, which is associated with lack of oxygen in the blood, is sometimes difficult to do through the intact skin. By keeping the right hand on the rebreathing bag, the anesthesiologist also can determine that the medulla of the brain is being adequately perfused with oxygenated blood, the rate and depth of respiration, and the airway resistance.

The standard monitors are blood pressure and pulse rate which are charted every five minutes; electrocardioscope which may have a digital readout for pulse rate, high and low rate alarms, and a means of printing the tracing; and auscultation with a stethoscope for breath sounds and heart sounds, which the anesthesiologist listens to with an ear piece. It has become the standard of care to monitor inspired oxygen concentration from the anesthesia machine. Even if this monitor is functioning properly, it does not indicate the alveolar oxygen concentration and tells nothing about the blood flow.

The defect in all these monitors is that the heart, which is a muscle and can beat anaerobically, does not respond to anoxia until the brain has been damaged. The fact that breath sounds are heard through the stethoscope does not prove that there is adequate oxygen in the inspired gas mixture.

There are devices to observe percutaneously oxygenation and even carbon dioxide levels. These are subject to error and, in 1990, are still experimental.

Temperature is monitored when indicated in infants and in persons suspected of being susceptible to malignant hyperpyrexia.

Intra-arterial pressure monitoring and blood gasses are reserved for special procedures or high risk patients.

One of the very best potential monitors is the electrocardioscope, which can be interpreted on an ongoing basis by a computer. It is, however, expensive, subject to artefact, interfered with by cautery, and its scalp electrode needles may serve as an alternate ground for cautery current, and thereby result in burns.

The very best monitor is the capnogram, which indicates breath by breath carbon dioxide excretion. No doubt in a short time its use will become the standard of care. It is so good that the anesthesiologist can actually administer safe anesthesia by its proper use.

Fluids, Electrolytes, Blood, and Other Agents to Maintain Circulation

A primary responsibility of the anesthesiologist is to maintain homeostasis, which includes administration of the substances listed above. A patient may be brought to the operating room for elective surgery fasting and somewhat dehydrated, a significant problem in infants. Emergency surgery patients may be suffering from many disturbances which have not been or cannot be corrected before anesthesia and operative intervention.

Before induction of anesthesia and often before any pre-operative medications are administered, a secure intravenous route must be established. Through this route, the anesthetist can administer the substances listed above and any other drugs, such as muscle relaxants, needed to obtain satisfactory operating conditions.

Electrolytes are determined pre-operatively. Of these, low and high potassium can cause cardiac arrest. Pre-operative measurement of red cell mass, circulating blood volume, and extracellular fluid volume are research procedures which are never performed in the pre-operative evaluation of a patient. Pre-operative passage of a Swan-Ganz catheter may produce valuable data in the management of very poor risk patients.

The anesthesiologist relies on the medical history, physical examination, and laboratory results to estimate the need for blood and volume expanders pre-operatively, during surgery, and in the recovery room. The hemoglobin and hematocrit are concentrations and do not necessarily correlate with the red cell mass or the circulating blood volume. If the patient's systolic blood pressure is lower than the pulse rate, usually the patient is suffering from at least a 20% decrease in circulating blood volume. If this condition is permitted to persist for several hours, depending on the decrease in blood volume (50% is particularly grave), the patient may develop irreversible shock. As blood is being administered, when the systolic pressure and pulse rate cross, the patient is still about 20% behind in circulating blood volume.

Ringer's Lactate, or so-called white blood, will increase circulating blood volume, but after a few hours, only about 20% of the volume administered remains in circulation. The anesthetist administers whole blood for its oxygen-carrying capacity and its oncotic effect. Packed red cells may be administered in place of whole blood if only an increase in oxygen-carrying capacity is required, since the healthy body will replace albumin and globulins in just a few days, while red cells require up to three months.

Fresh frozen plasma will increase circulating blood volume and tend to restore normal coagulability. Platelets and white blood cells may also be administered. Hemophiliacs are given factor 8. All of these blood products can transmit AIDS.

Substances like dextran and hespan increase circulating blood volume, but have no oxygen-carrying capacity. Active research is now being carried out to develop substances that will take up oxygen in the lungs and give it up in the tissues.

Fear of AIDS and other blood-borne diseases has resulted in an intensified and expanded effort to remove a certain amount of blood in advance from a patient contemplating elective surgery, and then administering it during the operation.

Cardiac Arrest

Cardiac arrest is a loose term and is often found on death certificates. It is a meaningless term, since every death ultimately entails a cardiac arrest. Cardiac arrest has many causes, not all of which are necessarily reversible; nor should an attempt be made to reverse the arrest when the underlying condition is incompatible with life. Among the causes of cardiac arrest, defined as inadequate cardiac output to keep the brain alive, are asystole, ventricular fibrillation, electro-mechanical dissociation, failure of venous return, obstruction of the outflow of the heart, herniation of the heart through the pericardial sac, infarction of the myocardium, and various underlying states, such as electrolyte imbalance, acid-base disturbances, profound temperature changes, and anatomical disruptions, which can result in cardiac arrest.

Every anesthetizing suite must have nearby a cart on wheels with everything necessary to resuscitate a patient who develops cardiac arrest. The cart should have a board to place under the patient, a means of establishing the airway, an electrocardioscope and defibrillating paddles, drugs such as epinephrine, calcium chloride, sodium bicarbonate, and others, and several devices such as an Ambu-type bag.

However, it is crucial to realize that the airway can be established by bring-ing the mentum of the jaw forward and upward (provided there are no foreign bodies which must first be removed by a suction machine), that ventilation can be accomplished by mouth-to-mouth, and that closed chest massage can be performed successfully with the patient on the floor. The point is that resuscitation should be initiated immediately, and help and equipment sent for after resuscitation has begun.

A successful resuscitation should be defined as one which results in no loss of brain function, and not as one in which only heart and respiratory functions have been recovered, but the patient remains in a permanent, irreversible stupor or coma.

Cardiac arrests due to anoxia are not likely to result in successful resuscitations because the brain will have been destroyed before the heart has ceased to function. Those arrests due to reflexes, severe dysrhythmias, and relative or absolute overdose of anesthetic agents are most likely to result in successful resuscitation, if promptly recognized and treated.

Problem Anesthetic Drugs

Because it may require several hundred thousand administrations of a newly approved drug before major complications occur due to the drug, the problems due to its use may not be recognized for several years after its introduction. Anesthesiologists like to be on the cutting edge of technology because it reinforces, they feel, their status as professional specialists. They tend to shift to new drugs from old, tried and true ones as soon as a new drug is approved by the Food and Drug Administration. Drug houses promote with vigor new drugs for which they hold the patents, and resist strongly any suggestion, anecdotal report, and conclusions based on animal research (which is the only kind that can be performed) that may indicate the new drug is responsible for a newly discovered complication. The safest practice is not to use new drugs until they have been around for four or five years, unless they offer a distinct advantage not produced by an older, well-understood drug.

Bupivicaine is a local anesthetic with a significantly longer duration of action than lidocaine. It was approved in 1973, but by 1979, it was clear that it might be more cardiotoxic than the shorter duration local anesthetics. It also tended to produce cardiac arrest from which successful resuscitation could not be achieved, in spite of prompt recognition and proper treatment. In 1990, the drug houses which market this local still do not warn adequately, in spite of FDA prodding.

Succinylcholine was introduced in the early 1950's. It is now clear that it may produce cardiac arrest if administered to patients who have been severely traumatized, have suffered extensive burns, or are recently para or quadriplegic. It also will trigger malignant hyperpyrexia. It causes vitreous fluid to extrude if the globe of the eye is open.

Halothane was introduced in the late 1950's. Although the precise mechanism still has not been elucidated, this compound, as well as the other non-explosive, non-flammable, halogenated anesthetics, can result in liver failure and death. It can also trigger malignant hyperpyrexia.

Methoxyflurane was introduced in the 1960's and is seldom used today. It can cause renal failure.

Damage Associated With But Not Necessarily Caused by Anesthesia — Major Damage

Death
Stupor or Coma
Paraplegia or Quadriplegia; Adhesive Arachnoiditis
Loss of Vision; Loss of Vitreous
Brachial Plexus Injury; Other Nerve Injuries
Perforation of Trachea; Perforation of Esophagus
Aspiration
Burns

Minor Damage

Vocal Cord Injury; Pneumothorax; Sore Throat
Injection Site Phlebitis
Chipped, Cracked, Avulsed Teeth
Nausea and Vomiting; Anorexia
Headache; Backache; Shivering; Spasticity; Muscle Pain
Memory of Surgery; Dreams; Anxiety; Disorientation; Drowsiness

NEUROSURGERY

Introduction

Head trauma is a common cause of morbidity and mortality. Somewhere in the neighborhood of one-third of the patients brought to emergency rooms for head injuries are unconscious. Of this group, approximately 8% go on to die. In a classic, retrospective study of individuals who suffered a head injury and talked following the injury, and who subsequently died, it was estimated that approximately 50% of these patients could have been saved, based upon autopsy findings.

Care at the Scene (Pre-Hospital)

There is obviously an urgent need for pre-hospital patient management by trained individuals in instances of accidents involving the central nervous system. Competent care at the accident scene can often mean the difference between significant permanent neurologic injury and minimal sequelae. The sequence of pre-hospital management is predicated upon the life threat to each patient. The airway must be rapidly established, bleeding controlled, and obvious fractures stabilized. While waiting for help to arrive, use can be made of available materials in order to stabilize the victim. A trouser leg can be ripped off and used to tie an injured leg to an uninjured one. Neckties and small tree branches can be used as tourniquets, and shoelaces can be tied to wide pieces of cloth to stabilize limbs.

Victims who complain of neck and back pain, or who are unconscious, should be assumed to have vertebral column injuries, and should be stabilized until x-rays can confirm such injuries. The head, neck, and vertebral column can be fixed on make-shift backboards of wood or aluminum, so as to minimize and/or avoid damage to the spinal cord during extrication from a vehicle. The use of vertebral collars to support the head and neck is mandatory. Straps and bandages must be used to fix the head and neck to the board.

Although there is great temptation to use chin straps to support the head, this often proves to be a dangerous practice. Should a victim vomit, there is no way to open the mouth so as to permit either the egress of vomitus or prevent aspiration from the oral cavity. Thus, when chin straps are used on a victim, aspiration of vomitus is a potential pitfall in this method of stabilization. A heavy neck collar and strap placed across the forehead, both of which are tacked to the backboard, will minimize the risk of aspiration of vomitus, while ensuring head stability.

Communication — Lack of It

In the process of transferring a patient from one physician to another, there is often a gross inarticulation of the exact nature and extent of the clinical picture. As such, important information may be lost between the two physicians. It is imperative that not only should a thorough examination be conducted, but a detailed note outlining observations must appear in the chart so that a change in the patient's condition can be quickly and skillfully identified.

Evaluation

At the hospital, the key elements in the management of the head-injured patient are a rapid assessment and appropriate specialty consultations. An area of mismanagement of head-injured patients involves a failure to elicit a thorough history of the antecedent events. The least accurate historian is the patient who has sustained a loss of consciousness, despite the perceived brevity of such an event. Most practitioners in the emergency room mistakenly ask the patient how long he or she was unconscious. The treating practitioner fails to be aware that an unconscious patient has no time perception and is totally incapable of determining the length of time of loss of consciousness. To assess loss of consciousness in a most accurate way, the examining physician should question the patient about the last event he or she can recall prior to the trauma. By asking the patient to relate a series of sequential events prior to the trauma, the physician can more accurately determine the length of time of unconsciousness. A witness might also be a better judge of the time frame, although it should not be someone directly involved in the traumatic event. Moreover, the determination of a period of loss of consciousness represents an area in which serious errors in judgment, though frequently made, are so easily avoidable.

A patient must be assessed using a standard such as the Glasgow scale, which stresses objective descriptions of the patient's reaction. A CAT scan, now readily available, can be easily and quickly obtained and interpreted. It is generally accepted that a lumbar puncture is contraindicated in the presence of a head injury. The removal of spinal fluid or continued seepage through the dural rent, combined with high pressure within the cranial vault, will only increase the likelihood and occurrence of brain herniation and death. Often, an overzealous, inexperienced emergency room physician will trivialize a head injury and might attempt to perform a spinal tap.

Neurologic Examination

Another pitfall in the care of a head-injured patient is a failure to search for and/or recognize a Battle's sign, hemotympanum, or a depressed skull fracture that might not line up automatically with a scalp laceration. Often, a patient's head is simply not palpated, and a complete neurologic examination is not done. A complete and thorough neurologic examination is generally reserved for those who, due to loss of consciousness, are perceived as seriously injured. A key to the mismanagement of the head-injured patient is often the failure to order or conduct frequent neurologic checks to determine a worsening or deteriorating clinical picture. Thus, a patient often dies simply because of a lack of close observation.

A neurological exam must be performed concurrently with other evaluations to establish the patient's baseline status. A very rapid neurological evaluation will include assessing the functions of the following:
- cerebral hemispheres;
- upper brain stem;
- lower brain stem.

Pathogenic toe signs from the Babinski test indicate definite cerebral embarrassment or damage.

Cerebral Hemisphere Injuries

Cerebral hemisphere injuries manifest as one of several syndromes:
* cerebral concussion;
* cerebral contusion;
* cerebral hemorrhage;
* subdural hematoma;
* epidural hematoma;
* acute vascular injury to the brain.

It is beyond the scope of this Primer to detail these various conditions. The trainee is reminded that these disorders are insidious in nature with overlapping manifestations. A lack of suspicion and evaluation, resulting in delayed diagnosis or misdiagnosis, is fraught with great medical and legal consequences.

Although it rarely occurs, subarachnoid hemorrhage due to trauma, or as a spontaneous occurrence, must be considered under these circumstances.

Management Protocol

The overall management of patients with a head injury, with or without other systemic injuries, is complex and challenging. Careful input from a variety of health care personnel, such as intensive care physicians and nurses, neurosurgeons, trauma surgeons, and respiratory therapists, is essential. The specific care of the injured nervous system is best directed by the neurosurgeon, who acts in concert with the patient's other physicians to outline a total management plan. Careful attention must be paid to preventing secondary injury from inadequate ventilation or perfusion, unrecognized and inadequately treated infection, or suboptimal nutrition.

Ventilatory and Pulmonary Management

There are a number of pulmonary abnormalities. The commonest abnormality is a lung arteriovenous shunt and reduced oxygenation. Usually, this can be treated by increasing the patient's inspired fraction of oxygen (FiO_2). The method used to increase oxygen will vary, depending on the patient's condition.
* In the lethargic patient, a mist-mask with an FiO_2 of 40% or greater should be used.
* In comatose patients, an endotracheal tube should be in place. If the patient is breathing adequately, an increased FiO_2 can be delivered via a T-piece.
* Many patients with severe head injury exhibit some hypoventilation with accruing atelectasis (lung collapse), a condition that will require positive pressure ventilation. In addition, particularly when intracranial hypertension might be present, ventilation is controlled to reduce CO_2 below normal. In all of these instances, appropriate management is dictated by knowing the arterial blood gas values and by adjusting ventilation appropriately.
* In the multiple trauma patient, thoracic injury also may compromise ventilation and may be an additional reason why a controlled volume ventilator should be used.

On admission, the physician must record the following:
* Blood pressure: initally, this should be taken every 15 minutes for four to five hours, then every hour.

- Pulse and temperature: these should both be taken every hour; temperature may possibly be elevated because of a spinal cord injury.
- Respiration: is it normal or labored? Is there abdominal breathing? A patient may be breathing with the abdomen because the intercostal muscles are not functioning due to a spinal cord injury.
- Pupil size: are pupils equal in size? If not, which one is larger? Inequality in size suggests cerebral damage. If, within a few hours one pupil becomes much larger than the other and the patient's stupor deepens, this could be a prime warning of possible extradural hemorrhage from a meningeal vessel.
- Consciousness: the staff should note any changes. Is the patient becoming less or more responsive? The immediate loss of consciousness after the accident indicates cerebral concussion. Even a period of amnesia is sufficient to suggest this diagnosis. Extended periods of unconciousness or lengthy post-traumatic amnesia usually indicate severe injury.

Circulation

There is a tendency to overlook the importance of monitoring circulation to administer fluids to the point of overloading the system, particularly in the presence of incipient, and even true, shock. The parameters must be noted and followed vigilantly and diligently.

Airway

An important, but often neglected, key item of medical management for a head-injured patient is to secure and maintain a patent airway. A comatose patient is at great risk for the development of an obstructed airway and aspiration. An adequate airway potentiates hypoxia and dysplasia. Hypoxia acts as a negative feedback, which results in further destruction of brain tissue and a rise in the intracranial pressure. Therefore, a treating physician should never overlook the need to establish an adequate airway.

Endotracheal Intubation (ET)

Endotracheal intubation begins early and continues until the patient can adequately guard his or her airway. Physicians rarely resort to a tracheostomy, except in a few instances of severe craniofacial injuries that preclude ET intubation. With the current use of soft, low-pressure cuffs on ET tubes, the complication rate of intubation (if in place for less than a month) is probably less than that of a tracheostomy.

Consciousness - An Enigma

Unfortunately, head injuries tend to be trivialized if a patient is in a conscious state. Individuals who are unconscious receive priority attention, although there are often needless delays in obtaining consultation by a neurologist or neurosurgeon.

A concussion is a loss of consciousness, regardless of the length of time. Generally, following a concussion, there is no permanent brain injury. A concussion is easily diagnosed.

Comatose Patient

In the early stages of managing the comatose patient, arterial carbon dioxide pressure ($PaCO_2$) is kept in the 28 to 32 mm. Hg. range. Additional hyperventilation is not used generally unless the intracranial pressure (ICP) is above 20 mm. Hg. Although arterial oxygenation (PaO_2) of 80 mm. Hg. or greater may be entirely adequate for the normal individual, in the head-injured patient, the PaO_2 should be kept above 100 mm. Hg. Since focal areas of an injured brain may have local ICP increases and reduced perfusion, the oxygen extraction may be abnormally high in some brain regions, justifying a higher oxygen content with a raised PaO_2. Ensuring a PaO_2 above 100 mm. Hg. may require positive end-expiratory pressure (PEEP) to prevent or reverse atelectasis and improve oxgenation. The application of PEEP has variable and unpredictable effects on ICP. When PEEP must be used, its effect on ICP must be noted and other appropriate adjustments must be made.

Diminished Cognition

Lethargic or comatose patients with intact brian stem functions require stabilization, rapid assessment of the chest and abdomen, and emergency treatment of life-threatening disorders. These should be followed by an immediate computer tomographic (CT) scanning in order to diagnose extra- or intracerebral hematomas that will require surgical evacuation. Patients with external injury or pre-hospital evidence of head injury, who also have signs of transtentorial herniation (coma, pupillary abnormalities, and motor asymmetry) are taken for immediate burr hole exploration (a hole drilled through the skull) for subdural or epidural hematomas. CT scans are obtained for such patients at most hospitals. Lethargic patients who open their eyes to voice or painful stimuli, or who follow commands, may be observed while their general examination and resuscitation are completed.

If the patient is unconscious and his or her urine is bloody, the physician must insert a Foley catheter.

Paralysis

In the case of paralysis, there are several questions the ER physician must ask: Is the patient moving his or her arms or legs less or more since admission? Was the patient able to move his or her arms and legs at first, becoming paralyzed only later, or was he or she paralyzed immediately after the injury?

If there was a delay in the onset of paralysis, then swelling of the cord or a hematoma could be the cause and surgery may be required. If paralysis occurs immediately after the impact, destruction of the cord is probable, and the patient's prognosis is poor.

Latent Symptoms

While loss of consciousness and paralysis are obvious symptoms, there may be subtle changes that either contribute to a diagnosis or alert the examining physician to latent symptoms. Memory loss or amnesia, difficulty in speaking distinctly or dysarthria, and impaired verbal expression or aphasia are all warning signs of a cerebral injury, resulting from brain swelling or subdural hematoma, an injury that may not be apparent until days later.

Bleeding

If the patient is in shock, the physician must look for a source of bleeding, particularly in the lungs, kidneys, or viscera. It must be remembered that a concussion, or even hemorrhage of the brain, does not cause shock.

Intoxication

Intoxication is common in head-injured patients, which makes interpretation of the examination findings more difficult. Patients who can be aroused and who have intact brain stem functions may be followed with sequential examinations, as may patients who have had a witnessed seizure and are postictal in the emergency room. In both of these cases, however, the patient should improve within one to three hours if the neurological status is related to seizures or intoxication. If such a patient fails to improve, reassessment is imperative, and CT scanning should be done. Patients who show neurological deterioration should have a CT scan immediately. Throughout this period of physical examination and CT evaluation, the patient receives ongoing support of blood pressure by IV fluid administration and arterial blood gases by supplemental oxygen as necessary.

Depressed Skull Fracture

Another key diagnostic error is a failure to appreciate a depressed skull fracture because there is a lack of scalp laceration. Any patient who gives a history of head trauma must have a careful inspection of the skull to determine the presence of such an injury. A depressed skull fracture can be identified on an AP and lateral series of skull x-rays.

Compound Fracture of the Skull

When a compound fracture of the skull has occurred, the physician should give antibiotics at once and make sure the wound is clean. It is acceptable to let some hours pass until the physician arranges for proper debridement under optimal OR conditions. Unskilled debridement and inadequate or improper equipment can enhance and extend the damage. If bone has been driven through the dura or into the cortex, the attending physician should have a neurosurgeon perform the debriding procedure.

Surgical Intervention

The clinical circumstances which require immediate surgical intervention are those in which there is a large bony defect through which the brain may eventually herniate, or when there is a shard of bone seen to be penetrating the brain. The patient who presents with either of these two clinical circumstances is at greater risk for the development of meningitis, and thus warrants immediate surgical repair. Only in the face of an obvious meningitis should surgery be deferred. However, in any event, a neurological consultation must be obtained.

Multiple Injuries

The physician must look for multiple injuries first, and then determine the period of unconsciousness and how it relates to the time of impact. He should immediately note if there is paralysis of the extremities, respiratory difficulty, obstructed or shallow breathing, paresthesia of the extremities, history of amnesia, and what body area the patient complains of pain in.

Further Evaluation

As soon as the patient is stabilized, the physician should perform a rapid evaluation to facilitate the decision on the appropriate treatment of thoracic, abdominal, and extremity injuries. The following are primary elements of this evaluation.

- A general physical examination often can determine the presence of cardiac tamponade, hemothorax, tension pneumothorax, or a hemorrhage into the abdomen.
- A chest x-ray can be used to assess the presence or severity of chest lesions or a lung collapse, which can be treated immediately with chest-tube insertion and lung re-expansion.
- An abdominal examination may suggest intra-abdominal trauma. However, in the head-injured patient, this examination may appear entirely negative, even in the presence of severe intra-abdominal injury. In such a situation, diagnostic peritoneal lavage should be performed immediately to determine potential hemorrhaging, unless the patient has an unstable blood pressure and is taken immediately to surgery for a laparotomy.
- Extremity fractures, when found, must be splinted to reduce the risk of hemorrhage and neurovascular injury subsequent to fracture movement.
- A Foley catheter should be inserted if there are no contraindications, and the urine should be tested for blood. The presence of blood requires further genitourinary radiographic evaluation.

Cerebral Perfusion

Systemic circulation is carefully monitored to assure adequate systemic and cerebral perfusion. However, because of the association of cerebral edema with craniocerebral trauma, there is a tendency to dehydrate patients to a modest degree, not at the expense of reduced perfusion, but rather, to raise serum osmolality (concentration in solution) in the setting of an adequate circulating volume. Simple fluid restriction may achieve this, and patients generally receive about 75% of their calculated maintenance volume. This treatment differs from the treatment of general trauma patients, whose fluid administration is kept at or above normal replacement values to ensure that third-space losses in the abdomen or soft tissues are adequately replaced and to ensure high urine output.

Cerebral Edema

To reduce cerebral edema in the head-injured patient, mild fluid restriction often will keep serum osmolality in the range of 295 to 300 milliosmoles. Steroids such as hydrocortisone should be given in 100 mg. doses intramuscularly, twice-a-day for three to five days. However, the physician should administer steroids cautiously, since corticosteroids are contraindicated in patients who have a history of ulcers, diabetes, or hypertension. Osmolality can be further elevated through intermittent use of mannitol (a diuretic), which produces an osmotic diuresis, or use of a colloid solution such as albumin or aggregated starch solutions. Two to 3 gm. of mannitol per Kg. of body weight is suggested. The use of colloids allows maintenance of good circulating volumes, but with a somewhat elevated serum osmolality to reduce cerebral water content.

Dehydrating agents are used, predominantly in response to increased intracranial pressure. Since they monitor ICP regularly, physicians rarely give routine infusions of mannitol; rather, they restrict its use to treatment of specific ICP elevations.

If there is any question about adequacy of perfusion, measurements of pulmonary wedge pressures will assure the physician that there is adequate cardiac filling pressure. A monitoring catheter will allow determination of cardiac output, which should be kept at or just below normal levels.

Catheterization

The physician should use a Foley catheter when giving diuretics to comatose patients to avoid overfilling the bladder and to check urinary output. Catheterization is repeated in eight hours if necessary. The physician must be alert to watch for electrolyte excretion.

Nutrition

Nutrition can often be started fairly soon after head injury in the absence of intra-abdominal trauma. There is no particular advantage to parenteral (intravenous) nutrition, and a gastrointestinal route is preferred.

Intravenous intake should be restricted to 1,500 cc. during the first 24 hours after injury.

Infectious Complications

Infectious complications are common in the head-injured patient. Antibiotics and tetanus toxoids are indicated for deep, contaminated wounds. Antibiotics are used prophylactically in patients who have evidence of otorrhea or rhinorrhea.

Prolonged intubation, some degree of systemic dehydration, and multiple monitoring lines subject a patient to an increased risk of sepsis. Removing and replacing all IV lines started in the field or emergency room should be a matter of routine, since a high infection rate is found in these lines when left in for longer than 24 hours. It is important to use sterile technique for ET suctioning to reduce the risk of contaminating a patient's airway, a condition that can lead to pneumonia.

Dressings around ICP catheter entry sites must remain dry; any leakage of CSF along a catheter dramatically increases the risk of infection. Central lines must be inspected daily, and a fresh dressing placed at the skin entry sites every 72 hours or when soiled. Although Foley catheters are used during the initial phases of managing the head-injured patient, because of substantial fluid shifts, they are usually removed within four to five days, and intermittent straight catheterization is begun to reduce the risk of urosepsis.

Antibiotics are used routinely for compound depressed skull fractures or penetrating brain wounds. High-dose penicillin is given for five days. Positive sputum cultures are not treated in the absence of x-ray evidence of pneumonia. Spiking fevers should trigger ordering cultures of blood, sputum, urine, and a careful inspection of all wounds. If there is neurological deterioration, a lumbar puncture is performed after a CT scan has excluded a focal mass lesion and brain shift that might increase the risk of herniation following lumbar puncture. If a patient becomes clinically septic, with an unstable blood pressure and high fever, multiple cultures can be taken, and the patient can be started on a broad-spectrum antibiotic regimen (usually Vancomycin, Gentamicin, and Cefotaxime). If there is a clinical response, the antibiotics are continued while cultures are pending. If all cultures remain negative and the fever persist, the antibiotics are stopped after 48 hours to search further for sources of infection.

Post-Traumatic Meningitis

Post-traumatic meningitis may ocur in up to 25% of all patients with basilar skull fractures, and usually results from organisms that enter the CSF through a dural tear. Leakage of CSF after a basilar skull fracture has long been recognized.

Basilar skull fractures account for about 25% of all skull fractures, and thus represent a significant proportion of head injuries and potential for meningitis.

Diagnosis is usually based on one or more of the following: radio-graphic evidence, plain film or computed tomograms, CSF otorrhea or rhinorrhea, hematotympanum, raccoon eyes, and Battle's sign. CSF leakage ceases spontaneously in the vast majority of patients.

The peak incidence is seen in patients between 11 and 20 years of age, and the male:female ratio is approximately 2.5:1. Injury is caused by a motor vehicle accident in about one-half of patients, and a fall in about 40%.

Fractures of the parietal and temporal bones are seen equally as often in about half of the patients, with fractures of the frontal bone in 20% and the occipital bone in 15%.

The remaining patients have clinical findings of basilar skull fracture. No fracture site is determined only occasionally.

Pneumococcus is the most common infecting organism, followed by Hemophilus infuenzae and Enterobacteria aerogenes.

Because of increasing evidence against the prophylactic use of antibiotics for basilar skull fractures, observation alone is advocated as initial management, rather than antibacterial intervention. If clinical signs of CNS infection appear, a lumbar puncture should be done to confirm or exclude the diagnosis. When the results of the lumbar puncture are positive, therapeutic antibiotic coverage is instituted and altered appropriately as sensitivity data are obtained. In any event, the dura is closed surgically in all patients who have persistent CSF leakage.

Many antibiotics do not penetrate the blood-brain barrier well in the absence of meningeal irritation. This may explain why antibiotics that are often successful therapeutically fail prophylactically.

Seizures

Seizures commonly occur in association with a head injury. A seizure which occurs immediately when the head is struck is most likely due to a sudden cortical contusion eliciting a contemporaneous electrical discharge. Seizures may be a sign of a subdural hematoma. Therefore, the examining physician should have a high index of suspicion when a patient experiences a seizure with a head injury.

Retrograde Amnesia

Retrograde amnesia is the loss of memory of events which occurred prior to the actual trauma. Generally, the period of retrograde amnesia relates to the magnitude of the head injury. Therefore, the more significant the head injury, the longer the period of retrograde amnesia. It is often difficult for the practitioner to determine retrograde amnesia because a patient in the emergency room may be flustered and frightened and may simply be exhibiting discrepant recall.

Radiologic and and Monitoring Procedures

X-ray Studies
X-rays at the time of admission can be deferred if the patient is in shock. However, as soon as possible, roentgenographic studies should be done to determine the possibility, site, and size of a depressed skull fracture, fractured ribs, or flail chest (a loss of chest wall stability from a rib fracture), pneumothorax (air between the chest wall and lungs), fractures of vertebrae and possible cord injury, and fractures or obvious deformities of extremities.

Computerized Tomography (CT) Scanning
Repeat intracranial studies, specifically repeat CT scanning, are considered whenever ICP remains above 25 mm. Hg., despite appropriate medical management. In some instances, delayed subdural, epidural, or intracerebral hematomas will develop after an initial normal or unremarkable scan. Generally, the natural history of head injury is one of improvement.

A patient's failure to improve neurologically over the first several days should prompt a repeat intracranial study. Any neurological deterioration needs to be evaluated crefully and, in many instances, will necessitate a repeat CT scan. Acute hemorrhage is readily apparent on CT scanning, even without intravenous contrast enhancement.

If intracranial injury is suspected, especially if the patient arrives in a coma and has fixed pupils or other signs of intracranial damage, neurosurgical consultation and CT scanning should be requested simultaneously.

If neurologic symptoms develop, or if there is a marked change in the patient's mental status after a CT scan has been obtained, the scan should be repeated.

Subdural hematomas have three evolutionary stages: acute, subacute, and chronic, each of which can be distinguished by its different density on CT scan.

An acute subdural hematoma, when viewed by CT scan, appears as a high-density white area at the periphery of the brain. It usually extends over a larger area than an epidural hematoma ansd has a convex medical border directed centrally. A large mass may be seen, with a shift of midline structures to the normal side. The ventricle is compressed, and a "hematocrit" effect (separation of blood cells from serum) is seen; the white area represents the red blood cells, the blacker area represents the blood serum. Angulation of the head, which occurs because of the way a patient is positioned in a CT scanner, causes a red blood cell-fluid level. This can be compared with the air-fluid level seen in the stomach on upright radiographs of the abdomen.

The definitive diagnosis of subacute subdural hematoma often requires the use of an intravenous contrast CT study. In the subacute stage of a subdural hematoma, the injured area is isodense; it cannot be distinguished from the normal brain on CT scan.

Chronic subdural hematoma appears as a low-density, extra-axial hematoma on CT scan.

On unenhanced CT scans, an epidural hematoma appears as an area of increased density (white on the film) in a peripheral area, with centrally directed (spindle-shaped) convexity.

If a fracture is present, it may not be seen on CT scan, even though it may be well-visualized on a plain film. This is because the CT scan may not "cut" through the area of the fracture. Any accompanying soft tissue injury overlying the area is easily seen on CT scan. Penetrating wounds may cause extensive intracranial bleeding. The "bleed" is detected with CT scan, but definitive demonstration of the bleeding site requires angiography.

Magnetic Resonance Imaging (MRI)

Magnetic resonance imaging is useful in the subacute phases after head injury to demonstrate small cerebral lesions, but, thus far, has no real role in the acute management of a head injury.

In the classification of head injuries of the minor and moderate type, according to the type of lesion visualized by MRI, this test may provide useful prognostic information.

MRI v. CT Scan

In patients with minor or moderate closed-head injuries, MRI can be used to predict deficits in frontal lobe function and memory related to the size and location of lesions. However, MRI does not reveal additional lesions that would require surgical management.

Subacute or chronic subdural hematomas are well-demonstrated with MRI. Because of the proximity of bony skull, small collections of blood can be missed with CT scanning, especially if they occur bilaterally. Acute subdural collections (those less than 72 hours old) appear isodense in both T1- and T2-weighted images on MRI, unless one has a strong magnet. This, as well as other considerations, such as imaging time, currently makes MRI less desirable than CT scan for acute emergencies.

It has been shown that patients with a moderate head injury had lesions visualized by MRI that were undetected by CT scanning, but in no case did MRI reveal an expanding lesion that necessitated surgical evacuation. Localization and sizing of lesions is best accomplished by MRI, rather than CT scan, which gives smaller estimates of the size and number of brain lesions. Detection of focal injury by MRI is especially impressive for parenchymal lesions in the frontal and temporal lobes.

Positron Emission Tomography (PET) Scan

A new advance in positron emission tomography (PET) of the brain can unquivocally confirm the clinical diagnosis of permanent unconsciousness. The PET study measures cerebral blood flow and cerebral oxygen and glucose metabolism. In a new study, this was done in seven permanently unconscious patients, three patients with the "locked-in" syndrome and 18 normal controls. The cerebral metabolic rate was 50 to 60% lower in permanently unconscious patients after at least 12 weeks of unconsciousness, compared with controls.

Miscellaneous Laboratory Procedures

A complete blood count (CBC) and urinalysis should be taken from the head-injured person as soon as possible.

A lumbar puncture should be done if the patient is comatose, or has possibly lost consciousness, to determine whether there is a subarachnoid hemorrhage. However, the physician should never do a Queckenstedt's test (compression of the jugular vein to cause rapid increase in CSF pressure) on a patient with a cerebral problem. He or she may have an aneurysm.

In addition to x-rays and a lumbar puncture, the following may prove useful: electroencephalography; a brain scan; angiography; pnuemoencephalography; echoencephalography to determine midline shift; ventriculography, rather than pneumoencephalography, for patients with papilledema; electromyography, or a nerve conduction study, for muscle and nerve injury; and myelography.

Patients with frontal lobe lesions are more likely to make perseverative errors than were those with temporal lobe lesions attempting to draw novel designs. In contrast, temporal lobe and frontotemporal lobe patients showed greater impairment of long-term memory.

Too Little, Too Late

In summary, a delay in neurologic assessment, i.e., having a patient examined by a neurologist or neurosurgeon; a failure or delay in obtaining or interpreting diagnostic adjuncts; the tendency to trivialize head injuries in a conscious patient; the misjudgment of the history regarding the length of time of loss of consciousness; the failure to secure a patent airway; the failure to correctly identify serious skull fractures; and the failure to order or conduct frequent and thorough neurologic checks, all represent common pitfalls in the management of the head-injured patient.

Head trauma encompasses a significant number and various types of injuries which fall on a scale ranging from mild to severe. The key to successful management of the head-injured patient represents a clinical challenge, the aim of which should be to stabilize the patient and minimize residual deficits.

Spinal Cord Injuries

From 10,000 to 20,000 spinal cord injuries occur yearly. At the present time, there is no means available to restore the continuity of central nervous system functions which are disrupted at the time of a transsection of the cord. Therefore, treatment must be aimed at preventing the progression of the injury, either through the relief of compression or stabilization to permit the cord to "heal" itself. The management of goals includes restoration of bony alignment and maintenance of stability.

Management Starts At The Scene

Proper management of spinal cord injury must start at the scene of the trauma. In the face of a suspected spinal cord injury, immediate immobilization is the most essential aspect of medical management. In one series involving cervical injuries in diving accidents, it was determined that the injury to the cord occurred after the impact, suggesting that improper handling of the patient at the scene injured the cord.

Mini-Exam

In any patient with spinal cord injuries, a detailed examination is an essential part of the care. Often, the physician erroneously conducts only a "mini-neuro examination" if there are no overt signs of injury.

Movement - A No! No!

The most common area of mismanagement of the spinal cord-injured patient occurs at the scene with a failure to recognize the injury prior to moving the patient. There can be no doubt that movement of the spine in an early cord-injured patient can aggravate the injury.

Spinal Column Injury

Spinal cord injury most often accompanies an injury to the bony spinal column. As with other bone injuries, they may be open or closed. The lumbar and cervical portions of the spine are mobile and, as such, are the most frequent sites of injury. It is important to remember that the intervertebral disk may also be fractured and/or displaced, and that such injuries may cause damage to the spinal cord. The spinal cord can be injured in the absence of visible structural bony abnormalities. Therefore, it is essential that, in the face of trauma, a thorough search be made to rule out spinal cord trauma, even if the x-rays are read as negative.

Spinal Cord Compression

Spinal cord compression represents a real emergency. Every physician should possess the skills required to diagnose this problem. A thorough and accurate history and physical examination are essential if the lesion is to be diagnosed and promptly treated. It is important to note that signs related to the dorsal columns, lateral spinothalamic tracts, and corticospinal tracts generally start at the most distal lower extremities and ascend toward the level of the lesion. Therefore, a common error is to conclude that the lesion is higher than it is in reality. For this reason, a diligent effort must be made to accurately localize the level of the spinal cord lesion.

Any patient who presents with progressive spinal cord compression should receive emergency spine films, myelography, and CAT scans. A myelogram will define the site of the lesion, either extradural, extramedullary, or intradural. Decompression of the spinal cord is nearly always accomplished by immediate neurosurgical treatment. It is a serious, but all too common, error to delay in obtaining a neurosurgical consultation when a spinal cord compression is suspected.

Cervical Cord Injury

An injury to the cervical cord presents unique difficulties. The interruption of the sympathetic outflow to the body will result almost immediately in hypotension and bradycardia. Additionally, the innervation of the intercostal muscles is lost. Therefore, these patients are dependent solely on the phrenic nerve innervating the diaphragm, and the cranial nerves innervating the accessory muscles of respiration. It must be borne in mind that a high cervical cord injury may knock out the phrenic nerve, either by direct injury or ascending edema.

Surgical Intervention

In the face of a spinal cord lesion, there is still great controversy regarding surgical management. Most authorities agree that immediate surgical intervention is indicated when there is significant, progressive neurologic deterioration. Therefore, it is imperative that, as in head injuries, thorough and regular neurological examinations be conducted.

Much controversy surrounds surgical procedures in the face of an acute traumatic cord impression. One series has reported that in a patient with an acutely injured spinal cord and vertebral column, there are clearly two situations that might benefit from surgical intervention, namely, stabilization and neural decompression. There is no disagreement that an unstable spine must be immobilized immediately. Though there is often disagreement as to the timing or need for surgical intervention, skeletal reduction with tongs or halo may be life-saving, and is often required in the emergency room. Realignment not only addresses comprehensive trauma, it also prevents ischemic insults to the cord and spinal nerve roots. It is imperative that the emergency room physician rapidly recognize an unstable spine to afford the patient the best chance for survival with preservation of neurologic integrity.

One of the grave pitfalls in the spinal cord-injured patient involves neglect in the emergency room in instances in which there are no obvious deformities of the bony spinal column. Therefore, the patient's injury tends to be trivialized to the ultimate detriment of that patient.

Spinal Cord Injuries in Children

Spinal injuries, fortunately, are relatively uncommon in the pediatric population. The prognosis in pediatric spinal cord injury is almost directly related to a high index of suspicion and quick diagnosis. As in the adult spinal cord-injured patients, a multidisciplinary approach to resuscitation and stabilization should guide the medical management of the pediatric spinal cord-injured patient. The emergency room physician must always remember that respiratory function may rapidly deteriorate, even in a child who initially presents with competent respiratory ability. Additionally, a patient with an upper thoracic and cervical cord injury may appear as if he or she had been sympathectomized, i.e., the onset of bradycardia and profound hypotension. It is imperative that these physiologic derangements be quickly and correctly addressed to save the patient's life.

X-Ray Interpretation

As in the spinal cord-injured adult, children require spine films. However, their proper interpretation is dependent upon knowledge of the broad range of normal anatomic variants of the pediatric spine. There are certain pitfalls in the interpretation of cervical spine films in children, including the fact that the vertebral bodies are not rectangular in children, as in adults. Therefore, these may be misdiagnosed as compression fractures. Reliance upon the appearance of the soft tissues might be quite helpful in interpreting adult spine films. However, this is not terribly useful in pediatric radiograph interpretation unless the "reader" fully considers the patient's condition at the time of the exposure. The retropharyngeal soft tissues, for example, may change drastically when a child is crying. Lastly, the cervical spine in the pediatric patient has a high cartilage content. The ligamentous structures in the pediatric patient are lax. Therefore, extreme angulation may be present, even in the absence of apparent bony or ligamentous derangement. In effect, infants and children can sustain very severe spinal cord injuries without any evidence of radiographic abnormality. Therefore, the absence of radiographic findings in the pediatric patient does not preclude a spinal cord injury.

Spinal Cord Injury - A Special Situation

There are many perils and pitfalls in the care of the spinal cord-injured patient. Improper care at the scene of an accident; lack of preparedness in the emergency room to handle the patient; a delay in obtaining specialty consultation; a delay in obtaining or interpreting ample diagnostic studies; and incomplete neurologic and orthopedic assessment — all of these can contribute greatly to a poor outcome for the spinal cord-injured patient.

The problems unique to the pediatric spinal cord-injured patient deserve attention by medical personnel particularly prepared in the area of pediatrics. It is a very common and serious error to try to fit the pediatric patient into the adult mode. While the mechanism of injury and potential sequelae may bear striking similarities in the adult and pediatric spinal cord-injured patient, it is erroneous to assume that symptomatology and radiographic findings will be identical. It is a dangerous practice not to have a pediatric radiologist read spine films of a potential spinal cord-injured child.

Conclusion

Medicine is far from an exacting science. There are neither two identical patients, nor are there two identical sets of clinical circumstances. All that a physician can do in caring for patients with neurologic injuries is to make a thorough physical and neurologic assessment, looking for constellations of symptoms which suggest various diagnoses. The physician then must proceed through an orderly and predictable sequence in which diagnostics and consults are employed that pinpoint the nature and extent of the injuries determined. What is perhaps unique regarding neurosurgery is that the physician often does not have the luxury of time; the patient's life is often dependent on speed as much as on skill.

OPHTHALMOLOGY

Introduction

As primary sense organs, the eyes obtain a special importance both to the patient and the physician. Although physicians usually have recourse to the ocular specialist (the ophthalmologist), many eye problems are handled on a routine basis by the primary physician.

Fortunately, there are few true ocular emergencies; however, when encountered, prompt, appropriate treatment is essential to improve the chance of maintaining ocular integrity. Ocular emergencies and urgencies will be discussed with special attention to measures to be avoided.

Pain/Anxiety

The emergency room physician or resident on call should have a basic approach to ocular conditions which, if followed routinely, will not only provide ease of diagnosis, but greatly improve the effectiveness of treatment. An ambulatory patient in pain and/or with sufficient anxiety must first have the pain/anxiety reduced to manageable levels.

Visual Acuity

Except in true emergencies, visual acuity should then be taken, either by Snellen wall chart or hand-held near acuity card.

Acuity in the normal individual can be affected significantly by refractive error. All patients should be asked whether they wear glasses or contact lenses. A myopic individual without refractive correction would be expected to perform poorly on a wall chart, but can often read the equivalent of 20/20 on a near acuity chart. The presbyopic individual can read the wall chart with ease, but would fail on the near chart.

The uncorrected hyperope and high astigmate often does poorly on both near and far charts, but the use of a pinhole usually results in dramatic improvement in visual performance. When literacy, language, or age limits testing ability, the use of the letter "E" can establish reliable if less specific visual performance levels. If all else fails, the use of a penlight will establish direct light reaction.

When visual acuity is found to be decreased and no cause is apparent, the patient should be specifically asked if the condition is longstanding. A personal history of an old injury or ambylopia can aid in establishing etiology. Bear in mind that many patients who have good acuity in one eye may be unaware that acuity is diminished in the fellow eye. A complaint of visual loss may actually represent unmasking of a prior condition by a coincidental ocular or periocular injury.

Evaluation

A careful history should be obtained with special attention to duration, time, and extent or intensity of the complaint. Family members may be invaluable in refining the history obtained.

Examination should first be external with as much light as possible. (Certain ocular conditions make patients extremely photophobic, so a dimmed room may be necessary.) When eyelid swelling prevents the patient from opening the lids, a lid speculum is quite useful. Forceful opening of the lids with the hands is advised only as a last resort, since this action places added pressure on the globe and increases patient discomfort and anxiety.

After the external exam is completed and an ocular condition is suspected, a slit lamp microscopic exam is indicated. In the absence of a slit lamp, a hand held direct ophthalmoscope can be useful, and in the case of abrasions, dye and a woods lamp are often adequate. Most injuries and conditions located behind the iris are best recognized by an ophthalmologist, who will examine by means of an indirect ophthalmoscope.

General Considerations

Topical Anesthetics

Topical anesthetics are frequently misused by the physician and are subject to significant abuse by the patient. These medications must be used sparingly and only as an adjunct to diagnosis and/or treatment. A physician should never prescribe such medications for patient use as topical anesthetics retard healing and, by reducing corneal sensitivity, may mask serious injury or infection.

Cyclopegics

Instillation of cyclopegics is highly recommended when paralysis of the ciliary muscle and accommodation is necessary. Thereafter, prompt referral to an ophthalmologist for further care should be made. Additional care required is beyond the scope of this presentation.

Antibiotics

When it is determined that topical antibiotic use is indicated for any ocular condition, the physician must weigh the need for a specific antibiotic with its side effects and potential to interfere with the healing process. For a minor injury where infection is not suspected and prophylaxis is desired, the use of Sodium Sulfacetamide, 10% drops or ointment, is an excellent choice. This agent has a broad spectrum of action and rarely affects normal healing. It is also useful in minor conjunctivitis and blepharoconjunctivitis.

Aminoglycosides (tobramycin and gentamicin) are good choices for corneal ulcer and purulent conjunctivitis, because they guard against pseudomonas and also have a broad spectrum of action. They do, however, retard corneal healing with extended use.

Neomycin, usually in combination with other antibiotics, is commonly used by non-ophthalmologists. While it is effective, it is the most likely to induce an allergic reaction and is most implicated in slowing the healing process.

Steroids

Antibiotics which contain steroids should generally be avoided by physicians who do not have access to a slit lamp biomicroscope, and who have limited familiarity with ocular external disease. These agents are often misprescribed for viral diseases. At best, they will mask the viral symptoms, and at worst, they will either accelerate the infectious process or prolong the disease. Herpes simplex can now be specifically treated wth several agents. The use of steroids on a herpetic infection can greatly increase morbidity.

Ocular Emergencies

Chemical Burns - Acids and Alkali

The most common "true" ocular emergency is chemical burns of the eye either by acid or alkali. The burning chemical agent should be identified not only to aid in treatment, but to help establish prognosis. Acid burns have a better prognosis in that acid is rapidly buffered by ocular tissues, and the damage, while often extensive, is limited to the area of contact.

Alkali burns are not adequately buffered by tissue, and the duration of the action of alkali is correspondingly longer, sometimes for days. In addition, alkali penetrates the eye more readily than acid.

The treatment for acid and alkali burns is the immediate and copious irrigation of the eyes with water for at least 20 minutes. Adequate exposure is essential, and the use of anesthetics, both local and topical, may be necessary to enable the physician to open the lids. This is most readily accomplished on a supine patient, and an IV pole, hanging bottle, and tubing provide the most convenient mode of continuous irrigation.

Vascular Occlusions

The only other "true" ocular emergency is the occlusion or impending occlusion of the central retinal artery. Unfortunately, the patient rarely presents to the physician until hours after the event when treatment is no longer effective. In those cases when the patient does so present, the physician often fails to associate the symptom of intermittent amaurosis with artery occlusion unless periocular trauma is suspected to have raised orbital pressure.

For the astute physician who suspects impending occlusion, the immediate treatment is having the patient breathe into a paper bag so as to rise blood carbon dioxide levels and dilate the artery. Breathing oxygen with 5% carbon dioxide is also useful.

If the artery is compromised by orbital pressure, a lateral canthotomy should be performed without delay. The canthotomy is easily made (clamp tissue with hemostat and cut with scissors or blade) and repaired later without difficulty. If the occlusion is found in conjunction with elevated ocular tension, anti-glaucoma medications are useful. In the non-nauseated patient, oral agents can be used, but if nausea is present, the use of intravenous diamox and/or mannitol is effective. If the intraocular pressure is significantly elevated, it may be necessary to have an ophthalmologist perform a paracentesis.

Ophthalmologists have been the subject of lawsits for failure to recognize or adequately treat central retinal artery occlusion. In one case, the ophthalmic surgeon encountered a retrobulbar hemorrhage after pre-operative retrobulbar anesthetic block. Despite the known complication of artery occlusion, the ophthalmologist only applied ice packs and failed to perform a lateral cathotomy. The patient subsequently lost the vision in her operative eye, and a lawsuit was filed.

Another retinal artery occlusion lawsuit was based on the repair of a blow-out fracture. In this suit, a carpenter who sustained a hammer injury to his orbital rim underwent inferior orbital fractive repair five days following his injury. Following the surgery, he had no vision on the side of repair. There was testimony that the physician must have failed to recognize artery occlusion due to bleeding during surgery. Of significance in this case was the fact that the patient claimed that after the injury but prior to surgery, his vision was normal. This illustrates not only the need to recognize intraoperative complications, but the necessity of obtaining preoperative acuity in any case involving the globe or orbit.

Critical Ocular Conditions and Injuries

Lid Lacerations
These external injuries are commonly seen in hospital emergency rooms, and their care is based on an understanding of lid structure. Since the lids are composed of skin, orbicularis muscle, tarsus, and conjunctiva (tarsus and conjunctiva are adherent), repairs should aim to meticulously approximate these layers. Whenever the laceration involves the lacrimal apparatus, the aid of an experienced surgeon is usually necessary to obtain both satisfactory cosmetic and functional repair.

All lid wounds merit careful skin cleansing and should be followed by prophylactic tetanus immunization. Animal bites should not be surgically closed due to the high risk of infection, and antibiotics should be strongly considered, as well as rabies prophylaxis.

Hyphema
This potentially serious ocular condition is most often associated with blunt trauma to the closed lid. The physician should carefully question the patient to determine whether the globe was traumatized. When suspicion is high, the globe should be inspected with careful attention to the cornea and anterior chamber.

Iris details are often obscured because the pupil is usually miotic, and if the injury is hours to days old, the intraocular blood may be layered. Intraocular tension must be determined as the exit of blood from the anterior chamber can often compromise the trabecular meshwork, resulting in increased intraocular pressure.

A patient with a hyphema should be hospitalized with bed rest. A clot will form at the area of the bleed, and the natural clot retraction at three to five days post-injury can result in a rebleed. Long-acting cycloplegic drops limit iris movement during the healing period, and when pain is present, anti-inflammatory drops are used.

Intraocular Tension
The pitfalls to avoid relate to failure to frequently monitor intraocular tension. A normal admission intraocular tension should not be allowed to lull the physician into a false sense of security. Pressure often increases to dangerous levels, despite the lack of a rebleeding episode. When pressure rises do occur, the physician should be cautious in the use of carbonic anhydrase inhibitors in blacks (sickle cell disease) and diabetics.

All discharged patients should be advised to avoid strenuous activity for one month, and informed that the likelihood of an angle recession with possible late development of glaucoma exists. Follow-up with an ophthalmologist is essential.

Corneal Abrasions

This injury is one of the most common ones seen in both the office and hospital setting. Almost any agent can abrade the cornea, with the most common being plant branches, paper edges, and fingernails. Contact lens use (or misuse) is often implicated.

History is important to determine the potential for corneal infection and will often guide the use of appropriate antibiotics. A "clean" abrasion should be pressure patched after installation of an antibiotic drop or ointment. Depending upon the extent of the abrasion, patching may be necessary for several days.

Patients usually become comfortable soon after appropriate treatment, but this comfort yields a false sense of security. Patients should be counseled to use lubricating eyedrops for several weeks, and contact lens wear should be delayed for several weeks following the injury.

Since all corneal abrasions have the potential to convert to corneal ulcers, patients should be given appropriate follow-up instructions and adequate precautions should healing not go as expected.

Acute Angle Closure Glaucoma

Patients with this condition will often present to the physician with severe pain, photophobia, and a decrease in vision. Since these symptoms are similar to those found in iritis, misdiagnosis can occur.

The physician should have a high degree of suspicion with patients over age 45, persons with a non-reactive pupil (usually in mid-dilation in the affected eye), and pain-induced nausea. Any patient suspected of having an iritis must be examined with a slit lamp and the intraocular tension taken.

The slit lamp exam in narrow angle glaucoma will show a narrow anterior chamber angle, whereas the angle in iritis is usually wide. Cells and flare are the hallmark of iritis. The anterior chamber reaction is usually minimal in angle closure. Intraocular tensions are often above 40 in angle closure and usually below 15 in iritis (although in some cases of chronic iritis, the pressure can be elevated).

Once the diagnosis of angle closure is made, attempts to rapidly bring down the pressure are performed. Pilocarpine, 4%, is used every 15 minutes, and both beta blockers and carbonic anhydrase inhibitors are administered. The attack can usually be controlled within one to two hours with such treatment. After breaking the attack, the patient should be given definitive treatment to prevent further episodes. This consists of peripheral iridotomy by laser.

Foreign Bodies

A common emergency room problem, foreign body injury has resulted in many lawsuits for indequate treatment and misdiagnosis. A careful history is essential. Many patients present to the physician several days following their injury, as pain is often initially minimal and slowly builds over time. This delay in seeking treatment can result in the patient having traumatic iritis, and occasionally, significant infection.

When examining the patient, the physician should bear in mind that ocular localization of foreign bodies by patients is usually poor. Almost all patients will report that the foreign body is under their upper lid, slightly to one side or the other of midline.

The eye should be anesthetized with topical anesthetic to allow a comfortable and adequate examination with the slit lamp. In those patients suffering from traumatic iritis, their photophobia may impair examination. In such cases, instillation of cyclopegic eyedrops will improve comfort significantly.

Industrial accidents involving drilling or chipping can result in injury by high speed missiles. While the high speed usually sterilizes the missile, it can also cause penetration of the globe and result in retained foreign body. X-ray evaluation of the globe in such cases is required. Failure to recognize retained foreign bodies has been the subject of many successful lawsuits.

While most foreign bodies can be easily found, those consisting of transparent plastic and glass are particularly difficult to locate. Use of fluorescein dye (as in abrasions) can demonstrate linear scratches of the cornea, which can mean the material is embedded in the superior tarsal conjunctival. In such cases, eversion of the eyelid is helpful. If no foreign body can be found, swabbing of the tarsus by a moistened cotton tip applicator may be the only method of removing the suspected agent.

Initial treatment of a non-perforating foreign body by the nonophthalmologist should consist of removal of as much material as possible and pressure patching when infection is not present. Antibiotic eyedrops should be prescribed, and prompt referral to an ophthalmologist for follow-up is prudent.

Follow-up is important since the injury caused by the foreign body can convert to a corneal ulcer if infection sets in. Most ferrous metals leave a rust ring, and the retained material is removed with a drill burr. As with any corneal injury, long-term use of ocular lubricants to aid healing is indicated.

Simple Conjunctivitis/Blepharitis

This condition, due to its frequency, is often trivialized. While the great bulk of this disease can be adequately treated with almost any topical antibiotic, the physician should take great care to examine the cornea prior to and during treatment.

A keratitis is often present, and blepharitis is often associated with immune corneal infiltrates. When unrecognized, these immune infiltrates can convert to sterile corneal ulcers, which then become infected after treatment is discontinued. This is especially common with contact lens wearers.

The general physician is well-advised to make sure the cornea appears clear with normal shine and no areas of opacity. If any opacities are present, prompt referral is necessary.

Ocular Floaters and Photopsia

After the age of 30, most people will experience liquefication of the vitreous body. Since the vitreous is a protein matrix, the more solid portions will clump together and float in the liquid portion, thus the floating opacity noted by the patient. The vitreous body is adherent to the optic nerve head, macula, and periphery of the retina.

A posterior vitreous detachment will often result in a non-floating capacity shaped like a "C" or comma. When the vitreous detaches from the retinal periphery, it may stimulate the retinal photoreceptors and create photopsia. While most (95%) episodes of vitreous detachment are without sequelae, it is important for the physician to know which patients to refer.

Photopsia, accompanied by a shower of 50-100 minute dots, indicates that a retinal vessel has been avulsed (the dots are blood). This should raise a suspicion of retinal tear, and an examination of the retinal periphery is indicated. Most patients who complain of new vitreous floaters and/or photopsia should be referred for examination within one to two weeks.

Retinal Detachment

Head trauma rarely leads to retinal detachment unless the globe is also traumatized. Even when the globe is injured, traumatic retinal detachments make up only 15% of all detachments and most occur as late sequelae.

A history of globe trauma, followed by photopsia and floaters, should raise a strong suspicion of retinal tear. Patients whose retinal tear has progressed to detachment often will describe a partial loss of vision. The portion of the visual field affected is usually "veil-like" or "filmy", and will involve the periphery unless the macula is also detached. The visual loss is never described as "black", for a newly detached retina still maintains some, albeit defective, function.

Traumatic retinal detachments should be promptly repaired, especially when a giant tear or retinal dialysis is present. The natural history of such detachments is progression and inappropriate delay can greatly increase both the difficulty of repair and the risk of postoperative morbidity.

Non-traumatic detachments account for 85% of detachments. There may be symptoms similar to those found in traumatic detachments, or the patient may be unaware of the problem until the macula is involved. Unlike the rest of the retina, which is served by both retinal blood vessels and those of the underlying choroid, the central macula (fovea) has no retinal blood supply. Consequently, when the macula is detached, surgical reattachment must be attempted within seven to ten days to achieve good results.

Traumatic Orbital Fracture

The globe rests in a cushion of fat within the bony orbit. A blow to the globe by a blunt instrument or fist can result in a sudden increase in pressure, which is released by fracture of the orbital wall. This most commonly occurs in the thin floor of the orbit into the maxillary sinus.

Orbital fat, along with the inferior rectus and/or inferior oblique muscles, can herniate through the fracture site. Muscle entrapment may result in a downward gaze with significant restriction of upward (and often downward) movement.

Enophthalmos, movement restriction, pain on upward gaze, anesthesia of the upper lip and/or side of the nose, and diplopia all suggest orbital wall fracture, and an x-ray examination is mandatory both to establish diagnosis and plan subsequent action.

Repair of orbital floor fractures is not an emergency procedure, although a blow of sufficient force to fracture bone can also rupture the globe. Emergency measures should be directed to assess the integrity of the globe.

All orbital floor fractures do not need to be explored and/or repaired. In certain instances, inappropriate exploration can cause more damage than good. The physician may safely wait up to two weeks to observe the patient for improvement. Keep in mind that soft tissue swelling, orbital hematoma, and nerve paresis can cause all of the symptoms noted above. Their resolution may make fracture repair unnecessary.

When enophthalmos is present and herniation of significant fat into the maxillary antrum is demonstrated, repair is indicated to prevent permanent enophthalmos. Likewise, when extraocular muscle entrapment results in gaze restriction or diplopia, repair is appropriate. Repair for muscle entrapment should not be attempted, however, until soft tissue swelling has subsided and forced duction testing is positive for entrapment.

Perforating Injuries of the Globe

A missile or other instrument can penetrate the globe, and when penetration is complete (goes through at least one wall), the injury is defined as a perforation. Perforating injuries are urgent situations, requiring prompt attention.

The external penetrating foreign body can usually be located by appropriate diagnostic means. The perforating object is more difficult to deal with due to the greater local destruction caused by the object as it passes through the various tissues, which often obscures visualization. Furthermore, a penetrating missile can be retained intraocularly or within the surrounding orbital tissues.

The nature of the missile will guide decisions as to whether to leave the foreign body in situ or attempt removal. Intraocular ferrous metals can cause siderosis, and copper metals can result in chalcosis. Both conditions can seriously threaten sight. Steps should be taken to remove these metals, unless the removal is likely to place the eye at even greater risk.

Glass and plastic are inert in the eye and can be safely left alone. Lead and zinc have a low potential for a toxic effect and should only be removed if readily accessible.

Since a perforating injury leaves a wound, the non-surgeon should direct attention to cleaning the site and preventing infection. Broad antibiotic coverage is indicated, since it is almost impossible to identify potentially offending organisms at first examination. The surgeon should culture all removed ocular and foreign material, as well as the wound, prior to closure.

Failure to culture material from a perforated eye can and does result in delayed, appropriate antibiotic treatment and greatly enhances medical-legal liability exposure. Many organisms have an indolent course, and the dreaded complication of endophthalmitis can present days to weeks following injury.

Vitreous Hemorrhage

This condition can occur from trauma, retinal vessel avulsion, retinal tears, spontaneous bleeding from diseased vessels (diabetes and sickle cell disease), and following vitreous body detachment.

Depending on the degree of bleeding, the patient may report a sudden loss of vision or stringy "cobwebs" with minimal loss of acuity. Treatment is supportive while waiting for the blood to resorb. Some authors recommend bed rest with bilateral patching, but this is rarely necessary as long as the patient remains relatively quiet.

The blood will usually clear within days to weeks, allowing the physician an adequate view of the retina and assessment of causation. If an offending blood vessel can be found, laser photocoagulation is effective in most cases.

When the patient has a profound loss of vision and the blood fails to clear within one week, ultrasonic examination of the retina and vitreous cavity is necessary to rule out retinal detachment. Even if the retina appears attached, serial ultrasonic exams may be necessary until direct visualization can be obtained.

Organizing vitreous blood can form traction bands on the retina and cause late detachment. Skilled vitreo-retinal surgeons can now successfully intervene when this complication occurs. Failure to recognize a retinal detachment obscured by hemorrhage has resulted in several lawsuits.

Conclusion

The eye is one of the most complicated organs in the body. Fortunately, nature has endowed the globe with an amazing toughness and resiliency. This property allows the trained physician time to act in a considered manner so as to preserve the integrity of the injured or diseased eye. As with any other branch of medicine, a broad knowledge of anatomy and physiology serve the physician well when care is rendered to the patient with an eye condition.

OTORHINOLARYNGOLOGY

Introduction

This discussion is designed to acquaint physicians with some of the more frequently encountered and potentially difficult complications arising out of the course of care and treatment of otolaryngological problems, and those legal doctrines that may impact upon such risks and complications.

Infections and Sequelae

Infectious diseases of the ear, such as otitis media and acute mastoiditis, today present much less of a management problem than in the era prior to the introduction of effective antibacterial agents. Today, the early treatment of acute infectious diseases of the middle ear and mastoid with appropriate antibiotics almost invariably results in resolution of the acute process with little or no risk of permanent damage to the middle ear, mastoid, or inner ear.

An area of potential liability can arise in the treatment of chronic otitis media and/or mastoiditis. Chronic otitis media manifests itself most commonly in the form of a tympanic membrane perforation which exposes the middle ear to the possibility of recurrent infection. With recurrent otitis media secondary to a tympanic membrane perforation, there is a small but real possibility of extension of the infection to the central nervous system. Therefore, a patient with a tympanic membrane perforation should be given the option of surgical closure of the perforation to minimize the possibility of recurrent infection. Failure to afford the patient this option of surgical closure, and failure to disclose the risk of otitis media leading to central nervous system infection, might, in certain cases, be grounds for liability based on the doctrine of informed consent.

The treatment of chronic mastoiditis currently involves conservative management with the use of debridement of an attic cholesteatoma with topical and systemic antibiotics when appropriate. Even with aggressive medical management, chronic mastoiditis can, on rare occasions, result in the spread of infection to the central nervous system. Therefore, as in the case of chronic otitis media with tympanic membrane perforation, it is advisable that the physician offer the patient the option of mastoid surgery to eradicate the focus of infection and minimize the possibility of a secondary central nervous system infection.

Diseases of the Accessory Sinuses

As in the case of otologic surgery, since the advent of effective antibiotic and anti-allergy therapy, the frequency and extensiveness of accessory paranasal sinus surgery has diminished dramatically. Yet, sinus surgery involving the sphenoid, ethmoid, frontal, and maxillary sinuses still is performed today, although usually in an elective setting as opposed to a situation involving a potentially life-threatening acute infectious process. Thus, more contemporary elective sinus surgery at the present time is done for the alleviation of chronic infectious disease and/or allergic nasal pathology.

Recently, there have been reported numerous cases of malpractice litigation involving serious surgical complications previously thought to be rare in the pre-antibiotic era. Specifically, these include the complications of inadvertent entry into the intracranial cavity, and inadvertent damage to the optic nerve occasioned by surgery on the sphenoethmoid sinus complex. It would not be unreasonable to postulate that this rather recent increase in serious complications following sinus surgery of this type may be due to a relatively limited number of major spheno-ethmoid sinus procedures carried out by otolaryngologists, both in their training phase as residents and following residency. With the recent increase in the number of residents being trained and a concomitant decrease in the amount of serious sinus diseases encountered during residency training, a strong argument could be made that many otolaryngologists have had marginal training in sophisticated sinus surgery and lack sufficient continuing exposure to maintain the critical skills necessary to do effective and safe major sphenoethmoid sinus surgery.

The complications of visual loss, along with intracranial complications, can and do occur in the absence of technical negligence, and the mere occurrence of these complications does not mean that a malpractice claim against the operating surgeon cannot be successfully defended. Many plaintiffs' attorneys will argue that the mere occurrence of these complications could only be the result of technical negligence (probably inexperience) on the part of the operating surgeon. However, in view of the complexity of the anatomy in these areas, along with possible alteration of the anatomy by the underlying disease processes of polyposis and chronic infection, medical malpractice suits can be won by the defendant-surgeon, particularly if he can produce evidence of adequate training and a reasonable ongoing surgical case load which would support his technical expertise and ability in doing procedures of this type. Surgeons who encounter significant sphenoethmoid pathology only rarely in their patient case load should refrain frcm embarking upon extensive sphenoethmoid surgery, and should refer these complex problems to surgeons with greater expertise and greater surgical case loads in this area.

Acoustic Neuromas

The majority of malpractice litigation involving the care and treatment of otologic disorders involves some type of instrumental or surgical intervention. However, a major area of concern which can lead to significant potential medical malpractice liability concerns the proper diagnosis of cerebello-pontine angle tumors.

With the rapid advance of audiological, electronystagmographic, roentgenological, and imaging technology, potentially life-threatening tumors of the cerebello-pontine angle can be diagnosed at a much earlier stage than ever thought possible even ten years ago. It is essential that all physicians confronted with otological problems be familiar with these rapidly developing techniques and their impact on the early diagnosis of lesions of the cerebello-pontine angle, such as acoustic neuromas. A delay or failure to diagnose an early acute neuroma can cause a lost opportunity on the part of a patient to have his treatment of the acoustic neuroma carried out at a stage where preservation of hearing, facial nerve function, and even life itself, are possible. It, therefore, behooves a prudent physician who is presented with an otherwise unexplained unilateral sensorineural hearing loss to carry out aggressive otological, electronystagmographic, neurological, and finally, roentgenological procedures to rule out the existence of an early acoustic neuroma.

Surgical Risks - Informed Consent

Most elective otologic surgery, including such procedures as stapedectomy, tympanoplasty, and mastoidectomy, involve similar surgical risks. These risks include temporary or permanent damage to the facial nerve, temporary or permanent balance disorders, and actual worsening of the patient's hearing as compared to the pre-operative level. The more elective in nature the surgical procedure is, the greater degree of disclosure and discussion is required in providing adequate informed consent. Certainly, all patients undergoing procedures of the type mentioned above need to be warned and to fully understand the complications of facial paralysis, dizziness, or unsteadiness, which may impact on the vocational and non-vocational aspects of their daily lives, and finally, the small but real likelihood that an operation designed to improve hearing not only may fail, but may result in further deterioration of what residual hearing is left prior to the surgery.

Even with the tremendous advancements in microscopic ear surgery, modern otologic surgery to improve hearing and eliminate infection is fraught with many potential complications. Failure to offer the option of surgery and disclosure of the attendant risks of medical management alone, as in the case of otitis media, might be the basis for medicolegal liability based on the doctrine of informed consent.

In performing a stapedectomy, the complications of facial nerve injury, long-standing balance disorders, and total loss of hearing, although rare, occur with some degree of frequency. From a defense standpoint, the complication that would be the most difficult to defend against is that of facial nerve injury. In the vast majority of cases of otosclerosis, the middle ear anatomy is relatively normal, and a physician would be hard pressed to adequately explain any facial nerve injury occurring pursuant to stapedectomy surgery which resulted in significant permanent facial paralysis. Unlike facial nerve injury, though, post-operative vestibular problems and total loss of hearing can and do occur in the range of approximately 1 to 3%. These complications, of course, occur because of the requisite entry into the inner ear necessitated by removal of the oval window footplate. Therefore, in the numerous suits filed because of persistent balance problems and total loss of hearing, a defense based upon a showing of no formal technical errors occurring in the performance of this procedure, in spite of an otherwise unexplained total loss of vestibular and auditory dysfunction, can result in a jury verdict in favor of the defendant-doctor.

As in the case of stapedectomy surgery, in most cases of tympanoplasty surgery, the anatomy of the middle ear has not been altered by disease process so much so as to make identification and preservation of the facial nerve difficult. Thus, as in the case of a stapedectomy, a permanent injury to the facial nerve producing facial paralysis would be difficult to defend against based upon the standards and techniques currently employed in modern tympanoplasty surgery. Similarly, if there is no violation of the oval or round window during tympanoplasty surgery, the likelihood of severe permanent post-operative balance symptoms and severe post-operative permanent sensorineural hearing loss is quite small, and the occurrence of either or both of these untoward events would create strong suspicion that the operating physician had inadvertently violated the oval or round window, thereby making a successful defense to a medical malpractice action quite difficult.

Finally, mastoidectomy surgery can produce these same three major complications. Unlike the case of stapedectomy and routine tympanoplasty surgery, in mastoidectomy surgery, disease or prior surgeries may have altered the anatomy of the mastoid cavity, and significant injury to the facial nerve in its vertical course can occur with some degree of frequency. Therefore, if it can be shown that there was substantial alteration of the normal anatomy by prior surgeries and/or disease processes, an otologic surgeon will stand a much better chance of a successful defense than in the case where the middle ear and mastoid anatomy was relatively normal. Also, mastoid surgery carried out with even a low-grade infection can lead to permanent loss of hearing and vestibular dysfunction, and these complications arising after mastoidectomy surgery performed in the face of a well-controlled but even residual middle ear and mastoid infection provide a reasonable explanation and possible defense should these untoward complications occur.

Major Head and Neck Surgery

This subdivision of otolaryngology includes an enormous number of both benign and malignant disease processes which can give rise to an equally enormous number of major and minor complications. Only a few of the more common and serious complications will be dealt with here.

Thyroid and parotid gland surgeries are surgical procedures carried out with relative frequency by head and neck surgeons of various specialty backgrounds. In both, the principle complication is that of nerve injury to either the recurrent laryngeal or the facial nerve.

Since both the recurrent laryngeal and facial nerves are at high risk during thyroid and parotid gland surgery, respectively, it is incumbent upon the head and neck surgeon carrying out a partial or complete thyroidectomy and parotidectomy to disclose in great detail to his patient the nature of the injury to these respective nerves. The patient must have a clear understanding as to the voice change problems which can occur, even during properly performed thyroidectomy surgery. Also, the catastrophic function and cosmetic deformities resulting from inadvertent section of the facial nerve during parotidectomy surgery must be made patently clear to all patients who contemplate undergoing this procedure. A failure to obtain informed consent regarding these procedures could give rise to a claim for malpractice following the development of voice and facial paralytic changes, which would be most difficult to defend in the absence of proper documentation that a complete discussion had been carried out with the patient regarding these complications prior to surgery.

The currently accepted standards of care regarding thyroidectomy and parotid gland surgery require the surgeon to expose both nerves prior to surgical removal of some or all of the respective organs. Failure of the surgeon to properly identify the nerves in order to protect them during the subsequent surgical dissection of the thyroid or parotid gland likely would put the nerves at a greater risk, and would make the defense of a claim of technical negligence in the performance of the thyroidectomy or parotidectomy most difficult to defend in the absence of proper operative identification of the recurrent laryngeal and facial nerves.

A listing of all the potential complications associated with major extirpative head and neck cancer surgery is impossible in a handbook of this size. However, a new doctrine has appeared on the legal scene in the past ten years which has particular applicability to the care and treatment of head and neck cancer patients. This doctrine has been referred to as the lost chance or lost opportunity for cure or for less radical treatment. The doctrine comes into play in a situation where there has been a failure of or delay in the diagnosis of a head and neck cancer. More specifically, the doctrine applies where the delay in diagnosis results in the cancer causing the patient great agony and death, or where the patient is forced to undergo a more radical ablative surgery than if the diagnosis had been made at an earlier time.

Facial Plastic and Reconstructive Surgery

The past 15 years have seen a tremendous development in plastic, reconstructive, and cosmetic surgery of the head and neck. In the past, the bulk of this type of surgery was performed by other specialties, in particular the specialty of general plastic surgery. However, with respect to both training and experience at the resident level and as part of the specialty board examination, facial plastic surgery has increasingly become a major subdivision in the broad field of otolaryngology.

There is probably no area of otolaryngology where the doctrine of informed consent is as important as in the area of facial plastic surgery in general, and aesthetic or cosmetic facial surgery in particular. In discussing cosmetic operations of the head and neck, one must keep in mind that this surgery is the purest form of elective surgery. Rarely are there severe deformities or disease processes causing morbidity or mortality as in other areas of otolaryngology. It, therefore, would not be unreasonable to describe a good deal of facial aesthetic surgery as being "frivolous" in nature. The term "frivolous" here should not be taken as being derogatory in nature, but merely connotes surgery for which there is no true medical necessity, or surgery for vanity's sake alone.

Because of the nature of this surgery, more informed consent is required in this area than in any other area of otolaryngology. Patients usually come to these physicians not because of deformity or disease pathology, but merely to improve what is otherwise a relatively normal appearance. It is of utmost importance that the prudent facial aesthetic surgeon carry out a complete discussion of all the risks associated with the contemplated procedure, including major and even relatively minor or inconsequential complications. Since the surgery in its purest form is not necessary for the physical health or well-being of the patient, if he or she develops a complication which has not been disclosed, a strong argument can be made that that patient and a reasonable person in the position of that patient, because of the unnecessary nature of the surgery, would probably not have undergone the procedure if they had been told of an even relatively inconsequential complication. Although this analysis may seem harsh, it is but one of the "facts of life" which the aesthetic facial plastic surgeon is exposed to on a daily basis in carrying out surgery of this type. Failure to recognize and deal effectively with this potential area of liability can result in numerous lawsuits being brought where otherwise there would be no clear-cut evidence of negligence in the actual technical performance of the procedure. Documentation in the form of legible notes in the patient's chart, audio tape recordings, and with some potentially problem patients even videotaping, are effective methods of providing adequate evidence that informed consent has been given should a claim for medical malpractice based upon this legal theory of liability be brought later.

Informed consent should always be carried out by the treating physician and not by one of his office staff. The discussion should be in terminology which an average lay person can understand and technical terms should be avoided. In summary, the key to carrying out successful aesthetic facial surgery and avoiding the incurrence of a large series of medical malpractice claims is establishing good rapport between doctor and patient prior to undertaking the elective procedure, and establishing that the patient has a keen understanding of any and all material risks which may occur, even in properly performed surgeries of this type.

One of the issues that frequently arises when claims are made that a physician was negligent in the technical performance of the facial plastic procedure concerns the issue of standard of care. In recent years, numerous specialties have begun to perform aesthetic head and neck surgery which in the past was almost strictly within the purview of the general plastic surgeon. With the competitive encroachment of other surgical specialties, such as dermatology, ophthalmology, oral surgery, and otolaryngology, local competitive political turf battles have arisen. Out of this can arise medical malpractice litigation in which a major issue will be to establish what the standard of care is as it applies to the respective surgical specialist who performed the head and neck aesthetic operation. The key here is that there is only one standard of care, and that is evidenced by the standard of a reasonable, prudent physician who holds himself out as being competent to carry out the aesthetic head and neck surgical procedure in question.

Another area of concern is the potential for a breach of warranty lawsuit based on a physician's alleged promise of results in this area. A physician should be optimistic and hopeful, but never guarantee, either directly or by implication, what the results will be as they relate to the patient's expectations. These conversations should be conducted in the same manner as discussions undertaken to obtain a proper informed consent.

Hearing Impairment

Hearing impairment is becoming more and more of a medicolegal problem. People are living longer and long enough to develop impaired hearing. This must be detected; otherwise, older people become isolated, depressed, and may even suffer dementia. It must be differentiated from Alzheimer's disease. Hearing impairment can occur from trauma, particularly to the head. Malingering is a serious medicolegal problem in this area. Hearing difficulties may come from exposure to noise, including music - symphonic, as well as rock. In any event, the detection of hearing disabilities has advanced, as have the availability of hearing aids. The otologist must be vigilant and diligent, and thus be able avoid successful suits for negligence.

Conclusion

This brief overview of medical malpractice litigation and its applicability to otolaryngology in general, and its subdivision in particular, should afford physicians with a clear understanding of the requisite elements of negligence and informed consent. With this knowledge, a practitioner should be able to better structure the physician-patient relationship based upon the disease process of a patient, the patient's needs and desires, the patient's understanding of risks and complications, and one's own training and experience, so as to minimize the possibility of a medical malpractice lawsuit subsequently developing, and so as to allow one to mount an effective defense if sued by employing the principles and concepts discussed in this chapter.

PLASTIC SURGERY

Introduction

The frequency and severity of claims against plastic surgeons are usually lower than those in some of the other "high risk" specialties. Why then does plastic surgery carry a higher risk than many experts feel it warrants?

Many, if not most, plastic surgical procedures involve "body image" surgery. This is true whether the procedure is cosmetic or reconstructive. A bad result, therefore, can be as devastating as physical injury. Even if the procedure is designed to improve a pre-existing problem, the patient can nevertheless be psychologically devastated by an untoward or unanticipated result. It follows that many complications and/or untoward results lead to *visible* defects. Unlike general surgery or neurosurgery, where a mistake may well be internal, invisible, or latent, a jury can more easily relate to a bad plastic surgical result because it involves the plaintiff's difficulties regarding his or her day-to-day activities, such as going to work or appearing in public.

Informed Consent

Plastic surgeons have traditionally been identified as having excellent skills in the area of informed consent. More than perhaps any other specialty, plastic surgeons remain continually aware of the need to inform their patients, and yet attempt to match the anticipated result as closely as possible to the patient's expectations. In addition, most plastic surgeons are aware of the ideal inverse relationship between a physical defect and the patient's concern. In other words, the ideal reconstructive or cosmetic patient is one whose defect is "severe", but whose response is minimal or moderate at worst. On the other hand, the antithesis of the ideal patient is one whose defect is small, but whose concern is great. The plastic surgeon should spend a lot of time and effort in attempting to distinguish between these two broad categories of patients, and should be prepared to consider avoiding surgery on the latter group. The plastic surgeon may "huff and puff", but never promise, guarantee, or warrant.

Domain

There are few procedures which are exclusively the domain of the plastic surgeon. As recently as a few years ago, many would maintain that cosmetic surgery was their exclusive domain, but as we are all aware, that is certainly no longer the case. Since there is much overlap between the boundaries of the plastic surgeon's role with those of other surgical specialties, e.g., otorhinolaryngology, significant questions concerning training, experience, and surgical philosophy can arise. It is incumbent on anyone working in or analyzing these areas to be aware of the potential concerns involving training, knowledge, skill, and expertise.

Specific Areas of Potential Risk — Emergency Rooms

In the past two decades, patients have begun using emergency rooms for routine care, and in many cases, they have also increased their demand for specialty care for injuries which might have been handled by a family physician or the on-call general surgeon in past years. There is now an increased demand for repair of injuries ranging from routine lacerations to back injuries to maxillofacial trauma. The marked increase in injuries requiring a plastic surgeon is due to motor vehicle accidents and trauma sustained in a work or play environment. There are significant medicolegal considerations arising from this, because a variety of physicians may answer the call for care and management, i.e., the standard of care.

Standard of Care

If a non-plastic surgeon chooses to treat complex facial lacerations, he may be held to a standard of care that would be applied if a plastic surgeon had been called. In many instances, acute care of the severe facial injury may require only conservative debridement, and reapproximation of severely traumatized wound margins with no "ideal repair" being possible. In this situation, if properly treated, it could be anticipated that a plastic surgeon would have achieved a better immediate result; long-term revision or reconstruction might have been necessary in any event. On the other hand, simple facial lacerations, especially in children, can present judgment problems.

Honoring Patient Requests

If the patient, or more usually the patient's parents, request a plastic surgeon, emergency room physicians are best advised to accede to the patient's wishes. If the emergency room physician elects to treat, in spite of the patient's request, and if a bad result is achieved, there is a significant increase in the likelihood that the patient will complain and sue. This, despite the fact that the plastic surgeon might not have been able to achieve a better result. It is important to remember that even a mere patient complaint causes the physician and the hospital a loss of time, expense, and anguish. This may very well have been avoided in most instances, if the plastic surgeon had been called.

Many plastic surgeons, to say the least, experience frustration when called to the emergency room, particularly on a Saturday night, to treat a small, simple (2 cm.) laceration of the brow of an infant or child. Nevertheless, that bother is miniscule compared to the difficulty the health care provider will face if the emergency room or primary care physician chooses to ignore the wishes of the patient, and a bad result ensues. If the plastic surgeon is called and refuses, the administrative consequences can be serious, and his reputation will be "mud". A similar scenario may be played out in the case of a major injury which is treated by a non-plastic surgeon, such as an emergency room physician, either by choice or because the plastic surgeon was not available. In treating a major soft tissue wound of the face, especially when tissue loss or necrosis has already occurred, the peril and risk occur as a result of severe criticism of the physician, usually the emergency room physician, if he debrides the wound too aggressively and extensively.

The plastic surgeon who ultimately accepts the patient's care should not be critical of the repair person if he "tacked" back tissue which was obviously not viable. However, the original physician can be open to severe criticism and potential liability if by trimming away the severely compromised tissue, he either removes something that might have survived, or compromises the long-term reconstructive effort.

An extreme, though illustrative example, involved a teenager who sustained a high velocity gunshot wound to his cheek. A general surgeon, rejecting a plastic surgeon's help, elected to treat the through and through cheek injury without assistance. He was dealing with a 4 to 5 cm., full thickness defect of the cheek, which invariably requires extensive reconstructive surgery. However, the general surgeon's short-term solution was to simply pull the wound margins together, instead of treating it more appropriately as a true reconstructive surgeon would have. In achieving a "closed" wound, he distorted all the facial landmarks, including the eyelids, nose, and mouth. By the time the plastic surgeon came into the picture, he had to contend not only with the massive soft tissue loss, but also with the resulting scarring and distortion of other structures, all of which severely compounded the problem.

"Stupid" Remarks

Sometimes, facetious remarks can be potentially troublesome for another physician, specifically a plastic surgeon. In one such scenario, a general physician told a patient, "I could take care of your problem (either laceration repair or lesion removal), but I would prefer for the plastic surgeon to do it since he will leave no scar." In this case, a laceration had to be repaired. It could have involved the removal of a small facial lesion. Imagine the consequences if a scar resulted, yet there was no negligence. It would have been simpler to suggest a plastic surgeon, because he is a specialist; then, the referring surgeon would be off the hook and would not be placed in a potentially compromising situation.

Emergency Room Physician v. Plastic Surgeon

Quite often, in an emergency room setting, the only real advantage offered by the plastic surgeon is that he has the training, inclination, and opportunity to spend the time required to give the wound optimum care, whereas the emergency room physician may have a number of patients waiting for him. In the less acute setting, the plastic surgeon's training allows him to often select the best incision orientation and wound closure. However, no amount of training or experience guarantees that the repair of a wound will not leave a scar. A physician should do the plastic surgical consultant a favor and not lead the patient to believe that the plastic surgeon always gets "perfect" results. And finally in this area, it is always reasonable that if a physician chooses to treat a patient in a questionable situation, he should at least obtain a telephone consultation from a plastic surgical consultant, and an agreement that he would follow-up on the patient if desired.

Breast Cancer

Breast cancer represents a growing area of shared responsibility in management of the patient. It is the standard of care and custom that when a primary care physician discovers a suspicious breast mass, the patient is referred to a specialist for definitive diagnosis and treatment. This is usually a general surgeon, but once the diagnosis has been made, a plastic surgical consultation prior to surgery, especially for a mastectomy, is appropriate in today's environment. It is the responsibility of the primary care physician, especially if he has a continuing relationship with the patient, to suggest in many, if not most cases, breast reconstruction as a sequence to the surgery. Formerly, many general surgeons were hesitant to "allow" early reconstruction for their mastectomy patients, but this philosophy seems to be on the wane, though it still exists in some areas of the country even today.

Even if it ultimately proves not possible or practical for a patient to undergo early reconstruction, the psychological benefit gained from her being aware of the possibility can be of help in this stressful situation. If the patient desires to consider reconstruction, this can also be helpful in planning the timing of the mastectomy. For example, the "saber-slash" oblique vertical mastectomy incision favored by many surgeons makes breast reconstruction more difficult. By simply altering the incision, reconstructive options are enhanced without jeopardizing the result.

Though still controversial, the question of immediate versus delayed reconstruction can also be a factor in planning the mastectomy. For this reason, it behooves the general surgeon or the patient's family physician to ensure that in appropriate cases the patient has been offered a plastic surgical consultation prior to the mastectomy. Of course, there are circumstances when this is not possible, e.g., when a mastectomy is required directly after a biopsy which was expected to be negative and which showed invasive carcinoma. No valid criticism can be leveled at the surgeon under these circumstances. The patient's record should document that such was the case. It must be remembered, however, that even though it is expected that everyone is aware of the availability of breast reconstruction, some patients are not willing to "overrule" their surgeon when he declines a request for reconstructive consultation prior to surgery. It is, therefore, the responsibility of the primary care physician to advise a patient of this option.

For the general surgeon who anticipates a patient opting for reconstruction, he should consider tailoring the incision appropriately, so as to aid in the ultimate reconstruction. However, the surgeon should not limit the breast or skin resection merely to make reconstruction easier if, in the surgeon's judgment, this may lead to any increased risk. Many general surgeons formerly opposed reconstruction because they were concerned about the possibility of local recurrence and its impact on the course of reconstruction. Although the incidence of local recurrence is low now, a surgeon does not want to do anything which will increase this risk, even if the required skin resection does make reconstruction more difficult.

Neither the primary care physician nor the general surgeon should suggest to the mastectomy patient that reconstruction will result in a breast "as good as the original". With the advent of tissue expanders and improved flaps for breast reconstruction, surgeons often can achieve incredible results. However, it is a disservice to the patient to lead her to expect that this can always be expected. A better approach should be that the results of reconstruction be characterized in terms of the building of a "breast mound", rather than a perfect "new" breast. One rationale for delaying reconstruction is that it allows the patient to "adjust to her deformity", making it theoretically easier for her to adjust to a less than perfect reconstruction result. Today, most surgeons believe that this "period of adjustment" can be obviated by extensive discussion with the patient preoperatively. It nevertheless remains difficult for any patient to have a totally clear image of the result; it is the physician's job to make this transition as easy as possible.

Prophylactic Mastectomy

There are a number of aspects to be considered vis-a-vis prophylactic mastectomy for conditions such as fibrocystic disease. However, there is no true "prophylactic" mastectomy, except with the most extensive simple mastectomy. If the nipple and areola are preserved, and if the axillary tail of the breast is not resected, significant breast tissue remains where cancer may develop subsequently. It is a disservice to the patient to "sell" her a subcutaneous mastectomy, leading her to believe that she no longer will have to worry about developing cancer. On the other hand, as long as she clearly understands that this type of operation may decrease her chances of breast cancer, and may allow her to avoid multiple biopsies, which bring many of these women to a plastic surgeon, then it is arguably a reasonable surgical approach. If the nipple is to be preserved, however, the standard of care requires intraoperative pathologic inspection of tissue from the base of the nipple and areola, and of any suspicious palpable masses within the tissue specimens.

Mastodynia

A common complaint following subcutaneous mastectomy/reconstruction is mastodynia. It is critical that the surgeon caution the patient that subcutaneous mastectomy may have absolutely no effect on her mastodynia and, in fact, it may worsen, even though in some cases, it does abolish the pain. A plaintiff's attorney could establish that the standard of care requires that the patient understand this before undertaking a subcutaneous mastectomy when her chief complaint is pain. Many patients may even forget much of the content of their pre-operative discussion with the surgeon. It is, therefore, critical that the discussion be carefully documented in the patient's record. An experience with a former patient illustrates this problem. At the request of her general surgeon, I assisted him in doing her subcutaneous mastectomy and immediately thereafter performed a subpectoral reconstruction. She had a superb cosmetic result; when she came for suture removal, my office nurse thought that she had undergone a cosmetic augmentation rather than the mastectomy with reconstruction. Her chief pre-operative complaint was mastodynia. As stated in my office records, I spent two hours pre-operatively discussing her problem, her complaints, the proposed surgery, and all the anticipated potential ramifications. Most of the time was spent discussing the fact that I could not predict whether her pain would be the same, better, or worse post-operatively. There was no doubt she understood and accepted this risk. Surgery was performed seven years ago, but when I talked with her recently, she told me her pain was still as bad as, and perhaps worse than, the pain which brought her to the operating room. Incidentally, she has completely forgotten the content of our extensive pre-operative discussion, as well as conversations which occurred immediately post-operatively. Although we have maintained a close, positive physician-patient rapport, her greatest comfort came from her review of her record, a copy of which she took when she moved from my area. It reminds her that her current situation was a likely possibility. But for this, I have little doubt that the misery experienced by her would have led to a lawyer's office door.

Cosmetic Surgery

Cosmetic surgery represents an attempt to improve a condition which to the reasonable observer would appear to be "within normal limits". Reconstructive procedures, on the other hand, are designed to improve a condition that lies outside these so-called reasonably normal limits.

Patient Selection

One of the most important aspects of cosmetic surgery is patient selection. Perhaps more than with a "reconstructive" procedure, the cosmetic patient must be evaluated in terms of the sliding scale of comparison of patient concern and defect. Thus, the patient with a practically invisible defect who characterizes it as having ruined his or her life, is not a good candidate for cosmetic surgery. Nevertheless, many patients will still want the procedure done.

Informed Consent

Many plastic surgeons have created specific informed consent documents. They often videotape the discussions, and have the patient read an informative brochure and sign a confirmatory statement which is included in the record. It is incumbent on the referring physician to be certain that the plastic surgeon has adequately informed the patient. Many cosmetic procedures are performed by non-formally trained "cosmetic" surgeons. These so-called surgeons must be prepared to respond to plaintiffs, attorneys, judges, and juries who question them as to whether their training is adequate and prepares them sufficiently to hold themselves out as adequate practitioners of that specialty.

Suction Lipectomy

Suction lipectomy has become one of the most commonly performed cosmetic procedures. Many of them are done by non-plastic surgeons, including but not limited to general surgeons, gynecologists, dermatologists, otolaryngologists, ophthalmologists, and family physicians, and probably other groups of which I am not aware. The majority of plastic surgeons have not had formal residency training in suction lipectomy or "fat suctioning". The procedure did not gain wide acceptance in this country until the early 1980's. Therefore, the dermatologist's (and others) two or three day seminar may well be as adequate as the plastic surgeon's seminar. However, the surgeon's overall training and expertise certainly make a difference. Even though the incidence of severe complications from suction lipectomy is extremely low, a disproportionate percentage of these complications have been experienced by patients of non-plastic surgeons. Anyone who undertakes a suction lipectomy must not only learn the basic procedure, but also overall patient management.

Breast Augmentation

There are a number of controversial aspects incident to this procedure. The most common complication following this relatively "simple" procedure, occurring in 25-50% of patients, is inordinate "firmness" of the breasts, sometimes literally "rock hard". This can occur with the best of care. There are few procedures that carry an anticipated complication rate of this magnitude. Yet, this is the second most common cosmetic surgery done in the United States. Patient satisfaction has been found to be about 95%. There are a number of approaches that limit this complication. Firmness, denoted as capsule contractures, is not a "rejection" phenomenon, nor can it be avoided by any currently accepted approach. Nevertheless, most plastic surgeons consider the procedure and the silicone implants to be "safe" within the context of current understanding.

Two questions have surfaced regarding breast augmentation. One, can silicone implants cause cancer? To date, no such association has been documented, and silicone implants have been in use since the early 1960's. Two, can breast cancer be diagnosed in an augmented patient? Most surgeons are of the opinion that the augmented breast can be examined as easily, and perhaps more easily, than the non-augmented breast, since small lumps cannot become "hidden" in the intercostal spaces as they can in the non-augmented breast. However, it is clear that mammography has some limitations in the post-breast augmentation patient. The mammogram beam cannot "see through" the implant. However, this does not mean that mammography is impossible in such patients; it simply means that special views must be taken in order to look around the implant and visualize the breast tissue. A standard two view mammogram in such patients is simply not adequate, and cannot be considered diagnostically reliable.

Smoking

It has been demonstrated that tissue loss is much more frequent in patients who are smokers in facelift, breast reduction and reconstruction, skin flaps, and any procedure which results in wound tension or wide tissue undermining. A referring physician is obliged to reveal this historical fact to the plastic surgeon, as well as to the patient. She should make a decision whether to stop smoking. The surgeon can also decide what he wishes to do with a smoker, particularly if he believes that it represents a sufficient compromise of the surgical result. Some surgeons prefer to avoid facelift surgery and abdominal flap breast reconstruction on smokers who will not stop smoking for at least a couple of weeks pre-operatively and continue not to smoke for a week or two postoperatively. The bottom line, however, is that currently, physicians cannot give a hard and fast rule in this area.

Conclusion

The plastic surgeon shares many of the same liability problems as are experienced by all physicians, plus special problems inherent in this specialty practice, primarily because they greatly involve the patient's emotional and social concerns.

SURGERY

One specialty for a physician does fit.
Total medical knowledge needs genius' wit.

Introduction

Equanimity in surgical practice is an acquired virtue. Over many years, it increases slowly. Virtue eventually becomes its own silent reward. To receive this deserving superior personal merit demands a certain degree of self-protectivism. Surgical residents about to enter the professional world of surgery must be alerted to berms that can impede progression toward achieving this objective.

In centuries past, the ancient surgeons pursued specific traditional guidelines that gave courage to themselves, and simultaneously bolstered the stature of surgery. It was axiomatic for surgeons to adhere to primordial tenets. Thus, it was taught that one could not be a master surgeon without a familiarity with the foundations and generalizations of medicine. An admirable surgeon was looked upon as being moderately bold, not prone to unwarranted disputations, and who only operated upon patients after much premeditated studies. Prior to every surgical procedure, the surgeon was obliged to be provided with every asset necessary for successful surgery. Signs of the master surgeon were a temperate, moderating disposition, plus a cautious utterance of prognoses.

Surgeons should be logical, and know their spoken language so as to be able to communicate and understand their patients in both speech and written words. Opinions must be supported by proper reasoning when needed. To fulfill the surgical credo, one must be learned in the specialty to the height of an expert. Added to this expertise is the need for ingenious creativity with the ability to adapt to either unforeseen situations or complications.

All these traits weld the surgeon to be stern in all sure surgical knowables and fearful of unanticipated situations. Surgeons are constantly aware of the reality that the operation itself is but one incident, no doubt the most dramatic, in the concatenation of events between the illness and expected recovery. With this awareness, the financial adherent to the practice of surgery is of tertiary concern that takes care of itself.

Compassion

Magnificent advancements made by this century's bioscientists have formed a system in which most standardized operative procedures are safe for patients. However, all patients are not totally prepared for their journey through the operation suite. The patient may know or have ascertained that the surgeon is capable, and has cool judgment, technical dexterity, and reasonable rapidity. All these fine professional praises do not complete the surgical portrait. Surgeons should comfort their patients by pleasantness, and accede to their requests if they do not interfere with the plan of therapy or impede proper hospital policy.

Empathy is laudable, but in the surgeon-patient relationship, that sentiment is transcended. Compassion is more desired by the ailing patient. Dissatisfaction with the American surgeon has been pronounced in words and written about frequently. Many believe that surgeons have been mesmerized by new biotechnology. In the process of adaptation to it, they have lost compassion for and appreciation of the patient as an individual and the family that is concerned with the patient's well-being. Surgeons should be tactful not to be looked upon as technocrats without human sensitivity.

This concept of understanding commences during the initial meeting between the surgeon and the patient. First impressions may be the only impression arrived at by the patient. For this reason, the history taking and physical examination of the patient remain essential, fundamental principles that traditionally establish or disrupt the professional patient rapprochement. The intrinsic value of a precise history and complete physical examination remains the benchmark legacy of medicosurgical practice.

History, Physical Examination, and Laboratory Reports

Via a history taking, a physician commences to know his patient. A plenary history includes information that is personal, familial, social, and occupational, plus any other necessary details required to properly arrive at procedural requisites that will aid the patient. A medical history is the preamble to performing a satisfactory physical examination. Both are equally important in order to arrive at a tentative diagnosis prior to instituting costly laboratory studies to verify the clinical diagnosis.

Acquiring a detailed medical history leads directly to the performance of an adequate physical examination. Each examination of a patient must be done painstakingly, for it is the foundation upon which is derived the affirmation or denial of the symptoms (except for those entirely subjective, which do not produce physical signs) presented by the patient. There is only one standard for the performance of a physical examination, namely, thoroughness with completeness that leads to a scientific, unbiased, deductive interpretation of all the symptoms and signs discernible. The surgeon's conduct during the physical examination is the patient's litmus test of the examiner. Via the history taking and the physical examination performance, the surgeon will merit confidence, create esteem, and display professionalism.

In the matter of utilizing laboratory tests, economic overseeing is in vogue. Discretion is laudable, but negligence is to be avoided. Single laboratory tests that indicate an abnormality must be verified by a repetition thereof. Deviations from accuracy may be due to human or mechanical sources of error. A repeated test can verify or sustain initial laboratory findings. Under legal scrutiny, two laboratory tests of similar reading are more persuasive than one.

Among the most common sources of errors in the laboratory are mechanical imperfection of instruments, human failure, misinterpretations, mixed-up specimens, improper labels, clerical non-medical mistakes, etc. Surgeons should never become so busy that they fail to study the many laboratory reports attached to the hospital record and those included in their office file.

Medical Records

Every clinical, laboratory, and research physician during a professional career will be compelled to either dictate or write medical reports in the medical record.

The socioeconomic reality of life prognosticates that many of these documents will be admitted as evidence in a court of law. Therefore, every medical report of all kinds must be written with care if the author is to avoid embarrassment.

In all contemporaneous or contemplative writings, errors in grammar, misused words, confusing phrases, and improper medical terminology can be legally perilous. Hospital records are notoriously deficient in legibility, consistency (nurses' notes contradicting physicians' progress notations), accuracy, completion, and totality. The full value of proper medical records is appreciated when they are a defense against professional liability. Flawed medical records are in themselves evidence of negligent professional behavior.

Professionalism

The surgical discipline is neither recumbent nor invisible. It is a dynamic, progressively learned, intellectual, dexterous pursuit dedicated to the amelioration of injuries and the treatment of diseases. Those who elect to participate in its activities are readily identifiable by their deportment. It is called professionalism, which is the mark of a singular social station. Such persons are held in high esteem. They gain social prestige because they serve communities according to their needs without striving for large monetary incomes. All those who are educated in medicine have as their primary motive active service to humanity. Service orientation is an egregious ascription of people in medicine.

During medical school, residency training, and as young physicians professionalism is developed. This is expressed by upright deportment with other persons, individual etiquette, and personal hygiene. These traits engender the impalpable marks of distinction that illuminate the professional person. Inherent in these elements is the concept of self-evaluation and self-correction for the ultimate improvement of personality. Although it is true that the laity, via the printed and electronic media, has been among the strongest critics of the medical profession, nonetheless, physicians have been, by far, the greatest critics of themselves. Yet, awareness and response to the justified criticisms of others is critical to the individual surgeon and to surgery as a specialty.

Medical professionalism has a deep significance because it sustains an interpersonal physician-patient relationship. It is intimate. Thus, it demands mutual respect of unquestionable moral rectitude. To behave otherwise is to be a recreant to Hippocratic idealism. Professional persons encourage respectful conduct as the indispensable ingredient for the harmonious exchange of admirable human interreactions. Respectful professionalism creates, sustains, and preserves the patient's confidential trust in their physicians.

In some ways, the surgeon has burdens over and above colleagues in other specialties. The professional life of a surgeon has additional constrictions outside the knowledge and practice of surgery. Surgeons are restricted by many medicolegal, governmental, and intra-surgical guidelines. Conformity to these regulations, which often are irritants, fashions in its own manner professional conduct. Thus, the surgeon's duties, responsibilities, and obligations extend to all levels of society.

Surgeons have crowned surgery as king of the specialties. If they consider it to be so, then surgeons must have nobler behavior to merit this self-imposed accolade. The neophyte surgeon is encompassed into this regality. Surgical residents should not concentrate on future economic stresses and the earning capacity surgery allows. Such distractions blunt or obfuscate the aim of gaining the basic knowledge that is available during the formative period of surgical training. Residents should not look so far ahead that their present assignments may be devalued.

Ethical Conduct

The wisdom and prudential restraint of surgeons is relied upon to do all that is rightly proper for their patients. Surgery is a science from its source of knowledge. The application of this learning is an art. In addition, it has its own indigenous ethical code of honor which is an eternal quality derived from life itself. This is the central core of surgical practice. Surgeons are privileged to be invited into the hearts and minds of patients (also those close to the bedside) at a time when they are most vulnerable.

Intrinsic to this fiduciary confidence is the requisite for surgeons to follow the mores of humanity, namely, to participate in human activities which have for their purposes the improvement of the health, welfare, and education of individuals as human beings. Because of personal relationships with patients, surgeons should assist in the social growth of society as an integral segment of the humanity they serve.

All these are of optimal significance, which have their origin in personal conscience formation during the residency period. Every physician/surgeon has a prime duty to seek scientific truth, to adhere to the truth once it is known, and to discipline his entire life in accordance with the demands of truth. Conscience thus becomes an internal or subjective guide for the conduct which is manifested outwardly in human relationships of every category. It becomes the standard by which the individual self-interprets personal obligations due to all humanity and to things to which it appertains.

An indispensable safeguard against medicolegal entrapment is an educated, good, moral conscience. By definition, it is the faculty of recognizing the distinction between right and wrong in regard to one's own conduct. Therefore, conscience is an awareness of the moral goodness or blameworthiness of each person's conduct, intentions, or character. It includes the sense of obligation to do and to be that which is recognized as good. Surgeons abhor any tinge of unethical behavior.

Malpractice Allegations

Sterling qualities of surgeons are their mental, mechanical, and moral attributes. The first is founded on knowledge acquired by education, prescribed training, examinations, licensure, personal studiousness, and intellectual inquisitiveness. The second deals with manual dexterity leading to individualized technical skill, which is learned, perfected, and embellished during residency training. Third and foremost is the moral attribute which equates with judgment that is gained in the vineyard of professional life. Of this trinity, the greatest is the last. From it arises ethical conduct, moral behavior, individualized judgment, and the need to avoid legal pitfalls. Without a moral sense, there is neither security, sanity, safety, nor salvation in surgical practice. It is the basis upon which valued decisions are made. Additionally, it is legally protective against the onslaught of unfavorable allegations of negligence.

Surgical Judgment

Surgical judgment is a priceless treasure. As a privilege, it is not acquired easily. It is sown in the field of honesty, grows in the soil of knowledge, and is watered by the perspiration of hard work. Being tempered in the heat of failure, it is nurtured into maturity by the wisdom born through the painful labor of sad experiences. Proper judgment breeds legal protectivism and ethical propriety, because good, rational judgment upholds proper norms that are morally correct and legally defensible.

Surgeon-Patient Relationship

Hazards in surgery demand an alertness against them. As an initial caveat, the surgeon should not remove the human element in professional relationships with patients, their relatives, and other inquiring friends. The surgeon is more educated on the subject of surgery than the patient, but that does not imply deportment in explanations that belittles the patient's intelligence for comprehension. To do so is to diminish respect for and proper courtesy to each side. Cordiality is a most salutary prophylaxis against a malpractice lawsuit. This implies allowing sufficient time to the patient, answering questions, and explaining anticipated diagnostic procedures, as well as programmed therapy, with their merits and demerits.

The Personal Touch

In the course of discussion, the surgeon should not convey the impression that he is dependent entirely upon mechanical equipment to arrive at a diagnosis. This eliminates human assets which consign surgeons to a secondary role, or labels them as mechanical technicians. With such misimpression arises the concept of absent compassion, which further lends credence to the dehumanization of medicosurgical care. When a sympathetic understanding exists between the patient and the physician, legal intransigencies rarely occur. What is of equal importance is the rise in confidence as the patient passes from the diagnostic phase to that of active treatment.

It's Not Justice And Right; It's Who Is Best In Court

A surgeon's appreciation of the medicosurgical art is purely subjective. How it is practiced is not absolutely free expression. Many medicolegal ombudsmen monitor what is done by renderers of health care, which may produce legal discord. Trial lawyers know that all cases tried before juries are not always lost purely on the legal or even the logical merits of the cause of action. Jurors enter the courtroom with a psychological, prearranged frame of mind. Their preconceptions are formed by biases, prejudices, perceptions (misguided or otherwise), and preconceived attitudes of class, social, and geographical (regional) persuasions. All these influence human behavior in arriving at a verdict for or against a defendant-physician.

Prophylaxis Beats Malpractice

Time hardened experience has proven that to be forewarned is to forearm. This dictum is applicable to medical malpractice prevention. The subsequent thoughts are conveyed as guides to keep in mind to avoid accusations of negligence.

1. When time, opportunity, and adequate medical facilities are available, the law requires the surgeon to employ those fact-finding modalities in common usage to arrive at a diagnosis.

2. A decision as to when to perform surgery lies within the realm of judgment. No surgical procedure should be delayed for the surgeon's convenience. Primary concern must be for the welfare of the patient.

3. Even with all the updated, state-of-the-art machinery, patients do die. This may be difficult for the laity to understand. People are unable or unwilling to accept the reality that physicians/surgeons are not guarantors of immortality. An ancillary truism is that which is technically feasible is not an imprimatur of success. Operative procedures may be performed masterfully with death as the victor. All probabilities must be explained to patients or their surrogates prior to commencing any complex diagnostic or operative procedure.

4. Improper communication between surgeons and patients can be interpreted legally as misinformation. If surgeons are considerate and listen to patients, they will be respected as persons and honored for professionalism. Patients will be reticent to think of a lawsuit. Subjective, recursive discipline is the solace of surgeons.

5. A surgeon not well-trained in his field of endeavor is not trained for any specialty. Surgeons must pay attention to their own personal identity, respect patients, and practice in the surgical terrain they know. Otherwise, the surgeon wastes energy in defensive mechanisms under the shadow of malpractice allegations.

When physicians are victimized by the mental strain of medical malpractice allegations, they must have the resiliency to return to the dynamic stream of medicosurgical practice. After arduous training to achieve a goal, it should not be abandoned whimsically as a result of bitterness or frustration. Transitory, temporary, legal impediments should not cause disillusionment with a chosen career. Surcease to personal sorrow in such circumstances is found by knowing that all dedicated physicians are driven by an esurience to help humankind.

Unnecessary Surgery

Even though modern surgeons have been criticized for performing unnecessary surgery (cardiac bypass, herniorrhaphy, endoscopy), the majority of surgical procedures have been indicated via second/third opinions. Performing unnecessary surgery nips at the conscience, which inevitably becomes defensibly disturbed.

Mechanical Aids

Machinery does not think. Surgeons must not fall into the trap that belies the idea that mechanical ancillary diagnostic and/or treatment facilities are infallible. Failure in diagnosis occurs even with sophisticated, complicated equipment. Upstaged medicosurgical talent is glorified by the mechanisms that are available. In haste, physicians/surgeons may grasp the opportunity to operate them in order to be *comme il faut* in professional stature. Thus, endoscopy has expanded from a diagnostic procedure to one that includes therapy.

Designed for new uses in treatment are endoscopic retrograde sphincterotomy, bilary endoprosthesis, and stone management. Perfected snares and hot biopsy forceps are employed for facile polypectomy. Sclerotherapy, cytology brushing, and removal of foreign bodies via selected retrieval forceps are within the range of endoscopists. Every medical encounter utilizing instrumentation poses a risk to the patient, even in the hands of an expert. All this must be disclosed to the patient as a legal precaution.

Prevention against negligence is preferable to a prepared work-discovery defense against it. General preventive measures reside in the concept that no physician/surgeon should perform a procedure that is beyond his ability. Adequate consultations with referral to a more knowledgeable colleague is not to be regarded as indicative of a milquetoast personality. An exchange of opinion with associates is a protection against alleged or actual malpractice.

Similar cautions are advised in the newer appeal of laparoscopy for the general surgeon. The rising popularity of laparoscopic cholecystectcmy, adhesiolysis, and laparoscopic laser appendectomy may give rise to a false sense of security that may tempt surgeons into a state of legal lethargy. An adage containing much wisdom is:

> Be not the first by whom the new is tried.
> Nor the last to lay the old aside.

When recommending gallstone lithotripsy, selectivity is essential until more experience in its usage is gathered. Although 30% of patients with gallstones qualify for gallstone lithotripsy, some restrictions exist based upon the size, number, and appearance of the gallstones. Acceptable criteria are founded upon:

1. Age — 18 or older;
2. Weight — under 275 pounds;
3. Cardiac soundness — no pacemaker, etc.
4. Blood study — no blood clotting disorder; and
5. Absence of pregnancy.

In the use of instruments, the hand that holds them is the control. They must be used for the purpose manufactured and in the manner advised. Limitations of usage as instructed are to be followed. If proper procedure and maintenance are proven when a misadventure occurs, then the manufacturer may be culpable under the law of products liability.

An instrument is not to be blamed for human error. Iatrogenic episodes or accidents are mishaps that may happen to individual patients during medicosurgical diagnosis and/or treatment. Such an unfortunate occurrence is independent of the natural course of the illness for which the patient sought relief. These iatrogenic episodes are random events. They are unpredictable, unanticipated, and similar to those accidents occurring in non-medical life. These experiences are not the result of discernible errors in either conception, design, or implementation of a medicosurgical practice.

An advisory is appropriate at this time. Instruments that have been used for ten years are considered to be old. This is a reasonable estimation that is acceptable both medically and legally. Monitors, laboratory equipment, and all other mechanical supplementary modalities must be tested periodically for accuracy.

Defenses Against Liability

Prophylactic awareness of medicosurgical liability with preventive programs will be adopted by surgeons in challenging allegations of negligence. Victory is achievable when preventative alertness diminishes the need for aggressive legal defense.

Competently trained, experienced surgeons are mindful of legal liability. They follow a course of surgical care consistent with the ability and skill of colleagues of similar stature. Such surgeons, when accused of malpractice, rarely lose in a court of law. Contrariwise, surgical errors, mistakes, major judgmental miscalculations, and obvious negligence are difficult to defend.

Continuing surgical education and repeated review of current scientific literature are essential contributions to the maintenance of lofty surgical peerage. The quintessential surgeon must pursue professional actions that are in the best interest of the patient. This prevails even if it demands personal inconvenience. Surgeons can never be excused for any erosion of their intellects by extraneous influences (of whatever nature) that can eliminate human feeling from medicosurgical practice.

Consultations

In the matter of consultations, it must be realized that certain culpabilities may occur. A consultant can become involved legally in a malpractice action, even when there was no active participation by him in patient treatment. This occurs when the treating physician follows the advice given by the consultant. Contrarily, the greatest protection for the consultant is his written consultation report, disagreeing with the therapeutic procedure performed, when liability is claimed. The consultant's report should remain attached to the hospital records, and a copy must be retained in the consultant's private office files.

A surgical consultation should be answered only when one is properly qualified to render an honest responsive opinion on the subject at issue. Consultants can be sued for mishandling a consultation request. Especially is it legally dangerous to participate in opinion rendering in a specialty beyond the consultant's expertise. Likewise, surgeons can incur legal involvement by failing to answer a consultation, even as they can be involved by answering it.

Before each surgical procedure, the anesthesiologist is an automatic consultant whose findings are to be considered seriously. As a specialist, his opinions are respected. Acknowledgement of the patient as a holistic human person is the preamble to safe physiologic conduction through intravenous, gaseous, or spinal anesthesia. Pre-anesthesia evaluation is an advisory respite examination that can warn against complications — even death. Anesthesiologists assess the physical, as well as the psychological, status of the pre-operative patient. A classical anesthesiologist is not only a specialist in his field, but also a risk evaluator, a respiratory physiologist, and a pharmacologist.

Safeguards Against Negligence

With all that has been written, it is fitting that a list of gleaned kernels of wisdom be presented. These medicolegal didacticisms assist in avoiding the allegation of medicosurgical negligence.

1. Every injury to the face, head, or neck demands a complete neurological examination to eliminate the presence of intracranial and/or spinal cord injury. In emergency departments, many facial, cranial, ear, and nose lacerations are repaired without written notation that a neurologic injury has been eliminated.

2. In neck surgery, injury to the internal jugular vein is a common vascular accident, especially in cancer removal. Hemorrhage and air embolism may occur. Suture needle injury to the carotid artery is not a rarity.

3. Pathologic disturbances within the abdominal cavity remain a challenge to surgical diagnosticians.

4. Appendicitis continues to be a frequent cause for acute abdominal signs and symptoms. It is still a difficult diagnosis in many cases. Approximately 4% die without care, and 25% have recurrences. It is for this reason that the Navy mandates that the health care provider ice down the patient and give antibiotics,

rather than operate under restricted circumstances, such as on a submarine. Women can have equivocal findings more frequently than men. The presence of cystitis can be confusing, but the dilemma can generally be resolved by urinalysis. Right-sided ovulation pain is not so easily differentiated. Pelvic inflammatory disease can be confusing, particularly in somewhat older females, but pain on uterine manipulation should alert the diagnostician to its presence. Renal calculi in the ureter can be confusing and should be strongly suspected if red blood cells are found on urinalysis, particularly in males.

5. Blunt trauma to the abdomen can produce perforations in the intestinal tract, as well as to solid organs (spleen, liver).

6. In the management of patients with severe trauma, especially to the abdomen and spinal column, diagnostic thought must be given to kidney injuries with/without retroperitoneal hemorrhage and hematomyelia.

7. The diagnostic importance of vaginal and anorectal examinations has been proven repeatedly.

8. Lymphadenopathy is not due to acute primary injuries.

9. Every traumatic derangement of bone has associated soft tissue damage of varying degrees. Often, the tendon, ligament, muscle, and skin disruptions may be more extensive than the bone damage warrants. Soft tissue injury may cause post-traumatic complications (including nerve impairment).

10. Pelvic fractures frequently are associated with injury to the urinary bladder or pelvic organs with accompanying bleeding.

11. Following accidental injuries to the lower extremities, a nonhealing, ulcer-ating wound may be due to cancer.

12. Vascular injuries are known to accompany injuries to bones, ligaments, and tendons, which should be identified and treated with other injuries.

13. In automobile accidents, the line of force striking the body does not have to be severe to produce serious injuries.

14. Narcotic addicts can have symptoms suggesting gastrointestinal diseases.

15. Neck node biopsies and excisions should be planned considering the pos-sibility of future radical neck dissection. The facial nerve needs identification when preauricular and parotid biopsies are performed.

16. With appropriate advice as to examination, mammography and biopsy of breast lumps are critical. All deserve careful physician follow-up. Mammograms are not infallible and should be repeated, along with a repeat physical examina-tion of any breast lump, a possible biopsy, and even second opinions. Breast sur-gery is emotionally traumatizing to all women; some even refuse a biopsy. Whether simpler procedures, such as a lumpectomy and node dissection, or a modified mastectomy with the addition of radiotherapy and/or chemotherapy, will replace radical surgery is debatable, according to some recent articles. The fear of recurrent cancer is as distressing as the woman's concern about disfigurement.

17. Statistics indicate that biliary surgical injuries occur in reverse frequency to the experience of the surgeon. A young surgeon or trainee should do as many cases as possible with an experienced senior surgeon, before assuming primary responsibility, particularly with less experienced assistance. There is no substitute for complete knowledge of the anatomy of the biliary tract and surrounding organs, particularly since there are frequently abnormalities.

18. Rectal surgery is fraught with medicolegal hazards, often resulting in sub-stantial awards when there is a bad result that can be traced to negligence, since the defects are so dehumanizing. At best, hemorrhoidectomy patients face their first bowel evacuation with anxiety over anticipated pain. Frequently, patients will avoid a bulk laxative, which could assist in needed dilation during the healing stage.

They will resist, procrastinate, or refuse helpful rectal dilation. The surgeon should leave sufficient columns of the uninterrupted mucocutaneous junction to reduce the likelihood of circumferential stricture.

Severance of the anal sphincter is extremely demoralizing to the incontinent patient, and causes many practical and social problems. If it occurs, it should be repaired. This has led to a continuing debate regarding the relative merits of a wet anal colostomy versus an abdominal colostomy.

19. Patients undergoing hernia repairs have been known to end up with an atrophic testicle. This can result from torsion of the testicle if it is not tacked down following repair of a scrotal hernia; or from making the ring closure too tight; or from direct injury to the blood supply with sutures or cautery. Arterial injury does occur incident to femoral herniorrhapy. Nerve entrapment should be anticipated and measures taken to avoid the problem, especially with ileoinguinal hernia repair.

20. Excised pigmented skin lesions should always be followed by microscopic evaluation.

21. Cosmetic surgery should be left to Board-certified specialists. Nevertheless, certain general surgery principles need to be considered. Incisions should be placed in skin folds, or along the natural skin lines and not across them, if possible. This is not possible with a median sternotomy and is considered to be the reason for scar hypertrophy following this procedure.

To be protected against medical malpractice, gynecologists must be pre-warned against those entrapments innate to their specialty. This includes obstetrics. Because of the high risk for malpractice allegations in obstetrics and gynecology, there are enumerated the following remembrances that can avoid legal entanglements.

1. The use of instruments such as the vaginal speculum should be accomplished with gentleness, care, and discretion.

2. Some patients may respond poorly to early ambulation. Thus, it should be ordered selectively.

3. Abandonment of the obstetrical patient is the legal way of charging the attending physician with not being present during delivery.

4. Failure to perform a Cesarean section when the indications are clear-cut and substantiated by consultation can be the source of malpractice if an unfortunate occurrence eventuates.

5. During the prenatal period, the obstetrician must advise the future mother against danger to the fetus from drugs, alcohol, smoking, viral diseases, etc.

6. Phlebothrombosis and thrombophlebitis still occur during and/or following parturition.

7. Amniotic fluid emboli are known to be a complication, either at the time of or after delivery.

8. Post-operative fat embolism, wound infection, and incisional hernia are not rarities in obese women.

9. During gynecologic procedures, flexion and fixation of the legs and thighs may produce compression of the peroneal, popliteal, or sciatic nerves, resulting in post-operative nerve impairment.

10. Diseases of the female genital tract are frequently associated with disturbances in the urinary system with/without low back pain.

11. Errors in diagnosis can be avoided by recalling that gastrointestinal symptoms, orthopedic complaints, and neurological diseases can produce a clinical picture which may be misinterpreted as being of gynecologic etiology and vice versa.

12. Ureteral injury during a hysterectomy unfortunately occurs, even without the tissues being bound down. Ureteral catheters can help identification at

the time of surgery.

13. Uterine perforation is not uncommon and needs to be recognized as a consequence of dilatation and curettage. A small or minimal instrumental perforation can be safely observed with diligent and vigilant observation. In one reported abortion case where the forceps avulsed the sigmoid colon, the question of lack of experience was raised as to the ability to determine the depth of a pregnant uterus, and the amount of traction required to clean out the products of conception.

14. Intestinal perforation and obstruction of the fallopian tubes incident to laparoscopic tubal ligation have also called into question the experience of the surgeon and the presence of malpractice.

15. A frequent dilemma is whether a Cesarean section should be recommended in preference to a vaginal delivery, or vice versa. This agonizing dilemma continues to haunt the obstetrician. A second opinion may be desirable, and complete documentation of the contemplated procedure should be recorded.

16. There are several orthopedic dilemmas that bedevil the orthopedist. Cervical spine fractures require careful traction and adequate x-rays with splinting before significant movement of the patient is undertaken. A missed diagnosis of a fracture is still significant in quality assurance and risk management of medical professional liability. For example, an untreated or inadequately treated navicular fracture can lead to prolonged disability, possible fusion, and permanent limitation and pain. Most orthopedic accidents require local or crash induction anesthesia in order to perform timely surgery. The popliteal artery is frequently compromised in fractures of the knee and, therefore, requires the orthopedist's direct attention.

17. As for the urologist, he is under the gun because of the possibility of iatrogenic perforation during instrumentation. This injury requires early diagnosis and treatment. For this reason in particular, the indications for the procedure should be well-documented, as well as advising the patient of the potential risks. Perforation during ureteroscopy in a patient without a typical story of calculi, or without a positive extraneous pyelogram, as well as a urinalysis, when no emergency existed, is hard to justify. Transurethral prostatectomy is another procedure associated with a significant amount of litigation because of iatrogenic adverse effects, such as bleeding and impotence.

Conclusion

To be a surgeon is a vocational gift bestowed upon a selected few when compared to the nation's population. It is a unique distinction which benefits other people, while sustaining an inner realization of accomplishment. Both increase continually, which is self-rewarding. Surgeons share with all physicians a life-saving dedication. They are worthy of honorable esteem. Concomitantly, to deserve this acclamation, they must be aware that excellency in surgery demands sacrifices, impeccable behavior, love of study, and eternal defense vigilance.

With physical enduring stamina to preserve his own health, a price is demanded for surgical supremacy. It is a maximum moral conviction to serve the sick wholeheartedly, while simultaneously adhering to ethical requirements and an awareness of existing legal dangers. As a paragraphic addendum, the reality of life dictates that with failing body health, surgical ability declines. The surgeon's honest conscience will be the guide into retirement.

Many social restraints affect the work and behavior of surgeons due to controls originating within professional ranks, from external government agencies, state board regulations, legislative statutes, and common law derived from court decisions. Again, special reference is made to medicosurgical malpractice.

While it is undoubtedly correct that medical malpractice allegations will not disappear, nonetheless medicosurgical progress far outweighs the legal threat of negligence. Such accusations are inevitable because it is a profession in which science melds with art. Often, it is a science of uncertainty (as to results) and an art of probability. As an artful science, it governs therapeutic efforts and prognostic utterings.

The aim of malpractice prevention is to eliminate this disease by avoiding incipiency. Prophylaxis against surgical malpractice is the goal to achieve rather than chase it with ephemeral attempts to cure it or go to court to defeat the accusation. Surgeons can ill afford to be indifferent to the crucial legal issues that pertain to them. They must orient their thinking toward the subject of legal medicine. The medical curriculum and residency training programs have focused exclusively on science. By dint of necessity, this tunnel-vision attitude has to change. In spite of the professional demands placed upon them, surgeons can no longer ignore the advantages available by instruction in and consultations with medicolegal authorities.

Since professional activities are not universally pleasing and accepted, surgeons must do what they believe is right, just, ethical, and morally proper. Every health care renderer should extend his best efforts to patients. By so doing, physicians/surgeons will please the majority of them, provided the motivation is compatible with high, noteworthy standards.

No matter what legal attempts are made to profane or diminish the dignity of the medicosurgical profession, historians will acclaim and not disclaim the transcendental truth that modern American medical personalities have built a bulwark against the ravages of disease, multiple systems injuries, congenital anatomical defects, and deformities. These accomplishments are unprecedented in the recorded annals of medical history. A tribute is owed them for past performances. With the advent of the 21st Century, greater medicosurgical feats are on the horizon. Fortunate, indeed, are the upcoming generations of surgeons who have been invited to partake of this future scientific banquet.

THORACIC SURGERY

Introduction

There are significant perils and pitfalls that befall a thoracic surgeon. These invoke a number of admonitions for the surgeon to heed in an effort to avoid medicolegal problems.

Diagnostic Problems

One source of malpractice is likely when an exploratory thoracotomy is performed, and no disease, particularly cancer, is found. Before surgery is undertaken, the surgeon should order a CT scan and needle biopsy to be performed in an effort to increase the diagnostic accuracy preoperatively, particularly if the mediastinoscopy and/or bronchial biopsy were not positive.

Common errors contributing significantly to professional liability losses are errors in diagnosis, failure to provide continuous, acceptable, quality medical care, and attempts at procedures or treatments beyond the training, experience, and skill of the physician.

Wrong Side Surgery

Operating on the wrong side is simple human negligence that is inexcusable. One example is the exploration of the wrong side of the chest due to improperly marked x-rays. The surgeon should have verified the x-rays with the other medical information. Another example, with a reverse twist, involved a trainee anesthesiologist and a nurse who put a patient on the table wrong side up, while the surgical resident was otherwise occupied. Only because the surgeon was methodical and reviewed the records—chart and x-rays—was the patient spared an unwanted and unneeded thoracotomy.

Vascular Injuries

Vascular injuries are rarely due to negligence, but vascular compromise due to delayed correction is inexcusable. This can only be decreased by a high degree of constant suspicion. When it is considered, a prompt arteriogram is indicated and early intervention mandated.

Biopsies

A biopsy should never be performed if that procedure will compromise future care.

Cardiopulmonary Bypass

Central nervous system anoxia or toxic injury can occur during a cardiopulmonary bypass from underperfusion or embolization of the aortic or mitral valves by a calcium plaque or a left atrial/left ventricular clot. The brain-blood barrier may be injured by injecting medications into the vascular system while the patient is on a cardiopulmonary bypass system. There is still controversy over whether penicillin should be given before or during a cardiopulmonary bypass procedure. The danger of clot embolization is always present when resecting a left ventricular aneurysm or an atrial myxoma, and anticoagulation is always in order incident to these procedures.

Transecting an internal mammary artery or functioning vein graft is fraught with irreparable myocardial injury. Therefore, placement of bypass conduits distal to the obstruction is fundamental. Having Polaroid photographs accessible of significant lesions of the arteries can serve as a valuable road map in the operating room.

Surgery involving first rib resection has been debated for decades. Two approaches are available and have been the source of debate by recognized authorities. Injury of the brachial plexus can occur with either approach. Reduced nerve velocity, proven by conduction studies, is a prerequisite to surgical decompression. The subclavian artery and vein are not an uncommon source of injury. Such injuries are readily recognized, and these vessels must be restored to normal function before closing the patient.

Medical Care Before Surgery

Before surgery, particularly when an elective procedure is undertaken, the indication for a surgical procedure requires close scrutiny and evaluation. If possible, remediable medical intervention should be tendered before deciding surgery is the best or only way. As an example, it is known that bradycardia that comes with the use of beta-blockers can aggravate coronary artery disease, with resultant angina, and even myocardial insufficiency and infarction. Another such precaution is that hyperpotassemia should be corrected before determining whether a permanent pacemaker should be installed. Evidence of right heart strain on an electrocardiogram interposes an objective contraindication to pulmonary resection. It has been shown that otherwise the procedure may alter the patient's prognosis by increasing the work load of the right ventricle as a result of smaller pulmonary vascular system capacity.

Infections

Infectious problems should be cleared, or at least controlled, before elective surgery is undertaken. As an example, a cardiac surgeon, with an exclusive hospital contract, first excised a pilonidal cyst, and then performed open heart surgery. The patient ended up with two infected wounds, which compromised the benefits of the heart surgery.

Anatomical Knowledge

It has been opined that a surgeon sees fewer congenital anomalies after he becomes proficient in anatomy. The operating room perspective of anatomy varies from that of medical school and requires considerable experience and adaptation of dissection techniques. This became particularly obvious with the advent of cardiac surgery. One difference is that the operating field of vision is quite limited. Every surgical approach has had to be tailored.

Timely Therapy

Many of the medicolegal problems faced by thoracic surgeons are not peculiar to surgeons in general. Timeliness of treatment is paramount. A surgeon must not delay treatment (surgery) because of a personal or professional problem. Problems generally occur during so-called off-duty hours; however, they require the same diligence, if not more, since support personnel are frequently less experienced, whether it involves x-ray or lab personnel, house staff, or nurses. Additional partners or shared coverage may be needed, if the physician's practice demands are overburdening. Competent, alternative coverage is important in times of such need.

Wound Problems

Wound infections occur with the best of efforts to prevent them, even in clean cases. When they do occur, the standard of care requires taking bacterial smears and cultures. This should be followed by a prescription for an appropriate antibiotic. These measures should be routine when early resolution does not occur with simple local procedures.

Foreign Bodies

Foreign bodies, as complications of surgery, usually involve broken instruments with retained pieces, needles, and sponges. In order to avoid this type of adverse incident when a major cavity is opened, a sponge count should be demanded before closing. A second count should be taken when the skin is closed. If there is an error, there is still time to remove the foreign body before the anesthetic has worn off. If such a scenario occurs post-operatively, x-rays should be taken as soon as it is convenient after the patient is stable. The patient and/or family should be informed promptly, followed by appropriate documentation.

Neurological Complications

Complications involving neurological defects are unfortunately numerous and are not always avoidable. Hyperextension of both arms is rarely, if ever, necessary. Avoiding this position during surgery, if at all possible, is the key to avoiding the most common neurologic injury by eliminating the likelihood of stretch of the brachial plexus and its sequelae.

Rib Disease

When rib pathology is suspected, the surgeon must be careful not to biopsy the wrong rib. This can be avoided by inserting a needle into the suspected area and injecting a radiographic material to not only help determine the right rib, but also the site. The needle can be left in situ, and methylene blue can be injected to help to continue the identification of the diseased rib.

Recurrent Laryngeal Nerve Injury

Recurrent laryngeal nerve injury may be unavoidable in aggressive pulmonary resection for a pulmonary malignancy, or when the nerve is incorporated in an aneurysm of the aorta. If the lesion is unilateral, the opposite cord often migrates across the midline, resulting in a functional speaking voice. Other corrective procedures are successful if the diagnosis is made and the procedure implemented promptly.

Mediastinoscopy can also injure the recurrent laryngeal nerve. The procedure may disrupt the carotid artery, particularly if cancer has invaded its wall. Needle aspiration biopsy is recommended prior to any surgical procedure. The surgeon should be sure to blow air out the needle after aspirating, so a plug will not mislead him the next time he attempts aspiration.

Carotid Endarterectomies

An accepted standard of care in performing carotid endarterectomies does not include the use of shunts; however, juries almost always rule against the surgeon if there are less than ideal results when they are not used. Similarly, shunting may not be necessary in managing traumatic aneurysms; however, juries are also not sympathetic to end results that are unsuccessful, even when they are beyond the control of the surgeon. The rationale for not using shunts in both of these situations should be well-documented and fortified with concurring data.

Esophageal Surgery

Esophageal procedures are fraught with problems and potential liability losses. It is well-known that perforation during an esophagoscopy may be unavoidable, particularly where there is an impacted foreign body that is sharp (e.g., pin, bone, etc.), that may have already penetrated the wall when intraluminal pressure has compromised the blood supply. The surgeon should remember that unrelieved, violent vomiting leads to spontaneous rupture.

Esophageal anastomatic leaks are common following an esophagectomy. They are more common with colon interposition. It is believed that through and through permanent sutures are said to facilitate a leak; therefore, many surgeons advise at least a two layer anastomosis. Some surgeons use absorbable sutures internally and permanent sutures in the serosa.

Tracheostomy

A tracheostomy is rarely required nowadays unless there is a major injury to the airway above. Midline jugular venous tributaries are not uncommon and need to be ligated, leaving two ligatures on each end. Before incising the third or fourth cartilage during the procedure, aspiration should be performed and yield air. Although a tracheostomy is a relatively simple procedure, dire consequences causing injury to the carotid vessels or loss of control of the trachea may occur, unless the procedure is performed with precision by knowledgeable physicians.

Tracheal Intubation

Tracheal intubation can result in death when the tube is wrongly placed, either into the esophagus or too far down the respiratory tract, ending up usually on the right side of the bronchus and obstructing the left-sided flow. Portable x-rays should not be needed to make the diagnosis. Auscultation of the chest should afford immediate diagnosis if there is reason to suspect a catastrophe during an emergency.

Insertion of Subclavian Lines

Subclavian lines should be placed with the patient's head down, if possible, to reduce the risk of an air embolization. To be certain that the lines are properly installed, a portable chest x-ray should be taken, even if one aspirates venous blood easily, in order to be certain that the line is not in the pleural space. Blood and parenteral feedings have been given into the pleural space with disastrous results. If a Swan-Ganz is being used, the pressure recording can provide a clue as to the proper location of the line. It is probably preferable to insert more lines than needed under sterile conditions, as the unnecessary line can easily be withdrawn. If the x-ray shows the line to be in the mid-zone beyond the hilar artery shadows after passing through the heart, it can be assumed that the line is intravascular. If in doubt, installation of a dye should tell where the line is.

Venous cannulas should be sutured and anchored to the skin to avoid embolization. Embolized catheters can interfere with tricuspid valve closure, causing death in the form of thrombus of both lower lobe pulmonary arteries. Extravasated vasopressor areas should be appropriately observed and treated so as to reduce the likelihood of a slough. If a small pneumothorax occurs in an uncompromised patient, the patient can be safely observed with frequent chest auscultation and repeat chest x-rays. If there is no increase in the pneumothorax over a couple of hours, nothing further need be done.

Chest Stab Wounds

A stab wound of the chest can be the source of a liability suit for the physician serving in the emergency room. One such situation led to the settlement of a wrongful death action. The victim had been shot with a .22 caliber bullet. A university thoracic surgeon with limited emergency room experience inserted a chest tube and ordered four units of blood, but allowed the patient to die before the operating room was ready. He failed to note that an intercostal artery had been injured. The bleeding could have been controlled with a simple clamp and ligature. Although bare hands emergency surgery has saved many lives, gloves are recommended today because of the high incidence of Hepatitis-B and AIDS.

A good rule of thumb dictates that consultation be secured early in emergencies, particularly when lack of proper care can lead to extensive, permanent, adverse results.

Informed Consent

Informed consent is critical, particularly in surgery. In emergencies, if time permits, the next-of-kin should be informed if the patient is incapacitated.

Informed refusal is mandatory if the patient refuses care and management. In both situations, the patient needs sufficient information to make a knowledgeable, intelligent decision. The surgeon needs to indicate the risks of the procedure, the reasons why it is recommended, the alternatives and their risks, and the prognosis, as well as the diagnosis, and the differential diagnosis. The surgeon should indicate that the patient comprehends what he or she has been told. This can be difficult when an interpreter is required.

Record Keeping

Proper, timely recording of events as they unfold is good medicine. It aids the defense, if that unfortunately is required. This kind of record is certainly better than a rewritten, sanitized accounting.

Cardiovascular Surgery

Cardiovascular surgeons, in particular, should be aware that perfusion errors during cardiopulmonary bypass procedures are not an infrequent basis for a malpractice action, and include allowing air to be perfused following infusion of the reservoir blood upon completion of this type of surgery. Interestingly, this was the fate of one of the first human cardiopulmonary surgical procedures performed. Automatic alarm devices are incorporated to obviate this situation, but human attention is required. Failure to monitor activated clotting times during a cardiopulmonary bypass is also a malpractice problem, and again, requires diligence to prevent it.

Valve replacement has been complicated by iatrogenic conduction catastrophes, frequently due to septal defects at both the mitral and aortic annulus. An accident can occur involving mitral valve replacement when the prosthesis has been sewn in upside down, even by an experienced cardiac surgeon. Mitral sutures placed too deep have encircled the circumflex artery in the atrioventricular groove, causing an infarction. Excessive calcium plaque debridement, while excising the mitral valve, has caused defects to the atrium and delayed left ventricular rupture. A formidable event suddenly becomes apparent when there is an arterial injury during a laminectomy, if the surgeon bypasses through the annulus anteriorly.

Vein Stripping

Saphenous vein stripping can be complicated by an avulsion of an adjacent artery. The surgeon is charged with knowing the anatomy and the proper identification of the various structures at the time of surgery.

Professional Liability

Professional liability lawsuits against a physician for alleged malpractice may be filed for any of a large number of thoracic injuries. What gets a physician into difficulty is an incomplete, inappropriate, inaccurate, or delayed medical record maintenance. Although a patient's care may have been exemplary, the written record is what endures and what is relied upon by insurance companies, attorneys, consultants, experts, and all others in judging the quality of care rendered. The importance of complete and accurate records cannot be overemphasized.

Comments concerning an apparent conflict between nursing notes, consultant notes, and the primary physician notes must be concise and reflective of the true course of treatment. Operative notes and documentation of complications must be dictated or written in a timely manner, not days or weeks later.

A physician must always keep in mind that patient dissatisfaction with a result may occur. Although the result may be acceptable to and even expected by the physician and the medical community at large, if the patient and his or her family believe a "better" result could or should have been achieved, consultation with an attorney usually occurs.

Iatrogenic and missed thoracic injuries pose potential for a lawsuit. At times, such misadventures are not possible to avoid. Aggressive therapy is mandatory, and the time for a "fishing expedition" workup is simply not available.

A surgeon may become a victim of transferred liability for actions taken by another physician before transferring a patient. Transferring patient care responsibilities to other disciplines when treating a patient with chest trauma is asking for complications and delays in diagnosis and therapy. A significant number of lawsuits against surgeons taking care of patients with thoracic trauma involve situations where the patient had been transferred to the surgeon, which resulted in delays or iatrogenic complications created by non-surgeons.

Who Is In Charge/Continuity Of Care?

One of the causes of malpractice action involves who is in charge. Unfortunately, this occasionally becomes obfuscated in a chest trauma situation, resulting in a "Tower of Babel" situation. The surgeon, not the radiologist or other consultant, should decide about the need for an arteriography in a patient with chest trauma. Angiography, not computed tomography (CT) or magnetic resonance imaging (MRI), is the standard for determining the presence of vascular injury requiring operative repair. CT and MRI create further delay and only document the presence of mediastinal hematomas, rather than the specifics of a great vessel injury.

Trauma is a surgical disease. From the pre-hospital phase through rehabilitation, the surgeon must direct the care of a patient with thoracic trauma. Surgery is the only specialty that trains its residents to be involved in the total continuum of care. Invasive acts, such as tube thoracostomy, thoracotomy, crycothyroidotomy, and insertion of a Swan Ganz catheter, as well as decisions with regard to arteriograms, surgery, and the necessity of invasive monitoring, must be under the control of the surgeon. Emergency physicians, intensivists, and other consultants must never be primarily responsible for triage, decision-making, or specific treatment schemas.

The patient with a chest injury has multisystem problems, including cardiac, fluid and electrolyte, infectious, renal, hepatic, pulmonary, metabolic, immunologic, wound, nutritional, and many others. There are valid differences in the use and non-use of synthetic vascular grafts, appropriate monitoring techniques, protection of distal circulation when aortic clamping is necessary, and the length of time the spinal cord, kidneys, and liver can endure hypoperfusion. Yet, the choice of one may later return to haunt the surgeon.

Although the surgeon must directly manage the primary care of the patient, consultants invariably are necessary. Especially in the chest trauma patient, it is important that only one physician write orders and orchestrate the treatment program. Consultants must not a priori impose their orders, but rather cite their opinions in the progress notes.

In chest trauma particularly, controversy exists with regard to techniques and devices used in thoracic trauma. This creates a peril which hangs over the head of the physician. Retrospectively, should it have been done the other way? A good example involves paralysis. Paralysis is the most common condition following thoracic injury which results in a lawsuit. The circumstances that lead to paralysis after blunt trauma are exceedingly multifactorial and complex. Considerable debate exists as to the exact cause of paraplegia and how to prevent it. Indeed, in patients with major aortic injury, no treatment schema has reduced paraplegia to zero. The patient with severe injury requires longer and more extensive repair and has more associated injuries. In such a patient, all complications, including respiratory insufficiency and paralysis, are not uncommon. Disagreement about clamp times, monitoring techniques, shunt vs. clamp/repair vs. pump, and others exist. At the time of surgery, they are diversionary tactics, and the physician may ignore the more important issues of early diagnosis and location and timing of operating on a critically injured patient who may not be in any condition for transfer and meticulous evaluation of the multisystem injury. Yet, after it is all over, what was done at the critical time may be quesioned and be the basis for a lawsuit. The only defense is to completely document the rationale for having done it that way.

Standard of Care - National Standards

The physician who is involved in the case of a chest trauma patient has to recognize that because of the nature of the trauma, he is vulnerable to committing an act of negligence that may later make him a defendant. He must comply with the standard of care for the treatment of this problem. It is likely that he will be judged according to a national standard. Negligence by the physician/surgeon in this type of situation can be defined as the failure to do something that a reasonable specialist in the field, guided by those considerations that ordinarily regulate the conduct of a reasonably prudent specialist, would have done.

The more specialized a physician becomes, the more likely he will be held legally liable for professional acts based on national standards. Thus, a specialist needs to be aware of the standards established by his professional organizations and organized specialty groups.

In the past, courts recognized a standard of care as applying to practices in the same or similar locality or community. However, national standards recently have been invoked for health professionals and hospitals. Increasingly, specialists are being held to a national standard of care, defined as that ordinarily exercised by reputable members of their specialty under similar circumstances. Legally, "doing the best you can" is not a plausible defense.

A professional source for standards of care may be a publication of the American College of Surgeons (ACS). During the past dozen years, the ACS has developed a course for general surgeons and others as well. The purpose of the course is to instruct practicing physicians in trauma management. The course is entitled Advanced Trauma Life Support (ATLS). A certification of completion is awarded if the course is passed. Frequently, possession of such a certification may be a prerequisite to employment at a trauma center.

The ATLS manual describes in detail the management of a patient with trauma. In general, patients with thoracic trauma have multiple injuries, and although the manual is cautious and describes the system of trauma management as one of many possible techniques, the ATLS way is fast becoming a standard of care. The obligation in time to come will increasingly rest on the physician to prove that deviation from the ATLS standards was actually an improvement. This is especially true in those situations where things have gone wrong. The physician will have a difficult time if he fails to follow ATLS guidelines. Thus, ATLS is similar to the PDR (Physicians' Desk Reference), in that it provides a notice to physicians about an acceptable mode of clinical practice, deviations from which require considered judgment on the part of the physician.

The Team Approach

Organization and a team approach are crucial in trauma management in general, and chest trauma in particular, whether the trauma team consists of a physician and nurse in a small rural hospital, or a host of emergency room physicians, surgeons, thoracic surgeons, and critical care nurses in a regional trauma center. Team members must know their responsibilities and be prepared to carry them out with skill. The overall goal is to stabilize the patient, while simultaneously evaluating injuries sufficiently to allow his or her transfer from the emergency department to the appropriate site for definitive care, usually the operating room.

Timely Critical Interventions

The physician must always remember that complacency sometimes kills. When the physician thinks he is aware of all the injuries present, he should re-evaluate and think again. What else could be hidden away in the battered body? There are plenty of surprises to go around.

The early and rapid team management of trauma produces better results. If this "golden hour" is lost without effective resuscitative and stabilizing efforts, the patient is unlikely to respond to similar efforts undertaken at a later time. In the primary survey of the patient, the critical considerations are whether the patient's airway is patent, whether he is breathing, and whether circulation is normal. A number of procedures are available to preserve the trauma patient's airway. Another critical part of the initial assessment in ATLS is restoring the circulation. Another dilemma is whether the patient can and should be moved for diagnosis and treatment.

Patients who are confused, disoriented, and agitated must be controlled according to the circumstances. The JCAHO manual requires the emergency department to have a specific policy on the management of the belligerent patient with altered mental status. Frequently, the etiology behind the abnormal behavior of a patient involved in trauma cannot be ascertained. The physician's first obligation is to be certain that this "altered" mental state is not due to a life-threatening medical problem. Treatment of potential etiologies precedes diagnosis, especially where that treatment has a minimal risk of causing harm. Belligerence and refusal to accept medical therapy are most often due to a head injury, drug or medication abuse, alcoholism, electrolyte imbalance, hypoxic state, and drug overdose. Which of these are present can be determined easily by the laboratory, predicated on a high degree of suspicion on the part of the physician. In these situations, acquiescence by the physician to the patient's refusal of care may result in the death of the patient with all its legal consequences, particularly an action for wrongful death.

All of these actions fall within the accepted and required standards of care. If there is a deviation from these standards that caused the patient harm, a successful lawsuit may follow. It must be stressed that the physician must document his actions. To that end, he can then show that he merely made a mistake or an error in judgment, which is a human frailty, and not reckless disregard of the standards of care.

Specific Treatment

The standards for treating specific chest injuries of the patient have been established by the medical profession. Some do happen to be controversial. As soon as the patient has achieved cardiopulmonary stability, it is critical to attempt to get a thorough medical history, paying particular attention to the factors that determine the type and severity of the patient's injury. The physician must also find out as much as he can about the accident. The details of the accident may be a tip-off to associated injuries, such as blunt abdominal trauma, that may go unrecognized in all the excitement. Family, friends, and the emergency crew are all helpful sources. An outreach effort may be necessary to seek and search for people who may provide valuable facts.

In the physical examination, the first priority is to assess the level of consciousness. Determining the baseline neurologic functions heads the list, because if the patient survives, the ultimate concern is whether the physician is going to be left with a patient in a chronic vegetative state. Because hypothermia affects the body's response to resuscitation and supportive measures, a special low-reading thermometer may be required. The accepted standards for history taking, doing a physical examination, and ordering appropriate tests should be followed.

Benefits Versus Risk Rule

Concomitantly, the physician must determine as best he can the nature, severity, and the extent of the chest injury. With the trauma patient, time is precious, and the evaluation must be performed as rapidly as possible. Under any circumstances, life-saving treatment and stabilizing measures must be initiated as soon as problems are recognized, and often before they are completely understood.

This is frequently fraught with great difficulty because of the nature, extent, and severity of the chest injury, which makes the evaluation difficult. Time may be of the essence, and yet the physician needs some time to make the evaluation. Therefore, the extent of the evaluation must be made on the basis of the benefit-risk rule, i.e., an evaluation of the path that was taken and why is critical.

UROLOGY

Introduction

In defining the specialty of urology, it is obvious that the urologist is concerned not only with the urinary tracts of men and women, but the sexual functions of both. Although urologists ordinarily confine their surgical and medical practice to the genitalia of men rather than women, they are frequently concerned with the sexual activities of women.

Informed Consent

Obtaining informed consent is a medical and legal requirement for all physicians. It has particular significance for the urologist in treating a male, because some of the care and management that urologists render is fraught with the danger of causing impotence. This is a serious problem for men, and its occurrence and management should be thoroughly discussed when it is a "material" risk.

As part of informed consent, a patient is entitled to be advised of alternative methods of treatment. This becomes significant in treating a patient with urolithiasis in whom intervention is required. The patient should be adequately advised that in addition to surgery, lithotripsy or extraction technique are now available for the patient's consideration.

Reportable Diseases

A urologist, as well as all physicians, is required by statutory law in every jurisdiction to report patients with a sexually transmissible disease. In many jurisdictions, there are provisions for protecting the identity, privacy, and confidentiality of the patient and his or her contacts. Failure to report any patient and known contacts may place a physician at risk for administrative (licensure), criminal, or civil liability.

Consultation

Although a urologist usually serves as a consultant, he occasionally requires a consultation. This may be the result of a patient's request. Certainly, a urologist should seek consultation when he believes he may be in "over his head".

The usual scenario has the urologist involved in a joint venture with another physician who has sought the consultation. Occasionally, it is the urologist who instigates the joint enterprise. In either situation, there should be an understanding as to the relationship between the two physicians, i.e., who is responsible for what. This should be thoroughly documented, and obviously, the patient must be kept informed. Generally, the law holds each physician to be sufficiently knowledgeable about the other's field, so that each should know whether the other is operating within the standard of care. Each will likely be held responsible for the negligent acts of the other.

Ureteral Injuries

A frequent source of consultation for a urologist involves a ureteral injury during a hysterectomy. This occurs even without tissues being bound down. Ureteral catheters can help anatomic identification at the time of surgery. It should be remembered that causing an injury may not constitute negligence, but failure to recognize and treat it can be dangerous.

A ureteral injury may result from either blunt or penetrating trauma, but the commonest cause of ureteral injury by far is iatrogenic. Surgical procedures most often responsible include difficult pelvic operations on the female reproductive organs or rectosigmoid colon. In certain types of radical hysterectomy, the incidence of ureteral injury may be as high as 10%, but it will be less than 1% in abdominoperineal resections. Ureteral injuries have also been reported with vascular reconstruction, lumbar disk surgery, sympathectomy, urologic procedures, such as ureteral instrumentation with baskets or catheters, and in rare circumstances, prostatectomy.

The ureter is infrequently injured by external violence, not only because of its small size, but also because of its position in the abdomen. In diagnosing a ureteral injury, a high index of suspicion is necessary for three reasons. First, the incidence of ureteral injury is quite low. Second, a ureteral injury may be - and often is - overlooked because of other serious visceral injuries. And finally, the urinalysis and intravenous urogram may be normal or non-diagnostic in up to one-third of injured patients. If the diagnosis is missed early, delayed symptoms, including flank pain, fever, ileus, and urinary failure, may develop. Unfortunately, delayed recognition of ureteral injuries results in nephrectomy in up to about one-third of patients.

A physician should suspect ureteropelvic disruption in cases of rapid deceleration injury and injury from penetrating trauma, if the tract of the wounding agent is at all in the area of the ureter. Close examination of the ureter at surgery may be required. When a physician strongly suspects the diagnosis, but cannot definitely see an injury, a useful technique at surgery is intravenous injection of indigo-carmine dye to see whether it will stain the tissues in the area of the suspected ureteral injury.

When ureteral injuries are found, several principles are important in their management. Early repair or diversion is essential to preserve renal function, and a primary watertight mucosa-to-mucosa anastomosis will have the highest rate of success. The adventitia of the uninjured segment of ureter should be preserved because the blood supply to the ureter consists of many freely anastomosing vessels from the renal arteries, aorta, iliac vessels, inferior mesenteric artery, gonadal vessels, the uterine arteries in the female, and vesicle arteries distally. A partial ureteral tear involving less than one-third of the circumference of the ureter may be managed expectantly with wide drainage, but a tear involving more than one-third of the circumference should usually be transected, debrided, and anastomosed, primarily to prevent secondary complications such as stenosis. High-velocity missiles will cause more tissue damage than low-velocity missiles, and more debridement of the ureter will be required.

The specific treatment of ureteral injuries depends on the nature and site of the injury. Proximal ureteral injuries are usually best managed with primary ureteroureterostomy. If the ureteropelvic junction has been disrupted, a dismembered pyeloplasty is required to restore the functional shape transition from renal pelvis to ureter. Mid-ureteral injuries are also repaired with primary ureteroureterostomy.

Mobilizing the proximal and distal ureteral segments, with care not to strip off the adventitia, will permit resection of up to 6 cm. of damaged ureter.

If primary reanastomosis is impossible, other alternatives include a transureteroureterostomy to the opposite ureter if the ureteral length is adequate and no contraindications, such as tuberculosis, transitional cell carcinoma, stone disease, or chronic reflux, exist. When a long segment of ureter is damaged, other alternatives include small bowel interposition, renal transplant, or use of synthetic graft material to serve as a template for ureteral regeneration. If the distal third of the ureter is damaged, alternative techniques for treatment include reimplantation of the ureter, which often requires a psoas bladder hitch to relieve tension from the reanastomosis. If the bladder is not damaged, but additional ureteral length is required, a bladder tube flap can be constructed.

All of these methods of treatment require that the patient be stable, so the physician can spend the necessary time to restore ureteral continuity. In an unstable patient with multiple serious injuries, fast temporary alternatives include cutaneous intubated ureterostomy and diverting tube nephrostomy. Both of those techniques create controlled fistulas that maximize preservation of ureteral length and renal function. After the patient's other injuries are controlled and the clinical status is improved, the ureter can be repaired.

Testing

A urologist is one of the physicians whose professional life is bound to the laboratory. He should obviously order tests when they are needed, but not to protect himself from possible litigation. This brand of so-called "defensive medicine" can become offensive medicine - unnecessary testing and procedures may be considered malpractice.

While a urologist is trained to recognize the pertinent anatomical landmarks encountered during a transurethral resection of the prostate (TURP), on occasion he may go outside the confines of those landmarks and damage the sphincter, resulting in incontinence. There is no greater, more miserable existence than having the constant leakage of urine from one's urethra. Not only is it socially embarrassing, but it also causes tremendous medical problems, such as skin irritation and fungus infections. All is not lost, however. Silicone injections into the external sphincter can be used to rebuild the muscle layer and make the patient completely continent.

Misdiagnosis

Like all physicians, a urologist is vulnerable to misdiagnosis. Because some of the surgical procedures used to correct urological diseases are devastating themselves, a urologist should not perform a procedure until the diagnosis is established, utilizing imaging and biopsy.

Intravenous Pyelography

An activity of particular concern to the urologist is performing an intravenous pyelogram (IVP) and retrograde pyelogram. An IVP is a series of x-rays taken while an iodinated compound is injected intravenously into the patient. The contrast media is highly concentrated by the kidneys. There is a significant incidence of allergic reaction to the iodine, and the urologist and/or radiologist must be extremely careful in performing skin tests and obtaining a thorough allergic history prior to this study. Questions to be asked should include: (1) previous allergic history of any sort; (2) family history of allergies, particularly to the iodinated compounds; and (3) any allergies to seafood or shellfish (which are high in iodine content). If there is even an oblique connection between an allergic reaction and iodine, the test is contraindicated. Unfortunately, the skin test is not infallible, and a negative result is no guarantee. Also, there are reports that pre-operative testing has caused an anaphylactic reaction. Some institutions allow patients who have had an allergic reaction to the contrast media previously to receive steroidal or anithistamine medications prior to injection of the IVP contrast media in an effort to forestall a possible allergic reaction. This could still prove to be dangerous medically and legally, and unnecessary. A retrograde pyelogram or renal ultrasound may give the same information concerning the kidneys without intravenous injection of the contrast media.

The pyelographic finding of a non-opaque filling defect in the renal pelvis is a difficult diagnostic problem. Many pathological processes, including blood clot, transitional cell carcinoma, and calculus, may present as an isolated defect in the opacified renal pelvis. Clinical findings, laboratory data, urine cytology, and serial urograms may provide helpful information. Not uncommonly, however, these studies are not diagnostic, and more invasive procedures, such as renal arteriography, percutaneous or retrograde brush biopsy, or surgery, are necessary. Arteriography and brush biopsy are frequently inconclusive, while surgical exploration of the renal pelvis when tumor is present risks spillage of tumor cells.

Intravenous pyelography, including a plain film of the abdomen and conventional tomography, is a prerequisite to detecting masses, renal or ureteral displacement, gross calcifications, or urinary tract obstruction.

Renal imaging is best first accomplished with an intravenous urogram. A mass discovered on an intravenous urogram should be subsequently studied by either CT or ultrasound to determine if it is cystic or solid. Cyst aspiration may then be done to confirm the cystic nature of the mass. Dimensions of the kidneys can be accurately determined by CT. Both cystic and solid lesions of the kidney are demonstrable by CT. Cystic structures are definable because of their low absorption coefficients, which approach that of water. Tumor-bearing tissues in the kidneys show an intermediate density between cysts and normal parenchyma when intravenous urographic contrast agents are used. Although cysts, and sometimes tumors, have been seen incidentally on CT, it has proved very useful as a supplementary procedure in the evaluation of a mass lesion identified by intravenous pyelography. The diagnosis may be confirmed by needle biopsy under CT or ultrasound guidance. CT can specifically identify hemangiomyolipomas, detect the minute calcifications of neuroblastoma, demonstrate the persistent opacification associated with acute tubular necrosis, and distinguish masses adjacent to but separate from the kidneys. Hydronephrosis and renal cortical atrophy are readily apparent. CT is invaluable to the radiotherapist to delineate the total extent of tumor for precise determination of treatment dosage. Abnormalities of the bladder, such as carcinomas invading the wall, are readily detectable. Although CT is not the primary diagnostic tool, it supplies excellent information for planning radiotherapy.

Labeling or rather mislabeling x-rays can cause formidable misfortune, e.g., right for left, etc. A physician must always remember to be absolutely sure of which side is which by verification. He should never trust the "R" or "L" marker.

Cystectomy

Bladder cancer is one of the more dangerous forms of cancer, with one out of four persons dying of the disease. Very often, the preferred form of treatment is radical cystectomy, the surgical removal of the entire bladder and neighboring structures. In these cases, the problem of creating a bladder substitute is an extremely significant one, both in terms of maintaining patient self-image and minimizing the risk of complications. In the past, the ileal conduit has been the procedure of choice. An alternative is the Kock pouch, which obviates the need for a stoma bag and has several other advantages. But the surgery required for the Kock pouch adds several hours to the already lengthy (six hour) procedure, a substantial drawback.

Recently, a urologist successfully created an artificial bladder, an ileocolic neobladder, as a potential alternative to the external pouch for about one-third of men with bladder cancer who are under 70 and otherwise in good health. Besides the obvious psychological advantage, the artificial bladder, made from segments of the large and small intestines, appears to be associated with few infections or urine leaks when compared to operations with external appliances. The artificial bladder provides near normal voiding for patients who have undergone nerve-sparing radical cystectomy.

In addition, there is now an improved cystectomy that preserves potency. The nerve-sparing surgical technique which preserves potency is now being used in bladder cancer surgery for the 20% of men with bladder cancer who require bladder removal. The procedure allows surgeons to remove the prostate and/or bladder without injury to the cavernous nerves in the pelvis that control erection. In addition, by keeping much of the nervous system intact, the functioning of the urethra and urinary continence may be improved.

In a related discovery, it is possible to control bladder function in spina bifida patients. In a technique developed in Europe, the urologist inserts a catheter connected to electrodes into the bladder through the urethra. By delivering a series of increasingly stronger electrical charges to the bladder muscle over a period of months, the bladder can be trained to contract normally.

Traumatic Injuries

Genitourinary injuries account for up to 10% of injuries seen, and associated bladder injury occurs in 5 to 10% of patients with a fractured pelvis. Intraperitoneal bladder rupture caused by blunt trauma without pelvic fracture is rare, and extraperitoneal bladder rupture from blunt trauma without pelvic fracture is rarer still, but a physician must be alert to those possibilities so he can order an appropriate diagnostic workup, as well as any necessary consultations. Pelvic fracture aside, the commonest findings in a ruptured bladder are hematuria, difficulty voiding, and pelvic discomfort. Taking into account the mechanism of injury, somatic complaints, physical examination, and initial laboratory data, the physician should be able to formulate a plan of radiologic evaluation that will permit the diagnosis of subtle or uncommon urologic injuries. If the physician does not consider the possibility of bladder rupture in patients who do not have pelvic fractures, he might only order an IVP and drainage films. Because of incomplete bladder distention, however, an excretory urogram alone will reveal only 15% of bladder injuries. For example, in one case, the IVP was normal, despite a rupture. In addition, any woman with bladder rupture should be given a careful gynecological examination to assess for urethral tear or vaginal injury. That step is sometimes omitted in the emergency setting.

Bladder injuries can consist of contusion, intraperitoneal rupture, or extraperitoneal rupture. Bladder contusion is a diagnosis of exclusion after an IVP and cystourethrogram have shown the urinary tract to be intact; in that case, when hematuria is seen, it is due to a partial-thickness tear of vesical tissues. Extraperitoneal rupture usually occurs on the anterolateral walls, and a physician will see a "sunburst" appearance of contrast after cystography. Intraperitoneal rupture occurs when intravesicular pressure rises suddenly from a blow to the pelvis or lower abdomen when the bladder is full. Rupture usually occurs at the weakest part of the bladder, namely, the dome, and causes intraperitoneal extravasation. Intraperitoneal rupture is commoner in children because a child's bladder is in a less protected, more intra-abdominal position.

Mortality from bladder trauma depends more on the extent of associated injuries and the age of the patient than on the type of bladder injury. If intraperitoneal bladder rupture goes unrecognized, however, reabsorption of urine from the peritoneal cavity may lead to hyperkalemia, hypernatremia, uremia, and acidosis, with significantly increased morbidity.

In evaluating a patient with blunt pelvic trauma, a physician must pay strict attention to the proper sequence of radiographic diagnostic studies, in order to avoid incorrect diagnoses or further damage to the urinary tract. If the mechanism of injury, physical examination, or presenting complaints indicate urethral injury, the physician should not insert a catheter until the integrity of the urethra is confirmed. In a female patient, the physician should let the dye from the intravenous pyelogram fill the bladder and obtain a voiding cystourethrogram; in a male patient, a retrograde urethrogram should be performed. Extravasation of dye indicates urethral injury.

Urethral injuries in women are unusual because of the protection provided to the urethra by the pubic arch and by the urethra's short course and mobility. On rare occasions, however, bladder laceration will extend into the urethra. If the urethra is intact, the physician should insert a catheter and do a three-phase retrograde cystogram. The physician can achieve an accuracy rate approaching 100%, if he or she adequately distends the bladder with contrast material and uses a drainage film. Lateral and oblique films may not be feasible in patients with major pelvic fractures or other associated injuries. Patients whose accidents involve direct blunt trauma or deceleration may also sustain rupture of the renal pelvis, so an IVP is also necessary for evaluating the integrity of the upper urinary tract.

Infection

When a urinary tract infection (UTI) is suspected, the important question to ask is: How sick is the patient? If the patient is critically ill, treatment with intravenous antibiotics should be started while diagnostic studies are performed. If the patient is clinically stable, the source of infection should be determined and therapy initiated.

Although UTIs do not usually require emergency treatment, they can cause cramping or even severe abdominal pain. Sepsis from acute UTI, commonly pyelonephritis, requires emergency measures, but even when there is no emergency, the sudden onset of symptoms calls for prompt diagnosis and treatment.

Antibiotics

Antibiotics are of medicolegal concern to urologists, as well as to all physicians. Before they are administered, a thorough allergic history is mandatory, remembering always that cross-sensitivity testing is available. In urgent situations or emergencies, the antibiotic should be administered by titrating the dosage (gradually increasing the amount and/or decreasing the interval).

Ideally, the sensitivity of the offending organism to the antibiotic should be determined. This is frequently not possible. A broad spectrum should be used. Non-sensitivity or resistance should be considered when there is no clinical response, and confirmed by laboratory studies. Meanwhile, another accepted antibiotic should be prescribed.

There is a tendency for physicians to think that if one antibiotic is good, a combination should be better. Multiple antibiotics may be harmful, rather than helpful. They should not be used in combination unless there is an indication.

It has been reported that tetracycline may no longer be an effective treatment for some urogenital tract infections. Before prescribing tetracycline, physicians should perform sensitivity testing of the infectious agent. Tetracycline resistance was found in bacterial strains isolated from the urogenital tracts of women who had not taken any antibiotics for at least two weeks prior to sampling. Tetracycline resistance determinants were common to many isolated microorganisms, including 82% of the viridans group *Streptococcus sp,* 79% of *Peptostreptococcus* isolates, and 55% of the *Gardnerella vaginalis* isolates. Tetracycline's spectrum of sensitivity is much more narrow than in the past because we are frequently exposed to this drug. Although tetracycline is still effective against some infectious agents, such as chlamydia, physicians should not assume that it will be effective against all the bacterial strains that it was used for in the past.

Macrodantin

Macrodantin is a marvelous drug and is used a great deal by urologists because it is highly concentrated in the urine. However, hepatitis and several instances of pneumonitis have occurred in patients taking this drug. Proper monitoring by the physician must occur when prescribing any drug, but particularly this one. The package insert which accompanies the drug and the *Physicians' Desk Reference* (PDR) indicates that there are potential complications, and puts the physician on notice that he must be alert to them when prescribing this drug.

Drug Monitoring

A malpractice lawsuit for wrongful death was brought involving the prescription of over 1400 Macrodantin pills to a patient over a period of one and one-half years, without any monitoring of the patient. This is not an indictment of Macrodantin, but rather an example of a situation in which a physician lost control of his treatment plan. While a tragic result occurred because of the use of Macrodantin, the object lesson to be learned is that no physician should prescribe any antibiotic, or indeed any drug, without proper monitoring. Even aspirin, a popular over-the-counter drug, can have potentially devastating effects when not properly used.

Nephrotoxicity

Aminoglycosides, such as Gentamicin and Kanamycin, are known to be nephrotoxic, and most hospitals now require that peak and trough levels be drawn periodically when patients are on these drugs.

A recent medical malpractice case concerned a patient with a renal transplant who came to the hospital because of a Klebsiella urinary tract infection. His renal function studies were slightly elevated, and he was begun on a low dose of an aminoglycoside, and peak and trough levels were drawn. Subsequent peak and trough levels revealed toxic values, consistent with known side effects. In spite of this, and probably because the physician did not review the chart, the same dosage was continued. He was also on immunosuppressive medications.

The patient had a past history of drug-induced hepatitis, which resolved after hepatotoxic drugs were discontinued. The physician had treated this patient for years; yet, his past medical history was ignored, and the patient was again given hepatotoxic drugs. Additional complications ensued, and the patient developed hepatorenal syndrome which led to his demise. Although the patient's prognosis was poor, the fact is that nephrotoxic drugs were given to a compromised patient, despite his past history, and continued, despite toxic blood levels. The physician did not adjust the dosage accordingly.

Diet

Results of a national study indicate that specific dietary changes and improved blood pressure control may help slow the rate of kidney failure for people with chronic kidney disease. Foods containing protein and phosphorus are the primary source of waste filtered by the kidneys. If protein and phosphorous intake is reduced, the kidneys will not have to work so hard.

Hematuria

Gross hematuria or microscopic hematuria may indicate urinary tract injury. Anuria or difficulties inserting a Foley catheter into the bladder, especially when associated with pelvic fractures, may indicate urethral disruption.

A rectal exam should proceed catheterization, since inability to feel the prostate in a male indicates complete urethral transection. Urinalysis is essential early in the evaluation of a trauma patient. Intravenous pyelogram and retrograde cystourethrogram will evaluate the complete urinary tract.

Minor contusions to the kidneys are treated expectantly until the hematuria clears up. More extensive injuries may need repair of the kidney or nephrectomy. Urethral injuries are best treated by debridement and repair. Fistula and stricture formation are common following undiagnosed uretheral injury. Bladder tears can be repaired in two layers and protected with a urethral catheter and/or suprapubic drainage. Associated pelvic fractures must be stabilized.

Radiation Therapy

The kidneys should be protected when radiation therapy in the area is not for renal malignancy. Radiation nephritis may possibly be associated with headache, nausea, and hypertension. The kidney may atrophy, and chronic renal failure can ensue.

Acute radiation cystitis from bladder radiation is manifested by dysuria (painful urination), frequency of urination, and reduced bladder capacity. Bleeding and bladder contracture may follow.

Manipulation

Manipulation of the lower urinary tract should be performed delicately and with respect. In the presence of urethral stricture disease, instrumentation of the male urethra is a fine art. However, urologists must comprehend the anatomy of the urethra, and the agility required to either bypass stricture disease or follow the tortuosity of the urethra. Authorities have admonished: "If it doesn't go, don't force it." They are quite correct.

Rupture of the urethra is another medicolegal peril and pitfall. Rupture can result from the urologist creating false passages into the surrounding tissue, or by forcing the instrument at the bladder neck under the bladder, or by perforating the urethra and passing the instrument into the rectum. There are recorded malpractice lawsuits predicated on urologists who did exactly that. They used excessive pressure and pushed a ureteral dilator through the urethra into the rectum. When they inserted a Foley catheter into the urethra and feces appeared, they recognized the error. The patients then required a diverting proximal colostomy, as well as further urethral surgery. The lesson to be learned is that gentleness is a prerequisite for the urologist. Obstructive lower-tract disease from causes such as prostatic obstruction or bladder-neck obstruction will be encountered, and again, gentle manipulation is a prerequisite in overcoming the obstruction.

Iatrogenic injury from perforation during instrumentation should be accompanied by early diagnosis and treatment. Perforation may be forgiven, failure to act never. The indications for the procedure and risks should be well-documented. Perforation during ureteroscopy in a patient without a typical story for calculi, and without a positive urinalysis or IVP, when no emergency existed, is hard to justify.

Epididymal Disease

Another frequent basis for urology malpractice lawsuits is the failure to differentiate between epididymitis, torsion of the testicle, incarcerated hernia, and testicular tumor. The most common disaster involves differentiating between epididymitis and torsion of the testicle. When there is trouble in a patient's scrotum, even with great technological advances, the most reliable approach is to take him to the operating room and explore his scrotum; the proper diagnosis will then be made.

There have been numerous lawsuits filed when physicians failed to consider torsion as a differential diagnosis of epididymitis; when they treated this complaint over the telephone, particularly after being called by the emergency room physician; and when they suspected the diagnosis of torsion, but treated the patient with antibiotics for 24 hours to "see if it will get better".

Torsion is a urological emergency and must be dealt with promptly, in order to save the testicle. The patient with classical manifestations, allowing for the differentiation of torsion from epididymitis probably does not exist, so every patient must be evaluated individually.

Testicular tumor is another source of misdiagnosis in attempting to distinguish it from epididymitis. The acute phase of epididymitis will usually resolve within 10-14 days, regardless of whether or not antibiotics are used. The critical aspect of management is that the patient be seen after an appropriate period of time for re-evaluation. A certain percentage of patients who do not manifest an underlying process which caused the epididimitis will be found to have a testicular tumor. Despite significant technological advances in urology, the best way to make a diagnosis is by "laying on of the hands".

AIDS

Prior to the AIDS epidemic, renal disease, i.e., focal glomerulosclerosis, was found primarily in intravenous drug users. However, in recent years, physicians have noticed an escalating number of cases of focal glomerulosclerosis in HIV-infected patients with no reported history of intravenous drug use.

The association of HIV infection and renal disease has been documented in two studies. However, the populations in both of those studies had large numbers of intravenous drug users and were primarily black.

The AIDS patients were mostly homosexual men, not intravenous drug users. Further, patients with acute renal failure are divided proportionately between blacks and other patients. A higher incidence of many renal diseases in blacks compared to other populations is well-documented, suggesting environmental influences.

Leaving Things Behind

A physician should not put things inside a patient, and then forget it was done. While vaginal packing of iodoform gauze or 4 x 4 gauze pads is done regularly by urologists to tamponade bleeding from the urethra, it is not uncommon to forget these packs. When the patient returns later with a foul, suppurative discharge, it can be a medical and legal problem. While tamponade is an acceptable approach to control simple and superficial bleeding, some urologists subscribe to the theory that a physician should not cover up what he wants to see! There is rarely only one standard of care.

The failure to remember to return for an indwelling ureteral stent inserted in a patient is fraught with consequences. There are a number of lawsuits where stents were left in patients for a period of six to eight months, resulting in encrustations that were so great that open surgery was required to remove them. In one instance, a stent remained in a patient for five years. In the interim, the patient had frequent urinary tract infections with pain on that side. Interestingly, two IVPs were performed during the five year period, and radiologists identified the indwelling stent. Nevertheless, the treating physician either never looked at the x-rays or read the report. He was unaware of its presence until it was removed by another urologist.

Since urologists use nephrostomy tubes or suprapubic tubes, it is important for the physician to advise the patient of the presence of the tubes, and also record this information in the chart. When the patient returns, the urologist's memory will be refreshed.

Proper record keeping is critical for continuity of care. Complete, intelligible, and timely entries should be made throughout the patient's hospitalization.

Venereal Diseases

House officers may have occasion to be involved in the treatment of patients with venereal diseases. The trainee must be cognizant that such patients frequently have multiple diseases. Furthermore, resistant causative organisms are not infrequent, and the physician must be knowledgeable regarding the various antibiotics and their properties. There are the duties of warning against sexual activity, reporting the disease(s) to the proper authorities under the state statute, and appropriate follow-up. Privacy and confidentiality otherwise pose serious consideration. The problem of contacts can be left to the public health authorities, although discreet involvement in this situation may be desirable.

III.
LEGAL

CONSENT AND INFORMED CONSENT TO MEDICAL TREATMENT

Introduction

Among the significant obligations flowing from physician to patient in the context of the treatment relationship is the physician's obligation to obtain the consent of the patient before undertaking treatment. Failure to properly obtain such consent may result in tort liability premised upon the legal theories of battery or negligence.

Generally, when a physician treats an individual without obtaining legally valid consent, there occurs a wrongful touching, which the law recognizes as a battery. Medical malpractice lawsuits based upon battery principles are seen infrequently. More often, lawsuits charging lack of consent to treatment are predicated upon negligence principles, i.e., that the physician failed to adhere to the standard of care in providing sufficient information to the patient to allow for a knowing or informed consent. Thus, although a patient may have voluntarily consented to treatment, it is argued that the patient's decision was made without sufficient data regarding the nature of the proposed treatment, the significant or material risks involved, the benefits reasonably to be expected, or the available treatment alternatives.

The following discussion addresses the physician's responsibilities in the context of obtaining consent to treatment. Emphasis is placed on the requirements for obtaining legally valid consent, as well as legally informed consent.

Consent to Treatment

It is a legal requirement that a patient's consent be obtained as a precondition to the provision of medical care and treatment. This requirement is premised upon the right of the individual to determine what shall be done to his or her own body. As early as 1906, the Illinois Supreme Court, in *Pratt v. Davis,* 79 N.E. 562, 564 (1906), emphasized that, "where the patient is in full possession of all his mental faculties and in such physical health as to be able to consult about his condition . . . it is manifest that his consent should be a prerequisite to a surgical operation."

This continues to be an accurate statement of the law throughout the United States. Thus, when there is a total lack of consent to treatment or when the procedure performed by a physician falls clearly outside the scope of a patient's consent, an action sounding in battery against the physician may be initiated for the unauthorized touching.

Consent to medical care may be express or implied. Express consent is an oral or written authority granted by the patient to render the proposed treatment. Consent also may be implied from the conduct of the patient in a particular case, or from the application of law to certain fact situations. A patient who voluntarily submits to treatment under circumstances that would indicate awareness of the planned treatment impliedly authorizes the treatment, even without express consent. For example, a patient who presents at the physician's office for a routine procedures implies his or her consent to treatment.

Generally, the courts will not find implied consent for a complex medical or surgical procedure that most patients could not understand without a careful explanation by a physician. In addition, the patient must have an opportunity to withdraw from the proposed treatment. In view of these considerations, implied consent, particularly in light of informed consent principles, should be relied upon only for simple, routine procedures.

Capacity to Consent

As a general rule of law, it is presumed that an individual is mentally capable of making reasonable decisions with respect to health care. In the absence of such mental capacity, consent to health care must be obtained from an individual who has authority to make such decisions on the patient's behalf. Such authority may be legally conferred upon a third party in the context of a legal guardianship proceeding or under the terms of a written power of attorney, sometimes referred to as a "durable" power of attorney.

A guardian of the person may be appointed by a court when it is judicially determined that an individual is incompetent or disabled, and thus unable to fully manage his or her person or estate. Typically, a guardian is a family member or friend who is interested in the welfare of the disabled person. To the extent ordered by a court, the guardian is responsible for making personal decisions for the ward, including decisions governing health care. The guardian acts in a fiduciary capacity, and thus is required to make decisions that are in the ward's best interests.

In the absence of a court-appointed guardian, a third party may be empowered to act on behalf of a principal under the terms of a written power of attorney. Such a document confers authority upon a third party to handle specific personal or financial matters on behalf of the principal. In recent years, these documents have been used to permit a third party to make health care decisions on behalf of a principal who has become functionally incompetent. Under numerous state statutes, these "durable" powers of attorney are legally effective until there has been a judicial declaration of incompetence or disability. In some states, recent legislation has authorized use of such documents, even after there has been a declaration of incompetence or disability.

As a practical matter, the greater number of cases involving mentally incapacitated patients arise in circumstances where there has been no written delegation of authority to make health care decisions, and where it is burdensome to initiate legal guardianship proceedings. Often, these cases involve elderly patients who suffer varying degrees of difficulty in making health care decisions. In cases of this nature, the physician should make every reasonable effort to communicate with the patient and to ascertain the patient's wishes, recognizing that the law favors a presumption of competence.

If a physician concludes that the patient is unable to appreciate the nature and scope of his or her condition and the recommended treatment, consultation with the next-of-kin is appropriate. Generally, it is this group of individuals who are most concerned about the patient's welfare, and who will act in the patient's best interests. Accordingly, in these situations, when family members consent to a proposed course of medical treatment that is reasonable under the circumstances, the physician may be guided by that consent in providing further professional services consistent with the proper standard of care.

If the patient's next-of-kin disagrees with the proposed treatment, or if the patient, although incompetent, takes a position contrary to the family's wishes, the physician must be extremely cautious. There is some indication that the courts will consider the wishes of the patient, even though he or she may be unable to give valid consent. In most cases, however, it is best to proceed with the treatment: (1) if the next-of-kin has consented; (2) if it is necessary to proceed quickly with treatment to protect the patient's health; and (3) if there is no applicable prohibitive statute.

In situations where treatment of a minor is contemplated, certain additional considerations must be kept in mind. As a general rule, the consent of a minor patient's parent or guardian is required before a physician may proceed with non-emergency treatment. There are many exceptions, however, which allow a minor to consent to selected or limited medical care without the advice or consent of parents. Because states vary widely as to the extent of medical care for which a minor may consent, the physician must be familiar with the relevant law in his or her area of practice. Among other things, state laws permit minors to obtain counselling and treatment for pregnancy, venereal disease, drug abuse, and alcoholism, as well as certain birth control services, without parental consent. Usually, state laws will set forth a minimum age (typically, between age 12 and 14) as a prerequisite to the provision of medical care in these situations.

Informed Consent

The doctrine of informed consent derives primarily from concepts of individual autonomy and self-determination within the framework of the physician-patient relationship. Historically, the informed consent cause of action sounded in battery, essentially as a form of unauthorized touching. As the informed consent doctrine continued to evolve, however, the focus of the cause of action became the quality of the consent rather than the unauthorized nature of the touching. This view rapidly gained acceptance throughout the country and today, except in cases where there is total absence of consent, the courts have adopted the now clear rule of law that informed consent actions are based upon professional negligence concepts.

Information Disclosure Standards

The primary component of the informed consent cause of action is the physician's duty to adequately disclose to the patient the nature of the proposed treatment or procedure, the significant or material risks involved, the available alternatives, if any, and the reasonable benefits to be expected. Two approaches have been adopted by the courts in delineating the scope of the physician's disclosure obligation — the professional disclosure standard and the reasonable patient standard.

Under the professional disclosure standard, a physician's duty to disclose is governed by the standard of the reasonable medical practitioner, practicing under the same or similiar circumstances. This disclosure standard, which is set forth either by statute or common law in a majority of U.S. jurisdictions, requires the physician to disclose information according to the prevailing standard of care, as established through expert testimony. Thus, in these jurisdictions, for a physician to be liable for a breach of duty in the context of obtaining informed consent, there must be expert testimony evidencing a failure to disclose information that would have been disclosed by the reasonable medical practitioner under the same or similiar circumstances.

The reasonable patient disclosure standard, which is set forth by statute or common law in a significant minority of jurisdictions, contemplates the existence of a duty on the part of the physician to disclose to the patient any information that would reasonably bear upon the patient's decision-making process. Thus, even in the face of contrary expert testimony, a physician may be held to have breached the proper disclosure standard in these jurisdictions if a jury were to conclude that specific information, which was not disclosed, would have been material to the reasonable patient in deciding whether to undergo a particular form of therapy or treatment.

Proximate Causation

As in other medical malpractice cases, it is essential for the plaintiff in an informed consent action to establish that the harm or injury suffered is the proximate result of a breach of duty or violation of the standard of care. In a medical malpractice case, injury is alleged to have occurred as the result of a treatment error or omission. In the informed consent context, however, litigation may be initiated even when there has been no treatment error or omissions, e.g., where a foreseeable risk of treatment materializes causing injury. The patient is thus heard to complain not that the treatment was negligently provided, but that, had there been full disclosure of the material risks or available alternatives, the patient would not have undergone the treatment, and thus would not have been injured.

Under the majority rule, which has been adopted by virtually all U.S. jurisdictions, causation in informed consent cases is determined by an objective standard, i.e., what a reasonably prudent person would have decided if adequately informed. The court, in *Guebard v. Jabaay,* 452 N.E.2d 751, 757-58 (Ill. App. 1983), offered a typical judicial explanation as follows:

> If disclosure would not have changed the decision of a reasonable person in the position of the patient, there is no causal connection between non-disclosure and (the patient's) post-operative condition; if however, disclosure would have caused a reasonable person in the position of the patient to refuse the surgery or therapy, a causal connection is shown.

In four states, a subjective causation standard is utilized. Under this standard, in order to prove causation, the *individual patient* must establish that he or she would not have undergone the medical treatment had the non-disclosed information actually been provided. In the few jurisdictions that have adopted this standard, the courts assert that subjective focus on the individual patient's informational needs is the only appropriate vehicle for complying with a patient's right of self-determination.

Practical Disclosure Considerations

In the context of obtaining informed consent to medical treatment, patients should be apprised of their diagnosis, differential diagnosis, the nature of the proposed diagnostic and therapeutic procedures, the material risks associated therewith, the prospects of success, and the details of alternative courses of treatment that are available. Material risks include those that are reasonably foreseeable, as well as those that occur frequently but constitute a significant threat to health or life. As the probability or severity of risk to the patient increases, the duty to inform increases.

It should also be emphasized that when a physician plans to treat a patient by a method that entails moderate risks, and the physician knows that an alternative, more risky treatment exists, there is an affirmative duty in certain jurisdictions to inform the patient of the more risky alternative. Similarly, a patient's right to know is not necessarily confined to a situation in which disease is present and has been conclusively diagnosed.

In one recent case, a 37-year-old man had seen his physician with symptoms of exertional chest pain of several weeks duration, and nitroglycerine therapy was prescribed. The court found that the physician had a duty to inform the patient that he suspected coronary artery disease, despite inconclusive tests. Thus, the duty of disclosure arises any time that a treating physician is aware of abnormalities that indicate risk of danger, and it is premised on the belief that a patient needs to know such information to make an intelligent, informed decision about the future course of medical care.

The right to know also extends to test results. If an abnormal test has clinical significance, as in a Pap smear that may suggest malignancy, the physician is obligated to notify the patient of such results.

Special Consent Situations

Spousal consent is not a prerequisite for treatment of a competent patient, even if the treatment involves procedures that may affect the patient's marital relationship. However, it is advisable to discuss thoroughly with the patient and spouse any procedure that may compromise the patient's ability to reproduce or to perform sexually. Although the husband's consent is not required for artificial insemination of his wife, a husband who is not consulted and does not consent may not be liable for support of the resulting child, and, in certain jurisdictions, a divorce may be based on adultery. As the welfare of the child resulting from artificial insemination may be at stake, the physician generally should not perform such a procedure without the consent of both husband and wife.

In the context of abortion, a woman's informed consent also must be obtained, without evidence of duress or coercion. Unreasonable restrictions may not be placed upon the woman's exercise of free choice in this regard, as set forth under the following standards prescribed by the United States Supreme Court: (1) for the stage of pregnancy prior to approximately the end of the first trimester, the abortion decision and its effectuation must be left to the pregnant woman and her attending physician; (2) for the stage of pregnancy subsequent to approximately the end of the first trimester, the state, in promoting its interest in the health of the mother may, if it chooses, regulate the abortion procedure in ways that are reasonably related to maternal health; and (3) for the stage of pregnancy subsequent to viability, the state, in promoting its interest in the potentiality of human life may, if it chooses, regulate, and even proscribe, abortion, except where it is necessary, in appropriate medical judgment, for the preservation of the life or health of the mother.

In the context of performing elective sterilization, informed consent is again one of the most important medical-legal considerations. The competent adult patient must make a knowing, intelligent, and voluntary decision after fully considering the nature of the proposed sterilization procedure, the available alternative procedures, the discomforts and risks associated with the proposed procedure, as well as alternative procedures, and the benefits reasonably to be expected. In addition, the patient must fully understand that while no guarantee of success can be made, the sterilization procedure is intended to be permanent and irreversible. The patient should acknowledge that if the operation is successful, the patient will be unable to produce a child.

Given the importance and finality of this decision, the physician must be certain to explain to the patient all lesser intrusive means of birth control and family planning. The patient also should be informed that a failure to undergo sterilization will not otherwise prejudice the patient's right to medical care and treatment.

When there is a question about the patient's competence to give a knowing, intelligent, and voluntary consent, the opinion of a knowledgeable consultant should be obtained and made a part of the record. In this regard, it should also be emphasized that absent clear statutory authority, the consent of a minor should not be deemed sufficient to authorize an elective sterilization.

Finally, the authority of the competent patient to consent to health care coexists with a well-established right to refuse treatment, even when such treatment is necessary to save the individual's life. This right has been recognized by numerous courts and is premised upon a patient's constitutional rights of liberty, privacy, and religious freedom, as well as the common law right of self-determination.

Members of the Jehovah's Witness religious sect, for example, refuse blood transfusions on the basis of their literal interpretation of the Bible's prohibition against drinking blood. However, some courts try to find grounds on which to order the necessary treatment. The courts usually will authorize treatment to protect the life or health of a child or fetus on the ground that the child will be "neglected" under applicable state statutes if treatment is refused, or that the state owes a paramount duty to protect its children. A number of courts have ordered necessary treatment over the objections of competent adult patients.

It is, therefore, necessary to evaluate each treatment situation carefully on the basis of available facts and circumstances in determining whether to honor a competent adult patient's refusal of medical treatment. In cases of deteriorating terminal illness, the refusal of an adult patient to accept further life-sustaining treatment presents an obviously less difficult determination than the decision of a seven-month pregnant woman to refuse blood transfusions that are needed to save her life and that of her viable fetus. Certainly, in cases of greater complexity, the physician should not hesitate to obtain prompt legal guidance.

Exceptions to Informed Consent Disclosure Requirements

Several exceptions to informed consent disclosure requirements have been consistently recognized throughout the United States. These recognized exceptions apply in the following circumstances: medical emergencies; lack of patient capacity to consent; prior knowledge on the part of the patient; waiver of the right of disclosure; and therapeutic privilege.

In medical emergencies, when the patient is unconscious or unable to communicate, or when there is a lack of time to obtain express informed consent, the physician may provide treatment under a theory of implied consent. The law presumes that the compelling need for immediate emergency treatment outweighs the requirement of obtaining informed consent. Similarly, if the patient is mentally incapable of granting express consent to treatment, the physician is not legally required to make a full and complete information disclosure to the patient. Under such circumstances, when possible, informed consent to treatment should be obtained from the incompetent patient's guardian or representative.

When a patient receives recurrent medical care, and thus has prior knowledge of the nature of the ongoing treatment, as well as the material risks and available alternatives, it is generally unnecessary to engage in duplicative disclosures of this information. Of course, if the patient requests further explanation or additional information, an appropriate response is indicated. Moreover, when considerable time has elapsed since previous treatment, or when there has been a change in circumstances, such as an increased risk during subsequent treatment, the patient's informed consent should be obtained.

Numerous commentators also have observed that risks which are widely known to the general patient population need not be disclosed in the context of obtaining informed consent. The physician should be cognizant, however, that speculation regarding which risks are widely known by the general patient population, or which risks are known to a particular person, can be perilous. Accordingly, a physician should not refrain from disclosing particular risks on the basis of the common knowledge or prior patient knowledge exceptions, unless the physician can demonstrate the basis for this determination.

Patient waiver is a more clear-cut exception. When the physician is specifically apprised that a patient does not wish to be informed of certain information relating to a course of treatment, such a waiver may be relied upon. It is advisable, however, for the physician to encourage the patient to explain the justification for the waiver. If, after discussing the waiver with the patient, the physician ascertains that the patient knowingly and intelligently insists on not being informed, and provides a reasonable justification for the decision, non-disclosure will be legally defensible.

The final exception to informed consent disclosure requirements arises under the doctrine of therapeutic privilege. Under this doctrine, a physician may refrain from disclosing certain information to the patient when it can be demonstrated that the disclosure would have a serious adverse effect on the patient or on the therapeutic process. As a general rule, however, courts have been inclined to look with disfavor on the therapeutic privilege, observing that, unless it is carefully circumscribed, the privilege may devour the disclosure rule itself. Physicians will bear the burden of justifying the medical legitimacy of any such failure to disclose.

Obtaining and Documenting Consent

With respect to obtaining and documenting informed consent, it should be noted that both the literature and the common law focus on informed consent as a substantive communication leading to a patient's knowledgeable consent to medical care and treatment. Too often, however, physicians view informed consent as the equivalent of a properly signed legal document. This view is erroneous. In actuality, a signed consent from is only as meaningful as the exchange of pertinent information that it memorializes.

The responsibility to obtain the patient's informed consent belongs to the attending or treating physician. This responsibility may be assigned to a third party, e.g., a nurse practitioner; however, any liability for non-disclosure of material information in violation of the professional standard of care ultimately will rest with the physician. Hospitals also have the responsibility to implement appropriate mechanisms with a view toward ensuring that informed consent is properly obtained.

It is advisable that the information provided to the patient include the following: a description of the patient's condition; the general nature of the proposed treatment; the reasonably expected results thereof, including an indication that treatment success cannot be guaranteed; the available treatment alternatives, if any, including the right to reject treatment; and the risks and benefits of undergoing either the proposed treatment or an available alternative treatment. When appropriate, the patient also should be informed of the identity and responsibility of other persons who will participate in the patient's treatment course.

Documentation of informed consent may be accomplished in a number of ways. A comprehensive written consent form can be utilized which specifically sets forth, in understandable language, each of the above-described elements of required information with respect to a particular course of treatment. The advantage of such an approach is that it offers a complete recitation of the information disclosed to the patient. A disadvantage of this type of form, however, is that it must be individually tailored and carefully reviewed to ensure that all material information is included on the face of the document. Any omission will be particularly evident in the context of subsequent litigation.

Another approach to documentation involves the use of a less detailed consent form. This type of consent document simply recites that the above-described elements of informed consent have been discussed with the patient. While this form will serve to evidence that some type of informed consent interaction did occur, it leaves open for jury consideration the precise details of the information disclosure.

Regardless of which type of form is used, the physician is well-advised to make appropriate entries in the medical record, documenting and describing the informed consent interaction. Such entries will provide a valuable supplement in supporting the sufficiency of the information disclosure to the patient. Moreover, in the absence of a signed consent document, these entries will constitute necessary evidence of the informed consent interaction.

Informed Refusal

When a patient rejects the physician's diagnostic or therapeutic recommendations, the physician must advise the patient of the potential adverse consequences of such a refusal. Reference to this discussion should be included in the physician's records along with the other informed consent material.

Conclusion

In the context of the physician-patient relationship, it is an important obligation of the physician to obtain consent to treatment, particularly informed consent, before embarking upon a course of treatment or therapy. Necessary information must be disclosed to the patient to permit a knowing, intelligent, and voluntary agreement.

Although two standards exist for determining whther the physician has disclosed sufficient information to the patient, it is clear that such information should include a description of the patient's condition, the general nature of the proposed treatment, the reasonably expected results thereof, available treatment alternatives, if any, and the risks and benefits of undergoing either the proposed treatment or an available alternative.

The most important consideration in the informed consent context is genuine communication between physician and patient. When the physician takes the time to engage in a thorough informed consent discussion with the patient, and the interchange is documented in the medical record and by a properly executed informed consent document, the physician will enjoy a particularly favorable defense posture in the event of informed consent litigation.

HOSPITAL COUNSEL

Introduction

From the outset, it is critical to identify the characters and their roles in the hospital health care-legal mosaic. One, there is the hospital entity represented by the Board of Trustees and its legal advisor and advocate - the hospital counsel. Two, there is the medical staff, who should have its own legal representative. Three, there are the individual attending physicians with hospital privileges, and they should have their own lawyers when necessary.

Why all the lawyers? The hospital needs a legal protector pursuant to its duties and responsibilities, predicated on the legal doctrine of "corporate liability". Its interests are not always identical to those of the medical staff and the individual physician; there are times when the various interests are in conflict. The physician must be aware of this and be alert to the time when hospital counsel is not only not his friend, but is actually a foe representing the enemy. You don't put the fox in the chicken coop! There are times when the medical staff alone, or together with the hospital administration, is in conflict with an individual physician. At such a time, the physician obviously should not rely on either the "friends" of the hospital or the medical staff. At other times, the relationships among the three parties is like a nonromantic eternal triangle - "each man for himself".

An employed physician is in a different position. The hospital counsel is an ally when the employee and employer see eye to eye. When their interests diverge, the physician needs his own counsel. There are situations when the employed physician also has medical staff privileges. In such circumstances, the script is the same as for the attending physician vis-a-vis the medical staff and/or hospital administration in a legal scenario.

The hospital trainee, e.g., house officer, intern, resident, fellow, must understand the role of the hospital's counsel. His client is the hospital. He will be the trainee's "friend", as long as the hospital's interests and the trainee's interests are in concert.

Although a trainee is a member of the hospital staff, he is not a member of the medical staff. The trainee is an employee working pursuant to an employment contract. Many of the services of the hospital counsel afforded to members of the medical staff are available to the trainee, and obviously can be extremely helpful. However, if the trainee is disciplined or his contract terminated, or he is treated in a detrimental manner by the hospital, or he is involved in a malpractice action, his legal resource is not the hospital counsel; he needs his own counsel. In truth, under these circumstances, the hospital counsel is an adversary or foe, not a friend.

Some of the legal concerns that are discussed in this chapter have little or no application to the hospital trainee. They are presented because the trainee should have a complete understanding of how the hospital functions - who is who, and to whom loyalty belongs. Furthermore, one day the trainee will become an attending physician and a member of a medical staff. Knowledge concerning such matters as medical staff bylaws, rules, and regulations, continuing medical education, and medical staff participation are for the trainee's future relationships. Legal problems involving antitrust, class action suits, and Medicare and Medicaid fraud will not very likely touch the trainee.

The hospital counsel is a member of the hospital team when a physician begins his practice in the hospital. Although counsel will not be joining in rounds or participating in case management conferences, he will participate in patient care through the establishment of protocols, policies, legal advice, and in-service education. To many physicians, the thought of association with hospital counsel in patient care practice may be foreign, or even intimidating. However, let's examine the ways and means in which this association can be helpful to a physician, and even enhance the care he provides to his patients.

Medicine and Law

The practice of medicine and the provision of patient care are not carried out in a vacuum, but rather are an integral part of our social system. Medicine is greatly affected by and impacted by the law. Therefore, it will be helpful for the physician to acquire an appreciation of hospital counsel's role, and how he can realize the full benefit from hospital counsel as his ally. How then does a physician identify with and relate to hospital counsel?

The hospital counsel is a professional member of the health care team, as is the physician. Although the hospital is the counsel's client, a physician, as a member of the medical staff, is a direct recipient of and benefits from the legal services that counsel provides to the hospital. Let's review some of the legal services that hospital counsel provides.

Patient Access

When we examine the areas of responsibility of hospital counsel, we find that they are very similar to many areas of the physician's responsibilities. For example, hospital counsel, just as is the physician, is concerned with patient access to health care, the quality of patient care, and with many other aspects of health care delivery. The main difference is that hospital counsel is responsible for and participates in the development of the corporate plan for health care, and the physician is responsible for and participates in the personal delivery of health care. However, the physician's respective interests and responsibilities are concurrent and not inconsistent. Indeed, hospital counsel is the physician's ally; and as with any other resource that the physician has in providing health care to his patients, it is in his best interest and the interests of his patients that he not only understand and appreciate the interface of law and medicine, but also develop an appreciation of the role of hospital counsel and utilize that individual as a resource and ally.

One of the first areas in which a physician and hospital counsel will be interrelating is the issue of patient care access. For example, hospital counsel will be very much involved in helping the hospital develop and articulate access issues pursuant to the hospital's mission statement. Hospital counsel will be involved in helping the hospital develop access policies providing that access is not conditioned upon race, color, national origin, sex, or other such factors. Hospital counsel will also be involved in helping the hospital structure and articulate its policy on access to patient care as it relates to the ability to pay. Although the physician will not, in most instances, be directly involved in articulating such issues, their resolution by the hospital will impact upon his practice in the hospital.

Patient Rights

Another area of great importance to practicing physicians in a hospital is the emerging concept of defined patient rights. For example, in the early 1970's, the American Hospital Association adopted a Patient's Bill of Rights that has been widely publicized. Copies are often distributed in hospitals. Although the AHA Patient's Bill of Rights is not legally binding, by adopting them, either expressly or implicitly, a hospital may have caused them to become standards in that particular hospital. Additionally, some states have enacted "Patient's Bill of Rights". Wherever a physician practices, he should ask hospital counsel to advise him regarding the issue of whether or not either statutory or adopted standards from the Patient's Bill of Rights apply at that institution.

Consent

Hospital counsel will also be directly involved with the medical staff and the individual physician as a member of the medical staff, in formulating and articulating hospital policy regarding consent.

Patients are entitled to know the nature and scope of their treatment, and the anticipated outcome and alternate treatment modalities, which are called "informed consent". As a member of the hospital medical staff, the informed consent policy of the hospital will directly impact upon the physician's practice in the hospital. Hospital counsel will also serve as a valuable resource to the physician in answering tangential issues arising out of informed consent protocols. For example, who gives consent if the patient is not emancipated, or the patient is comatose? How is consent obtained in an emergency? Who consents if the parents of a minor patient are separated? Such questions regarding informed consent go on and on, and a physician, as a member of the medical staff, needs access to an attorney well-versed in all aspects of health law to provide him with advice and counsel regarding such "legal issues" involving consent. Although issues of informed consent were first recognized decades ago, many of the current malpractice cases today rise or fall on the issue of informed consent. Hospital counsel will not only brief the physician on the hospital's policy regarding consent, he will also brief him on the prevailing law governing consent.

Confidentiality

In a physician's practice, he may be confronted from time to time with competing interests regarding the release of information gleaned from the physician-patient relationship. For example, what if a patient confides in the physician that he or she is planning to commit a crime or has, in fact, already committed a crime. Should the physician warn the law enforcement authorities and the identified victims? Or take another example, what should a physician do if in examining a patient, he finds that the patient is unable to physically operate an automobile safely, and yet the patient tells him that he or she plans to continue to drive? What should the physician do? He should call the hospital counsel. The counsel will provide the physician with recommendations regarding specific inquiries, and assist the physician in the formulation of appropriate protocols at the hospital that will protect the rights of patients to privacy in their medical records, and at the same time, comply with external requirements regarding the release of patient information, even when such information is gleaned from the physician-patient relationship.

Medical Records

Medical records is an area in which a physician will be directly involved with hospital counsel. Most states recognize the patient's right of privacy in his or her medical records. Information gleaned from the physician-patient relationship is subject to confidentiality. A physician can release patient information only pursuant to the patient's authorization, authorization by the patient's legal representative, a court order, or some specific statutory requirement. Hospital counsel will advise the physician that he should take a conservative approach in releasing patient information, and that he should never release patient information unless expressly authorized or required to release such information. Questions such as who can release a patient's records in the event that the patient is a minor, or is not emancipated, will often require the physician to review the hospital policy regarding the release of patient information, and obtain a consultation with hospital counsel in many instances. Always remember that a physician may get "fussed at" for not releasing medical records; however, it is highly likely that he won't get sued. If a physician releases medical records without authorization or pursuant to legal requirements, he may well get sued. Remember, a physician's first duty is to his patient to maintain integrity in his or her medical records against unauthorized disclosure. The physician should not view himself as a champion of social indignation for the release of medical records. Keep in mind that the physician is an advocate for his patients, and one of his duties as a patient advocate is to fight for the protection of confidentiality in medical records resulting from the physician-patient relationship.

Physicians should be aware of the fact that in almost all jurisdictions the patient has a right of access to his or her medical record upon proper request. In fact, the American Hospital Association adopted a "Patients' Bill of Rights" to this effect several years ago.

Peer Review

The physician will be confronted immediately after he becomes a member of the medical staff with the responsibility for peer review. Legally, peer review established the responsibility of medical staff members to observe, monitor, and help the medical staff and hospital to maintain the quality of patient care consistent with the standards in the hospital. For example, the physician may serve on utilization and review committees, quality assurance committees, or on a number of other committees that address themselves to issues of patient care in the hospital. Physicians, incident to their appointment as members of the medical staff, have peer review responsibility. Physicians and hospitals are experiencing an increasing number of complaints against medical staff members, alleging that they failed to meet their peer review responsibilities. It is not unreasonable to expect that there will be an increase in the number of verdicts and judgments following the increase of such complaints. Hospital counsel is instrumental in working with the medical staff to help it meet the responsibilities of individual members of the medical staff, and the medical staff collectively, regarding peer review requirements. Also, medical staff members may become involved in the PRO process either within the confines of the hospital, or at the regional or state level. Hospital counsel will serve as the physician's ally in helping him understand his responsibilities in peer review, both as a member of the medical staff and within the PRO requirements.

The trainee is intimately involved in the hospital quality assurance program

- peer and utilization review. He can be invaluable in helping obtain the goals of the program by noting and reporting deviations from the quality of care standards. The hospital counsel can be of great help to the trainee in this role. The relationship of the trainee, who is the subject of a quality assurance deficiency, is one of arm's length.

Incompetent Physicians

The Health Care Quality Improvement Act (HCQIA) of 1986 was enacted in response to concerns that incompetent or impaired physicians migrated from state to state to avoid disciplinary action. The Act contains two major provisions, one granting limited liability for peer review activity by professional bodies, and the other establishing a National Practitioner Data Bank for reporting of "adverse" information concerning health care practitioners.

The statute sets forth three general areas for which information must be reported to the Data Bank:
- Payments made on behalf of health care practitioners for medical malpractice suits or claims;
- Adverse licensure actions taken by state licensing boards; and
- Adverse actions taken against health care practitioners relating to clinical privileges.

All provisions of the Act are applicable to all physicians, including trainees. The hospital counsel can serve as interpreter and advisor for the hospital, medical staff, and physicians involved in the peer review process. He cannot be of help to a targeted physician; that would be a conflict of interest.

Risk Management

Another area in which a physician will become involved with hospital counsel is risk management or risk reduction. The malpractice crisis has focused attention on the need for physicians and hospitals to recognize, manage, and reduce the potential for risks from which malpractice suits can be filed. Hospital counsel will be actively involved in working with the hospital and medical staff in establishing a risk management or risk reduction plan that will apply to the hospital and to the medical staff.

The hospital in which a physician practices will most likely form a committee composed of hospital personnel and medical staff members to develop protocols for risk management or risk reduction. As a member of the medical staff, the physician will have an opportunity to participate in the formulation, monitoring, and review of his hospital's risk mangement or risk reduction program.

Not only has the malpractice crisis focused attention on the need for risk management or risk reduction programs in hospitals, it has subjected physicians to an increasing incidence of malpractice litigation. Statistics today are appalling regarding the escalating increase in malpractice suits against physicians. Concurrent with the escalating increase in medical malpractice suits being filed is an increase in the number and size of verdicts and judgments rendered against physicians and hospitals by patients alleging malpractice.

Incident Reports

Medical staffs and hospitals utilize incident reports as a management tool to monitor the quality of patient care in the hospital and to serve as an indicator of needed change. Incident reports are completed on untoward events in patient care; they serve as the basis for review of patient care and point out needed changes. Incident reports are not punitive in nature and should be viewed by physicians as a constructive tool, not only to monitor their own patient care, but also to monitor other members of the medical team in providing patient care in the hospital. The physician will be working closely with hospital counsel in reviewing incidents and formulating responses to avoid future incidents of a similar nature in patient care.

Discovery of Peer Review — Deliberations and Incident Reports

There appears to be a growing trend toward the patient's right of discovery of peer review deliberations and incident reports. Several appellate courts have held that it is within the trial court judge's discretion to permit such access upon proper presentation by the patient.

"Dumping" of Emergency Patients

Physicians must be aware of one of the "Miscellaneous Provisions" of the Budget Reconciliation Act of the 99th Congress, which governs hospitals with an emergency department wherein a patient with an emergency medical condition seeks medical care. If such a patient is "transferred" from that health care facility to another facility or is discharged, he or she may recover damages for "personal harm", if the condition worsens during or after such transfer or discharge, and the federal and state governments may impose fines. The patient must prove only that the condition was not "stabilized" at the time of transfer, and that the condition deteriorated due to the transfer.

In order to avoid liability, the physician or other medical personnel at the hospital must sign a certification that based upon the reasonable risks and benefits to the patient, and based upon the information available at the time, the medical benefits reasonably expected from the provision of appropriate medical treatment at another facility outweigh the increased risks of transfer. Presumably, if the patient is discharged to out-patient care at home, the benefits of these alternatives outweigh further care within the facility.

The transfer must be an "appropriate transfer". The criteria required to effectuate an appropriate transfer include all of the following: 1) the receiving facility has available space and qualified personnel and has agreed to accept transfer and to provide appropriate medical treatment; 2) the transferring hospital provides appropriate medical records of its examination and treatment; 3) the transfer is effected through qualified personnel and transportation equipment; and 4) such other requirements as the Secretary of Health and Human Services may find necessary. Presumably, the physician or other medical personnel who transfers the patient has the requisite knowledge of the staffing and competence of the receiving facility and has sought agreement for acceptance by the receiving facility prior to transfer. These requirements seem applicable whether the receiving facility be an out-patient clinic, nursing home, day care program, or a more intensive treatment center.

The hospital counsel can be extremely valuable in interpreting the law to the involved physician, help develop protocols to prevent infractions and the ensuing penalties, and give advice if an adverse situation arises.

Cost Containment

Hospitals are now increasingly beseiged by local, state, and federal cost containment requirements. Hospitals now demand that physicians provide care in an economical manner. The hospital counsel can be invaluable in analyzing and explaining the various legislation, rules, and regulations directed to controlling costs. One consequence has been the development of an adversary between the physician and the hospital, because the physician is costing the hospital too much money in ordering too many tests or keeping a patient in the hospital for a longer period of time than is necessary.

The hospital may decide to remove this "costly practitioner". Under such circumstances, the hospital counsel should not advise the physician. Hopefully, however, the physician's own lawyer can persuade the hospital counsel to use his good offices with the hospital and demonstrate that the practitioner's economic track record only appears relatively poor, because his practice consists of a large number of elderly patients, some of whom are economically disadvantaged and have multiple, chronic, complex medical problems. It is rare when some solution satisfactory to both parties cannot be worked out.

There are times, because of cost containment, when a hospital refuses to allow a procedure or tests, and requests that the patient be discharged. The physician knows that these hospital demands are not in his patient's best interests; historically, it has been the role of the physician to be primarily concerned with his patient's best interests and to look out for those interests. The physician's ethics and the court have told him that he must become a patient advocate. Allies become adversaries, including the hospital counsel. Hopefully, a resolution can be found, similar to the one when the physician is considered an outlier.

Trainees must be aware of cost containment restraints, and must learn to "stay their hands" rather than "go it alone", thereby creating problems for the hospital and the attending physician.

Malpractice

Malpractice is the failure of physicians to use due care in the treatment of their patients. Due care is generally defined as that standard of care that a reasonable and prudent physician would have used in like or similar circumstances and in like or similar communities. Some states have statewide standards, and some states have "local standards", which means that the standard of care is established community by community rather than by statewide standards. Hospital counsel will provide in-service training sessions for malpractice, including the elements of malpractice, to wit: duty, breach of duty, foreseeability, proximate cause, and resulting damages. Hospital counsel will, in helping a physician understand the elements of malpractice, assist him in developing protocols in his practice that will minimize exposure to risks that may precipitate malpractice allegations.

If a physician is involved in malpractice litigation, hospital counsel may be involved in the defense of the claim in representing the hospital or associating with special litigation counsel provided by the insurance company for the hospital, or by special litigation counsel retained by the hospital in the event that the hospital is self-insured. Hospital counsel will also serve as a resource for the physician in structuring his practice to minimize risk, consistent with good risk management or risk reduction techniques. Being named a defendant in a medical malpractice case is traumatic, time-consuming, and expensive. Malpractice litigation is protracted and often exacts a heavy toll not only on the physician who has been named as a defendant, but also on the physician's colleagues and the physician's family. In addition to serving as legal counsel to the physician as a member of the medical staff, the hospital counsel can also serve as a friend and confidant in matters involving the physician's practice and exposure to risks of malpractice claims.

Damages that patients may suffer in the event of malpractice are of significant interest to the physician, and hospital counsel will brief him on issues relating to damages. Compensatory damages may include economic and non-economic damages. Economic damages are definable and generally include lost wages, medical expenses, travel expenses, and other expenses directly incurred by the plaintiff. Non-economic damages generally include undefinable amounts, such as pain and suffering and loss of consortium. Many states, through Tort Reform Acts, have attempted to cap the amount of damages that patients may recover. Hospital counsel will advise the physician on the issue of damages in the state in which he practices. However, remember that punitive damages may not be covered by the physician's malpractice insurance.

Malpractice Insurance

Most hospitals now require that medical staff members maintain in force a defined amount of medical malpractice insurance coverage. Failure to have malpractice insurance is a recognized basis for denial of medical staff membership, and the failure to maintain medical malpractice insurance is an acceptable basis for termination of medical staff membership. Hospital counsel can be helpful to a physician in not only reviewing the requirements of medical staff membership, but also informing him of the adequacy of his coverage measured against experience and trends in malpractice litigation and damage assessments by judges and juries in the state in which the physician practices.

The issue of malpractice insurance will be vital to the physician in the current malpractice climate. Occurrence coverage, claims made coverage, and reporting endorsements are "household words" that will become familiar to the physician. He will receive information from his liability carrier, the medical staff, and other sources. He should talk with hospital counsel about his malpractice insurance, including, but not limited to, adequate coverage and other relevant factors.

The hospital trainee must remember that if he commits an act of negligence and is sued, the plaintiff's attorney will probably sue both the trainee and the hospital, relying on the doctrine of agency - respondeat superior and vicarious liability. Under these circumstances, the hospital's carrier will defend and pay any judgment rendered against either or both defendants. However, the plaintiff's lawyer may decide to sue only the trainee and not the hospital. If this occurs, the hospital's insurance company is not involved because it agreed to be responsible only if the hospital is sued for the acts of the trainee. In the first scenario where both are sued, or on a rare occasion when only the hospital is sued under the doctrine of agency, and the hospital is held liable, it can successfully seek to recover from the actual tortfeasor, the trainee, under the doctrine of indemnification or contribution. Actually, the insurance carrier, who pays the judgment, can successfully seek to recover on its own under the doctrine of subrogation. The bottom line is that the trainee should have his own insurance coverage. It is not expensive and is worth every penny, if only for peace of mind. Judgments have a life of their own and may be extended for 20 to 30 years, depending on the jurisdiction.

Antitrust

One of the "hottest issues" that a physician will face as a member of the medical staff is that of the threat of antitrust claims. Recently, physicians have shown a propensity to file antitrust claims in federal and state courts against individual members of the medical staff, against the medical staff, and against the hospital when they are denied medical staff membership, or their status as a member of the medical staff is changed. Antitrust litigation is protracted, expensive, and exacting. Awards resulting from antitrust claims, as well as punitive damage claims, may not be covered under a physician's medical malpractice insurance. Therefore, antitrust claims are not only dreaded, but can be devastating to physicians. Damages are trebled in antitrust claims, and attorneys' fees for the plaintiffs may be awarded. Hospital counsel can be invaluable to a physician in reviewing the antitrust climate in the state in which he practices, and helping him avoid becoming involved in antitrust litigation.

Bylaws, Rules, and Regulations

Medical staffs in hospitals are organized pursuant to medical staff bylaws. Medical staff bylaws are complemented by a fair hearing plan and rules and regulations. The medical staff bylaws address themselves to the relationships of the members of the medical staff to each other and to the hospital. The fair hearing plan addresses the procedural and substantive rights of members of the medical staff to due process, in the event that some deficiency exists or arises in regard to their request for reappointment to the medical staff. Medical staff rules and regulations address issues of patient care and are the product of departmental policies and requirements. The hospital counsel will be well-versed in medical staff legal issues and will advise physicians on medical staff governance.

In most instances, a physician will be provided with a copy of the medical staff bylaws, the fair hearing plan, and the rules and regulations of the medical staff when he applies for medical staff membership. He should carefully read these documents and understand them before he applies for medical staff appointment. After the physician is appointed to the medical staff, hospital counsel will be available to him to address concerns and issues regarding medical staff appointment and the granting of clinical privileges. Appointment to the medical staff is not a right but a privilege. The governing authority of the hospital has the inherent responsibility to appoint only those physicians to the medical staff who are qualified by education, training, experience, and demonstrated competence, consistent with the objectives of the hospital. The burden is on the medical staff applicant to clearly demonstrate that he possesses the skills to carry out the clinical privileges sought and is qualified for appointment to the medical staff. Remember, it is not incumbent upon the medical staff or the hospital to show that the applicant is not qualified.

Continuing Medical Education

The hospital counsel is a resource to physicians in providing continuing medical education. He is generally available for medical staff meetings, committee meetings, or discussing legal issues on ground rounds. One of the ongoing areas of responsibility of the hospital counsel is to provide the medical staff with information on legal issues impacting patient care in the hospital.

Training Program Approval

Of particular concern to the trainee is hospital approval by the JCAHO or a state agency, as well as a residency program by specialty. Otherwise, the training program will not be accepted for Board-certification. The hospital counsel can be of assistance to the trainee in completing the documents establishing his eligibility for Board-certification.

Medicare and Medicaid Fraud and Abuse Act

More issues about "kickbacks" and prohibited practice are surfacing under the Medicare and Medicaid Fraud and Abuse Act as the U.S. Inspector General continues his crackdown on violators, particularly as the entitlement programs of Medicare and Medicaid continue to expand. Prohibited payments are not clearly defined, and the punishment for violations is severe. Therefore, physicians should be concerned with the overall impact of the Medicare and Medicaid Fraud and Abuse Act in their practices and as members of medical staffs. Hospital counsel should be requested by the medical staff to provide them with ongoing information regarding the continuing increase in sensitivity to the Medicare and Medicare Fraud and Abuse Act.

Sexual Harassment

The incidence of allegations of sexual harassment against medical staff members is increasing and becoming of greater concern to medical staffs. Medical staffs are developing protocols to discourage sexual harassment and to deal with such allegations. Hospital counsel will have primary responsibility in working with the medical staff to develop such protocols and to monitor their effectiveness.

AIDS

The AIDS crisis has ushered in a new dimension of health care delivery. Because of the severe nature and consequences of AIDS, medically, socially, and economically, some jurisdictions have enacted safeguards to protect patients against the unauthorized disclosure that they have AIDS or test HIV-positive. Should all patients be tested for AIDS? Should members of the medical staff, hospital employees, and other patients be advised that a patient has AIDS or tests positive for HIV? Physicians should consult with hospital counsel to determine the hospital's policy on AIDS.

Recently, the AMA and other national medical groups have issued public policy statements calling for disclosure by a medical practitioner of his HIV infection to his patients.

Required Reporting Statutes

What about mandatory reporting requirements? The state in which a physician practices will have certain mandatory reporting requirements. The requirements vary from state to state; therefore, the physician should consult with the hospital counsel to determine what the reporting requirements are in his hospital. For example, the hospital will have a protocol on reporting suspected child abuse. Certain reports regarding communicable diseases are required. Certain injuries resulting from apparent violent acts must be reported. Hospital counsel will review the reporting requirements of the hospital, so that the physician can comply with them.

Right to Refuse Treatment and Die

Patients are becoming more sensitive to their right to a natural death. Hospitals are encouraging the dissemination of information regarding the right to a natural death and forms for patients to sign, requesting the right to a natural death. States vary on the requirements regarding the right of patients to execute an advanced directive indicating a desire for a natural death, i.e., a "living will" or durable power of attorney. Because of varying requirements, hospital counsel should be consulted to determine the controlling policy in the physician's hospital.

Organ Transplants

Legal issues involved in organ transplants and the donation of anatomic parts are very complex. Public policy encourages organ transplants and the donation of anatomical gifts. However, there are specific legal requirements regarding the harvesting and transplantation of organs, as well as anatomical gifts. The physician should consult with hospital counsel and review the legal requirements involved in organ harvesting, organ transplantation, and anatomical gifts. Every state has some version of the Uniform Anatomical Gift Act, which controls the disposition of person's body parts.

Medical Staff Participation

Medical staff membership carries certain responsibilities for members, such as attending meetings, participating in committee activities, participating in utilization and review, participating in quality assurance, corrective action against other members of the medical staff when needed, and in other medical staff activities. Hospital counsel will be invaluable in drafting medical staff bylaws, fair hearing plans, and rules and regulations. He will brief physicians on their requirements under the bylaws.

Hospital Liability

Physicians will be reading and hearing a lot about plaintiffs' attorneys attempting to expand the theory of corporate negligence by alleging that individual members of medical staffs, and medical staffs collectively, are responsible for malpractice committed by members of the medical staff in their practices outside of the hospital, as well as in the hospital. The theory of corporate negligence has been expanded over the past several years by plaintiffs' attorneys to include recovery under the theories of apparent or ostensible agency. Hospital counsel will keep physicians briefed on the attempts of plaintiffs' attorneys to expand the liability of medical staff members in their hospitals and in the communities in which they practice.

Hospitals and their medical staffs are facing an increasing widening of the scope of litigation that they are exposed to. An example is class action litigation. Recently, there has been an increase in the number of class action claims filed against physicians and hospitals. Class action litigation is complex and protracted. Physicians and hospitals involved in class action litigation are subject to substantial legal fees, and in the event of a recovery, physicians and hospitals may be without insurance coverage. In addition to being responsible for the payment of their own attorneys, physicians and hospitals, in the event that they lose or settle class action litigation, may be liable for additional legal fees. Class action attorneys argue for and quite often receive substantial attorneys' fees under the concept of a load star multiplier. Hospital counsel, in regular briefings to the medical staff, will address current issues and trends in class action litigation. In the event that members of the medical staff or the hospital are directly involved in class action litigation, hospital counsel will be involved in some cases in defending, selecting defense counsel, and coordinating the defense for the medical staff, individual members of the medical staff, and the hospital.

Ethics Committees

Hospital medical staffs are forming ethics committees to deal with various patient care issues. Ethics committees have traditionally dealt with questions of the right to a natural death and other similar patient care issues, but in today's increasing demands on the health care delivery system, ethics committees will necessarily be called on to consider additional issues involving patient care. Hospital counsel will assist and work with the medical staff in assuring that the ethics committee is properly structured and will address those patient care issues that should come before the ethics committee. If a physician serves on an ethics committee in his hospital, he will have an opportunity to work closely with hospital counsel in the structuring and formulation of agendas for the committee.

Investigation/Experimentation

Medical staffs of hospitals in which patient care investigations and experimentations are conducted are required to develop oversight protocols involving committees. If a physician is a member of such a medical staff, he will have an opportunity to be involved with the structuring and functioning of such committees. Hospital counsel will work closely with the medical staff in the structuring and functioning of these committees.

Conclusion

The above discussion of instances in which a physician will be involved, either directly or indirectly, with hospital counsel is not intended to be exhaustive or definitive. The physician should become aware of legal issues that he and hospital counsel will be concerned with in working together in formulating preventative protocols and taking whatever corrective actions that may be indicated. Hospital counsel can be a valuable professional ally.

HOSPITAL LAW

Non-Profit Hospitals

Hospitals are corporations. Throughout most of the Twentieth Century, the overwhelming majority of hospitals have been incorporated as non-profit institutions, enjoying tax exemptions under Section 501 (c) (3) of the Internal Revenue Code. Incorporation under this section of the IRC also permits individuals, corporations, and other legal entities to donate funds to these non-profit institutions, which these donor agencies may then deduct from their own taxable incomes, with certain restrictions. This recognizes what is still a long-standing and still firmly held belief that hospitals function as charitable institutions.

The Evolution of Hospital and Staff Physician Liability

In the early Twentieth Century, hospitals still enjoyed broad immunity from liability actions, being regarded as charitable institutions. Soon, the long-standing principles of vicarious liability (i.e., hospital liability for the negligent actions of its employees) began to apply with greater frequency.

Agency

Under the theory of agency (vicarious liability and respondeat superior), hospitals would be held liable for the negligent acts of all employees (including employed physicians, such as house staff), both for the employees' negligent acts and negligent acts performed under the supervision of employees (e.g., those of medical, nursing, or other types of health care "externs").

For some period of time, however, hospitals continued to escape from vicarious liability, if they could prove that the actions of one of their employees (e.g., house officers or nurses) were under the independent and complete control of an independently contracting non-employee medical staff physician at the time of the alleged negligence. This represented the "borrowed servant" doctrine, which held that the attending physican as "captain of the ship" should bear complete liablity, thus relieving the hospital. This doctrine was first abolished in a 1976 Pennsylvania Supreme Court case, which has been followed throughout the country. The case held that whenever an employee of a hospital committed a negligent act (whether or not while under the "complete and independent control" of an independent contractor, usually an attending physician), the hospital, as the employee's employer, was vicariously liable.

Ostensible or Apparent Agency

During the past 20 years, there have been a series of cases which have upheld the liability of hospitals for negligents acts performed by non-employee contract physicians in the emergency room, radiology, pathology, cardiology, etc. The theory behind this is one of agency and has been denoted as ostensible or apparent agency. Even though emergency room physicians may not have been employees, an increasing number of courts are holding hospitals vicariously liable for having "held out" physicians with whom they contracted to work in their various departments, particularly the emergency room, as working for or on behalf of the institutions. Furthermore, the courts have opined that patients receiving services in such departments have been denied a free choice of health care providers, and thus, the hospital is liable for the acts of these personnel as if they were employees. This theory has also been applied to attending physicians.

Corporate Liability

Another legal theory of hospital liability has developed, known as corporate liability. This doctrine originated with the landmark decision in a 1965 Illinois case, *Darling v. Charleston Memorial Hospital*. That case and those following it stand for the proposition that hospitals have an independent duty to their patients to ensure the quality of care practiced by their physicians, whether or not they are actual or apparent employees. Hospitals and their governing body members and executive management may be found independently liable for having failed to implement and oversee appropriate and effective medical quality management systems, designed to minimize the risk of negligent acts by both their employees and independent contractors. As to the latter, the hospital has a duty to properly credential and recredential its medical staff physicians, to monitor them on an ongoing basis, and to actively and affirmatively intervene on behalf of the patients when they fall below the standards of care.

Brother's Keeper Doctrine

Finally, there has been some movement by the courts in some jurisdictions to extend the net of liability for inadequate medical quality management to medical staff physicians themselves. The landmark case, which extended this potential liability to all physicians on a medical staff, was the 1975 New Jersey case of *Corleto v. Shore Memorial Hospital*. The theory was that every staff physician had a duty to ensure the quality of every other staff physician.

The theory behind *Corleto* was resurrected in New Jersey recently. In this later case, which involved an injured newborn, the court held that the Chairmen of both the Obstetrics and Pediatrics Departments were liable for not having previously recommended to the medical staff's credentials and executive committees appropriate restrictions of the clinical privileges of the negligent obstetrician and pediatrician.

Implications of Increased Health Provider Liability

As we move into the emerging era of greatly heightened public awareness of the quality of medical care and accountability for it, it is probable that other courts throughout the country will hold that key medical staff physicians (including chief residents) should be held liable for not having adequately "policed their ranks". This liability will probably extend to physicians sitting on key medical staff quality management committees (including the medical executive committee, quality assurance committee, utilization management committee, and the various medical staff ancillary services monitoring committees). To the extent that house officers are members of these committees, they, too, may be found liable for not having adequately monitored the quality of care practiced by staff physicians, as well as by house officers.

The Legal Status of House Officers — Employees or Students?

House officers occupy a unique position in the hospital. On the one hand, they are considered to be employees in that they are "on the payroll" of the hospital, with all the federal, state, local, social security, and unemployment insurance tax deductions which that status involves. They also enjoy the benefits of other employees, such as health and life insurance, disability insurance, and paid vacations. Also, as discussed above, they are regarded as employees for the purpose of holding their employers (i.e., hospitals) vicariously liable for their negligent acts performed in the course of their employment relationships.

On the other hand, house officers function as students (even when in their ninth or tenth post-doctoral years), because they are obtaining necessary training to become fully Board-eligible and certified specialists and sub-specialists capable of practicing their specialties and subspecialties independent of supervision in private practice settings. Although they are not typical students in that they do not pay tuition (and, in fact, draw salaries), they are not typical non-supervisory employees either for the following reasons:

1) They do not punch time clocks;
2) They do not get paid by the hour;
3) They do not get paid overtime for the 40 to 80 hours per week of "overtime" they log weekly; and
4) Most importantly, they have not yet been found to be distinct bargaining units to permit them to engage in collective bargaining and job actions, pursuant to the language of the National Labor Relations Act (although proposed regulations being debated at the time of this writing could change in the future).

Except in the case of house officers whose base teaching hospital is a federal facility or is located in the District of Columbia, the National Labor Relations Board has not yet held house officers to be employees capable of engaging in collective bargaining. The National Labor Relations Board has consistently held that since house officers' "primary purpose" is to obtain the necessary training for Board-eligibility, they are not employees capable of forming bargaining units and engaging in collective bargaining, pursuant to the language of the National Labor Relations Act. The proposed regulations being debated at the time of this writing, however, would permit all employed physicians (possibly including house officers) of hospitals to organize into separate bargaining units recognizable by the National Labor Relations Board. If these regulations are upheld, as currently proposed, there could be a significant increase in unionization among house officers in hospitals throughout the country, again assuming that previous rulings by the Board have not already precluded house officers from being regarded as hospital employees for this, or any other purpose.

Some State Labor Relations Boards, e.g., California, have held house officers to be employees under their laws.

Contractual Issues and Disputes

Despite the National Labor Relations Board's continued characterization of house officers as students, another indication of their status as employees is their contractual relationship with their "home base" teaching hospital. The contract that a house officer signs shortly after "Match Day" is a legally binding agreement, indicating an offer by the hospital to retain the services of the prospective house officer, which is understood and freely accepted by the prospective house officer. In exchange for the prospective house officer's promise to perform the duties assigned to him or her as part of the training program and service agreement with the hospital, the hospital (through its administration) agrees to pay the prospective house officer a specified salary with benefits (including paid professional liability insurance).

The house officer (at least prior to completing medical licensure requirements) may practice medicine only under the supervision and direction of fully licensed physicians. A first year resident will be granted a temporary license to practice medicine, which limits him or her to practicing only on patients in the hospital to which he or she is assigned, as part of his or her responsibilities pursuant to training program requirements. A first year house officer may legally only practice medicine on patients admitted to the hospital at which he or she has a contract, and which have been assigned to him or her as part of covering for a private staff physician's patients or a ward service's patients (where attending staff physicians rotate as "attendings"). He or she may also care for patients who are being covered while on call at particular times, or who are being seen in an assigned hospital out-patient clinic rotation.

Once a house officer has obtained an unlimited license to practice medicine and has obtained the Drug Enforcement Administration's (DEA) certificate to prescribe various controlled substances, he or she may practice medicine independent from his or her teaching program institution(s). If the house officer is still completing a training program, then such medical activities would be "moonlighting". Whether or not this is permitted, under what conditions, by whose permission, in what amount, where, and when should all be outlined in the contract between the house officer and his or her "base hospital".

As stated above, the house officer would have to purchase his own independent professional liability insurance to "moonlight" at a hospital, which is not part of his or her training program. Even if the hospital is part of the house officer's training program where he or she is moonlighting, he or she would have to purchase his or her own separate insurance, since this activity would not be pursuant to his or her training program contract. If involved in a professional liability action at another hospital where he or she is moonlighting, it is even possible that the moonlighting resident's base hospital might have to indemnify the hospital at which the resident was moonlighting for not having trained him or her sufficiently well.

Needless to say, these represent some, if not all, of the reasons why hospitals are increasingly restricting the ability of their house officers to moonlight.

Finally, there is the matter of suspension, release, or nonrenewal of a house officer's contract. There are many conditions which could give rise to this. In general, any breach by the house officer of any material terms of the contract (e.g., violation of a restriction on outside activities) could result in suspension, revocation, or nonrenewal of his or her contract. Other possible breaches might include gross insubordination, habitual tardiness, failure to complete medical records, or any other significant failure to fulfill the duties of house officers in a timely and reasonably effective manner.

House officers generally have yearly contracts. In the event that a house officer's contract is not going to be renewed, he or she should be given sufficient notice of this to permit him or her to obtain another appointment so as to not to interrupt or lengthen his or her training period. If a house officer has his or her contract suspended or revoked in the middle of the year, he or she has certain rights of due process (including routes of appeal), which should be thoroughly laid out in the contract.

House officers are considered to be members of the hospital's medical staff. As such, they must comply with the requirements of the medical staff's by-laws and rules and regulations in caring for the hospital's patients. Nevertheless, they are still not afforded the full "fair hearing" procedures available to other medical staff physicians whose staff appointment or clinical privileges are being curtailed. Still, they do have certain rights, as established in their contracts, including (but not limited to) notice of the reasons for suspension or dismissal, a right and opportunity to rebut these reasons, a right to a hearing and to confront any adverse witnesses, and a right to appeal at least as high a level as the medical director, director of medical education, and/or hospital executive director (i.e., chief executive officer), although probably not to the governing body.

MANAGED CARE AND PROFESSIONAL LIABILITY

Introduction

After a period in which unlimited application of health care resources was the expected standard, economic considerations now influence even routine clinical decisions. In the past, the primary issue in a medical malpractice case was whether the care provided by a physician complied with applicable standards. In the future, physicians may have to explain why they complied with new standards economically imposed and how such compliance affected their clinical judgment. Thus, a dilemma has emerged for physicians. Society has suddenly demanded economic accountability for health costs, yet juries do not look favorably upon a physician's explanation of how the care provided to a patient was influenced by economic realities.

The advent of cost containment of medical services has generated various utilization activities and review requirements such as "prior authorization", "concurrent review", and "second surgical opinions". A patient who is denied financial coverage for medical treatment, which, in retrospect, is determined to have been necessary, will probably seek some form of legal redress for being wrongfully denied necessary medical care, if the patient's resultant outcome is sufficiently compromised.

Discharge and Referrals

The objective of some payment-setting mechanisms is to make reimbursement correspond to all inpatient services associated with a specific diagnostic-related group. Therefore, discharges, transfers, and referrals of patients may pose certain problems for hospitals. The transferring hospital usually incurs a financial burden because inpatient costs tend to be greater early in the admission when the majority of expensive care is delivered. There is a financial incentive to resist discharges and transfers when the reimbursement rate will obviously provide inadequate reimbursement. Thus, to minimize a financial loss, providers may elect to continue to treat the patient in facilities that are less appropriate to treat that patient's particular condition than other available facilities.

A physician who knows, or who should know, that his patient's condition is beyond his knowledge, ability, or capacity to treat with a likelihood of reasonable success, is obligated to advise the patient of the necessity of other or different treatment. In addition, the *AMA Principles of Medical Ethics* requires a physician to seek consultation whenever it appears that the quality of medical services may be enhanced thereby. Thus, physicians who allow their medical judgment to be influenced by non-medical factors are at risk for liability for failure to refer and seek appropriate specialty consultation.

As in the case of the failure to transfer, the patient may suffer adversely if his physician discharges him prematurely simply to qualify for full payment and outlier treatment rather than transfer to another hospital. If, to avoid losing full diagnostic-related group reimbursement, a physician discharges a patient rather than refer the patient to another facility, the physician may be exposed to a charge of abandonment. Abandonment involves the withdrawal of care by a physician without justification when the patient's condition requires continuing attention. The physician's burden to satisfy a jury that the discharge was reasonably justified will be much more difficult if the patient establishes that economic considerations influenced the physician's clinical judgment. These considerations create an inherent conflict between ethical requirements to transfer and financial pressures not to discharge.

A physician's decision to admit, transfer, or discharge a patient may also be significantly affected by prospective payment systems, which attempt to generate "profit" by rendering services below the average rate of reimbursement set for a particular diagnostic-related group. Medical decisions influenced by economical considerations may compromise the malpractice defense of cases where the clinical outcome is poor or unexpected. Physicians who limit services to patients because of non-medical reasons will not be sympathetic defendants in a medical malpractice case.

Misdiagnosis and Miscoding

A physician may be tempted to classify a patient's case under a more lucrative diagnostic or therapeutic grouping to maximize reimbursement. This may expose him to allegations of diagnostic and therapeutic errors. The physician's manipulation of diagnostic classification diminishes his beneficial reliance on the medical record in defense of such allegations. Ordinarily, the medical record is the most important evidence of the reasonableness of the physician's conduct under the particular clinical facts and circumstances of the case. Discrepancies between a physician's testimony and the entries in the medical record will strain his credibility in the eyes of the jury. Even if the physician candidly admits that the medical records were prepared in a manner to support a reimbursable diagnosis, a jury would probably conclude that a physician who is willing to shade the truth in submitting a bill for services for montetary purposes would have a tendency to shade the truth about other matters in a malpractice case for similar reasons.

Failure to Diagnose and Defensive Medicine

Under a traditional cost-based reimbursement system, there was an incentive for physicians to utilize services. In addition, the increase in the frequency and severity of medical malpractice suits subtly encouraged "defensive medicine". Consequently, "over-utilization" of diagnostic services became embodied in clinical practice. Some physicians performed marginally unnecessary diagnostic procedures because of the perception that it would enable them to withstand retrospective scrutiny if they were sued for failing to diagnose the patient's problem. This attitude was reinforced by some courts which proclaimed that if a physician does not use all the diagnostic means available to obtain the best factual data upon which to make a diagnosis, such omissions may be considered evidence of negligence.

The practice of "defensive medicine", however, is at conflict with a prospective payment system which attempts to establish an all-inclusive rate of compensation or reimbursement by a diagnostic-related group in an effort to affect the "intensity of services" provided to a patient. Since medical procedures are not subject to separate reimbursement in a prospective payment system, in order for a physician to meet the diagnostic-related group rate, the number of diagnostic tests and procedures are more closely scrutinized and limited. If at trial, a physician admits that he would have ordered the diagnostic tests he did not order in a particular case, except for the payment system constraints, it is tantamount to admitting that the prior tests were unnecessary and only ordered to protect himself. Alternatively, if a physician concedes that the hospital exerted pressure on him to cut down on the number of tests ordered for a particular condition, it is unlikely that a jury will look favorably upon such compliance that could have a deleterious effect upon an individual patient of the physician. Although a prospective payment system is a powerful incentive to curtail the use of diagnostic procedures, the trend of courts to extend theories of liability and to increase damage awards intensifies the impression that physicians are expected to utilize every diagnostic tool available to diagnose a patient's condition.

HMO's and PPO's

As health care delivery became more expensive, employers who were required to provide health benefits to employees sought alternatives to encourage more efficient and appropriate use of health services by managing or controlling hospital admissions, ancillary services, and therapeutic procedures. Consequently, two alternative health plan mechanisms emerged: the Health Maintenance Organization (HMO) and Preferred Provider Organization (PPO). The HMO is a health plan in which patient care is prepaid, often on a capitation basis. The subscriber incurs no other significant charge for health services other than the prepaid fee as long as the subscriber complies with the provisions of the plan. The PPO is similar to traditional health insurance plans, except that an incentive is given to the plan subscriber to obtain care from a provider under a contract to the participant as a member of the PPO panel of providers. In turn, these providers agree to discount their services to the PPO.

The financial success of an alternative health care plan depends upon controlling health care costs by adherence to norms of care through contracting with and limiting the number of providers who are paid for health services. These norms address hospital admissions, length-of-stay, specialty referral, and utilization of diagnostic and therapeutic resources. Because the financial risk is borne by the HMO, it must enforce the concept that only services which meet the necessary and appropriate tests are covered by the plan.

The professional liability process, however, is concerned with the physician's application of clinical knowledge and skill in a duly diligent and careful manner. It measures physician performance and conduct by referring to the practice of qualified physicians under similar facts and circumstances. Managing a health care plan through effective utilization review requires ongoing determinations of medical necessity and appropriateness, a hybrid balancing of medical and economic factors. Since such determinations do not apply to criteria exclusively concerned with the patient's medical condition, a physician may now have the difficult task of demonstrating how medical necessity and appropriateness is consistent and compatible with the requisite standard of care.

Managed Care Program Activities
Pre-Admission Certification

Pre-admission certification is a process which attempts to enforce predetermined criteria for hospitalization for which the health plan will provide coverage. Participating physicians are expected to assimilate into their own medical admission criteria those standards of medical necessity and appropriateness of hospitalization utilized by the plan to avoid gaining the reputation as a "poor utilizer". The adoption of compromised standards for admission may require a physician to later admit, when questions about the health care he or she provided are raised, that a patient was not hospitalized primarily because of health plan affiliation.

Concurrent Review of Hospital Stay

A managed care program's use of stringent utilization control techniques may encourage the exposure of a physician to liability by declining to approve payment for necessary health services surgery or for continued hospitalization unless proper safeguards are incorporated within the program. Concurrent review is a process which assesses whether a hospital stay continues to be medically necessary and appropriate. If it involves clinical determinations by a third-party plan representative, it can result in prompting a premature discharge and consequential professional liability exposure. The physician's role and responsibility in these matters is beginning to be articulated. A physician is put in a conflict of interest situation. If he disagrees with the UR determination, his hospital may have to absorb the cost of any unapproved hospital days. On the other hand, if the physician complies with the UR determination and prematurely discharges the patient, resulting in harm to the patient, he may be liable for the patient's injury. A physician has the responsibility to appeal the third-party payor's decision to discharge the patient earlier than the physician has planned. The attending physician's failure to appeal will likely put the liability for the subsequent course of the patient's treatment on the physician's shoulders. Thus, physicians will be held liable if, against their medical judgment, they comply *without protest* with utilization limitations imposed by third party payors. The emerging principle is that physicians may be held liable if they fail to appeal or override cost containment-based insurance decisions they believe may be adverse to the patient. Therefore, physicians should be on notice that they have a duty to patients to appeal utilization review decisions when they believe that a utilization management decision will be adverse to a patient's health. The reasonable physician should not remain silent, but make calls, write letters, and convene a meeting of the hospital utilization review committee, using the appropriate scale of assertive tactics, depending on what will be the severity of the effect on the patient of complying with a utilization management decision. In light of recent legal, governmental and societal developments, the modern day physician must assume a more forceful role as an advocate of his or her patients.

Specialty Referral ("Gatekeeping")

Allegations of negligent failure to refer are likely to arise with increasing frequency of physician participation in a health care plan where specialty referral is limited by the requirement that specialty referrals must be coordinated through the utilization review staff. Under such circumstances, the traditional referral practice is encumbered by the imposition of economic considerations; the patient may not be referred to an appropriate specialist because the primary physician is mindful of and attempts to comply with the health care plan's desire to limit referrals.

Physicians should be alerted to an apparent legal trend in which HMO subscribers may attempt to sue their HMO and their contracted physician providers if insufficient care is rendered by the PCP whose financial considerations affect referrals and utilization of health care resources. Such lawsuits will attempt to blame the HMO's gatekeeper arrangement for the failure of its physician providers to deliver necessary and appropriate medical care. To the extent that it can be demonstrated that a specialty referral was refused for primarily economic reasons, a patient-plaintiff's case will be strengthened.

In one such case against an HMO and two of its contracted physicians, a primary care physician "gatekeeper" approach was employed to curb excess utilization. A patient subscriber of an HMO asserted that her primary care physician had a conflict of interest in his role as a "gatekeeper", and his financial incentives to reduce the volume of specialty services used by HMO had a detrimental effect upon her medical outcome. The patient contended that such an arrangement caused the failure of her HMO physician to properly diagnose that she had cervical cancer. As an HMO subscriber, the woman could only obtain specialist services upon referral by her designated primary care physician (PCP), who was entitled to a refund of excess money paid into a special "withhold" account for specialist fees, in the event that contributions to that account were not exhausted at the end of the contract year.

When the patient complained of abnormal vaginal discharge, the PCP treated the patient's "vaginitis", but did not perform a Pap smear. When the vaginal discharge persisted, the PCP referred her to a gynecologist designated as a plan referral care specialist provider (RCP). Since the referral authorized only treatment limited to the vaginal infection, a Pap smear would not be reimbursed by the HMO if it was performed by the RCP. Therefore, it was not performed.

When the patient was subsequently diagnosed by a non-HMO physician as having cervical cancer, she sued the HMO, contending that the "gatekeeper" system, which provided refunds to the PCP from the "withhold" account for restricting referrals, contributed directly to the PCP's failure to make a timely diagnosis of her cervical cancer.

The following significant issues are likely to be raised by similar cases in the future:

1) Will an HMO's capitated "gatekeeper" arrangement be considered a causative factor in a PCP's failure to order certain tests and to make referral in a timely way, when it is established that such failures caused a compensable injury to the patient?

2) Will an HMO's risk-sharing arrangement, in which funds are placed into accounts for specialty, laboratory, and hospitalization costs, be considered an actionable conflict of interest if money remaining in the referral pool at the end of the accounting period is split with the PCP and HMO?

3) Do the capitation and risk-sharing arrangements place a PCP in a conflict of interest situation similar to that created by the illegal practice of fee-splitting, but with the opposite incentive to not refer cases to specialists?

4) Does the contractual relationship between the HMO and its PCP encourage the PCP to ignore the accepted standards of medical practice for personal financial reasons?

5) Must a patient be told about the financial agreement a PCP has with an HMO subscriber so the patient can question the potential impact that such an arrangement may have on his situation?

6) Must a PCP make the patient-subscriber aware that the financial relationship of the physician and the HMO may affect the manner in which health

services will be delivered?

7) Will patients who are not aware of the PCP's capitation arrangement be presumed to think that their medical problem is not serious when they do not receive customary services for such a problem because of the financial incentive and arrangements of a prepaid health plan?

The modern physician should become adept at identifying situations that may give rise to conflicts of interest and resolve them to the patient's benefit in conformity with relevant public policies.

Thus, a physician who has contracted to be a "gatekeeper" in a managed care health plan may be exposed to greater liability for medical malpractice than his non-gatekeeping colleagues because of an apparent "conflict of interest" predicated on the physician's incentive to reduce utilization of specialty services. A patient with an adverse outcome or unsatisfactory result will likely allege that this conflict had a detrimental effect on that outcome. The patient will contend that the gatekeeper arrangement substantially interfered with treatment, thereby "causing" the alleged maltreatment. An alleged conflict of interest argument would be strengthened if the physician was entitled to a refund of excess money paid into a "withhold" account for specialist fees, in the event that health care plan contributions to that account were not exhausted at the end of the contract year. The patient's contention would be that a focal but potentially serious complaint was not given appropriate diagnostic procedures to avoid depleting the "withhold pool". Moreover, the patient may further contend that if, after persistence of symptomatology, he is finally referred by the primary care physician to an appropriate specialist for diagnosis, the specialist may be limited to performing only narrowly focused procedures specifically for the condition referred. Under these circumstances, the seriousness of that condition may have been missed or underestimated; or a certain specialty procedure may not be a service reimbursed by the HMO if not authorized by the primary care physician.

A capitated primary care physician himself may not be eligible to receive reimbursement for the performance of medical services which are considered by the HMO plan to be "specialty services". If a patient is subsequently diagnosed as having a serious preventable problem which was not timely diagnosed, the "gatekeeper" may be sued for restricting a proper referral, thereby contributing to the failure to reach a timely and correct diagnosis.

Physicians contracted to an HMO may be sued by HMO subcribers if substandard care is rendered by the physician, whose financial considerations affect referrals and utilization of health care resources.

Sentinel Legal Case in Managed Health Care
Wickline v. State of California

Five days after undergoing arterial bypass surgery, Ms. Wickline was required to undergo a lumbar sympathectomy for severe peripheral vascular insufficiency. Although she was scheduled to be discharged four days later, her vascular surgeon believed that she needed to remain in the hospital for eight days. Relying on information provided by a utilization review nurse screener, a physician utilization reviewer authorized only four additional days. Although the vascular surgeon knew that he could attempt to obtain a further extension of the patient's hospital stay by telephoning the physician reviewer, he did not do so. Acting within standards of practice based on length-of-stay norms, he discharged Ms. Wickline. Nine days later, Ms. Wickline was rehospitalized because of occlusive thrombosis of her leg. An infection in the graft site had developed, making it difficult for the surgeon to surgically remove the thrombosis because of concern that the surgery would spread the infection systemically. One week later, a below-the-knee amputation was required. Ms. Wickline sued, alleging that the failure to approve the surgeon's requested extension of her hospital stay led to complications that resulted in amputation of her leg. The vascular surgeon testified that had the requested eight day extension been granted, he believed that he would have observed the color changes in her leg, and that would have caused him to reopen the graft to remove the thrombosis and to control the infection with the vigorous use of antibiotics. The physician utilization reviewer testified that had Ms. Wickline's surgeon decided it was necessary to keep her in the hospital for a longer period of time than the reviewer had authorized, he would have expected the surgeon to make such a request. The court declared that the decision to discharge Ms. Wickline was the responsibility of her attending physician. The court pointed out that although the vascular surgeon may have been intimidated by the third-party payor, he was not rendered powerless to act appropriately if other action was required under the circumstances.

The court declared that the third-party payor did not override the medical judgment of the patient's vascular surgeon at the time of her discharge because the surgeon did not protest the utilization physician reviewer's decision. The court also declared that cost containment programs should not be permitted to corrupt the professional judgment of physicians, and that attending physicians should be encouraged to appeal adverse utilization management decisions with which they disagree.

The court pointed out that the physician who complies without protest with the utilization review imposed limitations when his clinical judgement dictates otherwise cannot avoid his ultimate responsibility for his patient's care. He cannot point to the third-party payor as the liability scapegoat when the consequences of his own determinative medical decisions go sour.

Although the main, if not the only, purpose in the world of business and commercialism is gaining a livelihood, in the medical profession such matters are said to be secondary. In medicine, the tenet that financial interests should not interfere with a physician's medical judgments on behalf of his patient is exemplified in Maimonides' Prayer: "Do not allow thirst for profit, ambition for renown and admiration to interfere with my profession, for these are the enemies of truth and can lead me astray in the great task of attending to the welfare of Your creatures."

Certain changes that are occurring in our increasingly enterpreneurial health system could undermine patients' trust in their physicians and society's trust in the medical profession. The progression of professional entrepreneurialism constitutes a compelling impetus for each physician to examine any financial arrangement that may interfere, or appear to interfere, with the exercise of his best medical judgment on behalf of the patient. The Institute of Medicine has noted:

All compensation systems - from fee-for-service to capitation or salary - present some undesirable incentives for providing too many services, or too few. No system will work without some degree of integrity, decency, and ethical commitment on the part of professionals. Inevitably, we must presume some underlying professionalism that will constrain the operation of unadulterated self-interest. The question is not to find a set of incentives that is beyond criticism, but to seek arrangements that encourage the physician to function as a professional, in the highest sense of that term.

Conclusion

Measures taken to control health costs may unavoidably affect the quantity and quality of care that a physician may provide a patient. The encumbering of a physician's clinical decisions with economic considerations expands the liability exposure for the practicing physician. Allegations of professional negligence against physicians will be magnified by questioning whether their professional judgment was unduly influenced by economic considerations.

ORGAN PROCUREMENT AND DONATION

Introduction

The traditional organ procurement policy in the U.S. has been one of "voluntarism", in which organs and tissues will not be used for transplantation unless the decedent or his or her next-of-kin volunteers or consents to the donation. The supply for organs and tissues, however, has fallen well short of demand. The chief impediment to organ procurement in the past has been the failure of the health care team to appropriately ask families for consent to organ and tissue donation.

Statutory Procurement Laws

State law in 44 states, the Joint Commission on Healthcare Organizations (JCAHO), and the Federal Medicare/Medicaid funding requirements now demand that families be approached for consent for organ and tissue donation. No longer can one presume that the family would not tolerate intrusion by such questions in their time of mourning, or that the family would say "no", or that the particular organs or tissue would not be used, or that it would be against the family's religious beliefs; nor can the physician fail to make a request because he himself or she herself might believe organ donation objectionable, or find it emotionally difficult to approach the family. Furthermore, federal law and many state laws call for sensitivity in the approach. It is unprofessional, ineffective, and certainly insensitive to simply declare: "I hate to bother you with this, but the law requires me to ask if you wish to donate any organs or tissues!"

The Procurer

In some states, the request is to be made primarily by the physician, while in others the request is intended to be made by a designated member of the hospital, or by representatives of the regional organ procurement agency. Appropriate training of the requestor is sometimes required.

Types of Requests

State statutes are divided into "required request" and "routine inquiry" types. The required request legislation requires consent to be requested of appropriate family members in appropriate cases; and the routine inquiry legislation, essentially a weak form of required request, is merely an insistence on a policy of routinely approaching family members to inform them of the option to donate, typically by requiring a hospital protocol to this effect. In 18 states, the request is specifically required, while 26 states and federal funding legislation have adopted the latter approach. Only one state, Kentucky, has an explicit penalty for failure to comply.

There are numerous exceptions to the requirement of request among the state statutes, such as exclusions based on medical criteria, known objections, or religious considerations. In Alabama, the attending physician in his or her sole judgment can determine that an inquiry shall not be made. In Massachusetts, exception is allowed if discussion would cause the family undue emotional distress. Lobbying efforts have exempted whole hospitals in several states.

Uniform Anatomical Gift Act (UAGA)

In the late 1960's and early 1970's, all 50 states adopted the Uniform Anatomical Gift Act (UAGA), many with minor variations, which authorizes persons or their families to make an "anatomical gift" of all or part of his or her body to take effect at death. This law continues to be the mainstay of organ procurement in the United States, specifically defining the legal mechanics of organ and tissue donations.

Any person 18 years or older and "of sound mind" may execute an "anatomic gift". An anatomic part which may be given includes: "organs, tissues, eyes, bone, arteries, blood, other fluids and other portions of the human body".

The decedent's own wishes, if known, are paramount and to be carried out. However, as a practical matter, if the family objects to removal over the express desire of the decedent to have organs and tissues harvested, it may be prudent to decline to accept the decedent's donation to avoid a public relations fiasco and possible clarifying litigation.

If a deceased has not indicated his or her intentions, then the UAGA spells out who, as next-of-kin, is to be approached for donation, specifically: the spouse; and if he or she is not available at the time of death, then an adult son or daughter; if they are not available, then a guardian of the person of the decedent at the time of his or her death. The statute is silent with regard to the status of divorced or separated spouses, stepparents, stepchildren, other dependents, etc. Consent by one next-of-kin (i.e., one brother) is legally negated by the objection of another of the same class of next-of-kin (i.e., another brother), although inquiry of all of a class is not required to exclude the possibility that someone might object. If no next-of-kin is available, then any other person authorized or under obligation to dispose of the body (for example, medical examiners or anatomical boards) may donate the body or body parts. Of crucial importance, the UAGA gives little guidance as to the time and diligence necessary in attempting to contact individuals before considering them as "unavailable", although the time limits for the harvest of the particular organs and tissues contemplated would clearly be relevant. The consent by other than the decedent must be timely, after or immediately before death. The specified individuals for purposes of consent for organ and tissue donation are probably, but not necessarily, the same as for general autopsy consent.

Any specified person, physician, hospital, accredited medical school or university, tissue bank, or procurement agency may accept an anatomic gift for education, research, therapy, or transplantation. The attending physician is the presumed donee, absent other indications. A donee may accept or reject the gift. The donee of the entire body may authorize embalming and funeral services. The donee of a part must remove the part without unnecessary mutilation, and then relinquish custody to the next-of-kin or other person under obligation to dispose of the body.

The gift may be executed by a will or other document. Such provisions in typical estate wills are discouraged because they are usually not immediately available at the time of death. The use of "living wills" is preferred because they are immediately available as a part of the medical record. Two witnesses are necessary to validate a gift during the donor's lifetime, but are not required in the case of a gift by a next-of-kin. The next-of-kin may make gifts by a signed document or by telegraphic or recorded message. Neither delivery nor public filing is necessary to effectuate the gift. The gift may be revoked or amended by a signed statement, an oral statement in the presence of two witnesses, or a statement to an attending physician.

The UAGA was amended in many states during the mid-70's to allow organ donation by the mere signing of the back of a driver's license. As a general rule, organ procurement agencies and transplant surgeons will not accept such a signature by itself, but rather will require the contemporaneous consent of the next-of-kin. They argue that the decedent may have changed his mind since the signing, and that they could not afford the negative publicity which might occur in the absence of affording the family an opportunity to object.

The physician who removes an organ in good faith is protected from civil and criminal liability by the UAGA. This act, on its face, appears to take effect only after death has been declared. Failure to comply with the provisions of the act may evidence bad faith. However, it is to be construed liberally to achieve its stated goal of promoting organ and tissue donations. Further immunity is provided by legislation in most states, which specifically holds blood transfusions and transplantations to be regarded as services rather than the sale of a product, and therefore, exempt from strict product liability.

To avoid conflicts of interest, the UAGA prohibits the physician who makes the determination of death from participating in the procedures for removing or transplanting a part, although he or she may communicate with the transplant team.

The UAGA does not apply to bodies within the purview of the medical examiner. Most vital organs are retrieved from brain dead individuals, usually from the neurosurgery service, in which case the body is likely to fall under the medical examiner's or coroner's jurisdiction as a case of suspicious, violent, or other non-natural death (e.g., death by motor vehicle accident). If so, consent and authorization for organ procurement must come from the medical examiner or coroner instead of the next-of-kin. The medical examiner is likely to refuse only in a few select cases where such might interfere with the performance of his or her post-mortem examination, particularly toxicology analysis. By local custom and as a public relations measure, many medical examiners additionally require the consent of the next-of-kin. Many states have explicit provisions for organ retrieval by medical examiners or coroners.

The UAGA also does not apply to organ procurement from living related donors. In such cases, consent is again the central issue, but the consent in this instance will be more closely scrutinized. The consent must be made voluntarily and after the party has been fully informed of the potential risks. In the typical case, an HLA-matched family member is asked to give one of his kidneys, or perhaps a sampling of his bone marrow. There is no legal duty to be a Good Samaritan and comply with the request. In fact, family and community pressures may significantly cloud the issue of voluntariness. In the case of minors and incompetents (e.g., mentally retarded sibling), a court order will usually be necessary for the organ harvest. Although parents may generally consent to the medical treatment of their children, they probably lack the same authority when the surgery will not directly benefit the child. The consent of the parents may additionally be sought, but it is not per se necessary, and the court may overcome their refusal. In most cases involving intrafamilial transplants, judicial approval has been granted, often in chambers as a simple judicial approval of parental consent. However, case law on this point has not been uniform, and although most decisions have upheld the donation based on best interests, parens patriae, psychological benefit, or by substituted judgment, some courts have found no objective reason for the donor to submit to the risk and bodily intrusion of an organ harvest, or that the court has no authority to so order in the absence of enabling legislation.

Brain Death Statutes

In the late 1970's, nearly all states enacted brain death statutes allowing pronouncement of death based on brain death criteria, without the necessity to await cessation of respirations and pulse. These statutes were generally patterned after the Uniform Determination of Death Act, in which the determination is simply made "in accordance with accepted medical practice". Despite significant concern and reservation on the part of physicians, these statutes were probably unnecessary as no court had ruled against a surgeon based on a premature organ removal.

National Organ and Transplant Act

The Federal Government, in 1985, enacted the National Organ and Transplant Act (PL 98-507). This act creates a national Organ Procurement and Transplant Network (OPTN) to match donor organs to prospective recipients. The national OPTN was contracted to the United Network for Organ Sharing (UNOS), a previously existing private network. Regional organ procurement agencies have now been designated in order to fully implement the federal system.

The act also prohibits the sale for valuable consideration of human organs for use in human transplantation. This federal prohibition is limited to transfers affecting interstate commerce. The term "human organ" is defined as the human kidney, liver, heart, lung, pancreas, bone marrow, cornea, eye, bone, skin, and any other organ included by the Secretary of the HHS for regulation. It is not intended to include replenishable tissues such as blood or sperm. The term "valuable consideration" does not include the reasonable payment associated with removal, transplantation, implantation, processing, preservation, quality control, and storage, or the expenses of travel, housing, or lost wages in connection with the donation of the organ. Several states have enacted similar legislation.

Legislation was enacted in 1986 (COBRA), which required that hospitals become members of the national OPTN and abide by the UNOS by-laws in order to quality for Medicaid and Medicare funding. These membership requirements essentially have the force and effect of governmental regulations. Therefore, many of the detailed aspects of transplantation, including recipient selection, will be dictated by UNOS.

Potential Liabilities

When drafting policies and procedures for organ donation, it is important to consider the hospital's legal responsibilities and potential legal liability in the procurement process. Once a potential donor is identified, the attending physician and the donor hospital bear the potential liabilities associated with determining death and obtaining consent for donation. Most states, however, have adopted the provisions of the UAGA, which eliminated such liability for actions taken in good faith and in accordance with the terms of the act.

Most states have specific statutes which maintain that strict liability does not apply to blood transfusions and organ and tissue transplants. However, liability for negligence might arise from failure to test a donor's serum for antibody, or otherwise to adequately screen for HIV risk factors. Arguably, serum from a prospective brain dead donor should be tested to ensure adequate time for completion and reporting of the test.

HIV Testing

The Public Health Service has previously recommended that all donors of tissue and organ allografts be evaluated for risks associated with HIV infection and tested for HIV antibody. All living bone donors should be retested at least 90 days after tissue is obtained, and only bone from living donors negative for HIV on this repeat testing should be used for transplantation. Bone from donors not available for retesting should be used only when bone from retested living donors is not available or appropriate.

The PHS has also recommended that donors of all organs and tissue allografts be assessed for risks of HIV infection, including reviewing the donor's medical record, testing the donor for HIV antibody, and interviewing living donors. The form on which the results of this assessment appear should be kept in the tissue bank with the donor's other records.

Sperm Banks

Physicians and sperm banks engaged in artificial insemination prefer not to work with fresh sperm. Since the AIDS test became available, it has become the practice of sperm banks to freeze the specimen and quarantine all donations. This protocol has uncovered people who test positive for AIDS, and who might have slipped by if such a protocol had not been followed. The question of efficacy for frozen sperm should not be a concern since frozen sperm is just as effective as fresh. The determining factor is the freezing method itself. Any physician whose patient is infected by contaminated sperm faces a tough time in court.

All sperm banks have stopped using anonymous donors, although the test for AIDS is supposed to be quite good. One clinician has come up with two solutions for avoiding problems. First, the source of the donor embryo should be limited to a woman who produced it by sexual intercourse with her regular sexual partner. In essence, the couple donates to a bank an embryo which later gets "adopted". This means that the donor is not inseminated with semen from a man she would not normally have intercourse with, so her risk of exposure to AIDS is lessened. The drawback is that the adoptive couple get a baby with no genetic link to them. The laboratory will still do AIDS testing, but it will not carry the nearly impossible burden of having to protect the woman from someone she does not know. The second method would be to use a relative or close friend as the egg donor. In such a case, the burden of responsibility for determining the donor's health status belongs to the woman and the man.

Bone Transplants

The Center for Disease Control has reported a case of HIV infection transmitted through bone transplantation.

Donor Transmission of AIDS

Several cases of the human immunodeficiency virus (HIV) have been reported in the medical literature following transplantation of various organs and tissues, including corneas. Although it is now a generally accepted practice to test for HIV antibody in donor serum, some cases of transmission have occurred, despite a negative HIV antibody test.

PHYSICIAN — ATTORNEY RELATIONSHIPS

Introduction

A physician can anticipate that he will occasionally be confronted by attorneys. Whether he likes it or not, their cards and letters will appear on his desk. Much of the contact will be due to the fact that the physician treats patients, and those patients have medicolegal problems. A patient may have been involved in an accident; he may have problems with insurance coverage; or there may be other reasons that will confound even the most experienced, legally astute physician.

The most important concept to remember is that an attorney, whether he represents a patient, an insurance carrier, or even, though unlikely, the physician himself, may have interests and motives that are in conflict with the physician's best interests. A physician should always consider what the attorney's motives may be, determine what is in the physician's best interests, and make decisions from that point of view.

General Principles

The nature of any relationship of a physician with an attorney will be dependent on a number of factors.

• Is the attorney investigating the physician's work for the purpose of a critical evaluation?

• Is the attorney requesting the physician's personal assistance for the purpose of critically evaluating the work of a colleague who treated the same patient, or another physician's care of a patient?

• Is the attorney requesting the physician's personal assistance for the purpose of representing a patient in litigation arising out of an accident unassociated with the practice of medicine?

An attorney dealing with a physician expects that there will be compensation required for the physician's time and effort. However, there are numerous instances when an attorney might have an arrangement with the client to pay the bills, and he or she may be unable to do so. Consideration must be given by the physician in requesting his fee in advance, if a substantial effort is to be expended, or if time is to be set aside for an appearance in court. The fee should reflect the time, effort, and expertise expended on behalf of the particular patient.

While many physicians deal with attorneys on a regular basis, some are far more effective than others. The degree of effectiveness is directly related to the physician's testimony in his area of specialization, and to the manner in which that testimony is presented.

Relationship With Plaintiff's Attorney

An attorney may become involved when there has been an adverse result during the treatment of a patient. This does not necessarily mean that there has been a diagnostic or therapeutic error. It is the duty of the patient's (plaintiff's) attorney to discover if there has been a diagnostic or therapeutic error, and attempt to have the treating physician commit himself to an admission or acknowledgement of that mistake.

If there is any question as to the quality of care rendered, the treating physician is better off not discussing that issue with the attorney. He should advise his insurance carrier of the contact. The physician should not, under any circumstances, rewrite his office records or any portion of the hospital records. Too often, there is a tendency to "improve" or revise what has already been said. Such actions do not come off well before a jury, and an otherwise defensible position may well become indefensible.

If a physician's treatment results in litigation, the plaintiff's attorney will want to take the treating physician's deposition, and may well call him as a witness at the time of trial.

If the treating physician is not the practitioner who caused the alleged diagnostic or therapeutic error, and is approached by the attorney for the patient, consideration must be given to what the effect will be of a verbal statement or written report rendered by this treating physician.

If the care and treatment rendered was incompetent or negligent, a private discussion with the plaintiff's attorney may be appropriate; however, a public discussion could have a deleterious effect to the testifying physician who continues functioning within the institution, because of the hostility among the members of the medical staff who may consider him a "traitor".

Any reports should be limited to the care and treatment rendered by the treating physician, the reasons for the treatment, and the patient's ultimate prognosis.

If a physician is approached to be an expert witness in a medical malpractice suit, or as a treating physician and expert in other litigation (automobile, construction, etc.), he should consider the following.

As a treating physician, he will be relying on his treatment records, as well as those of the hospital. As an expert, the physician will also be relying on the records supplied by the attorney. In either situation, prior to preparing the report requested, the physician should make sure that he has in his possession all the records that he feels are necessary to prepare the report.

The physician should have a discussion with the plaintiff's attorney to determine what should be included in the report. He should also discuss his fees for the time spent in the preparation of the report, as well as for future services such as a deposition and appearance in court at the time of trial.

The report should relate all the facts that have been garnered. The physician should make sure that there is accurate dictation and typing. Attorneys will often pick on small and relatively insignificant errors to suggest sloppiness in the preparation of a report.

The report is generally prepared in the same manner and fashion as any medical summary of a chart. There are some exceptions. The plaintiff's attorney will usually request that the prognosis be included, as well as the life expectancy of the patient. If the report relates to a malpractice event, the attorney will request a clear statement as to the deviations from the accepted standards of practice, a delineation of those deviations, and a statement that the deviations resulted in specific injuries suffered by the patient, based on "reasonable medical certainty or probability". In a simple accident case, there should be a statement that the accident caused the specific injuries suffered by the patient, and a delineation of those injuries, based on reasonable medical certainty.

Any report that is prepared will be used by counsel for both sides. It will be used by the plaintiff's attorney in an attempt to substantiate the case, and by defense counsel to discredit or challenge the same case. The testifying physician's role is that of an expert reporting the facts and interpreting the results without any concern for the interests of either counsel. He should not be an aggressive advocate. That is the attorney's job. Maintaining such a posture in the written report makes giving a deposition or appearing in court at the time of trial relatively easy.

Preparation is the key for giving a deposition or testimony at trial. An attorney who is prepared will know the following:

- What questions he intends to ask.
- How he will want the materials presented to the jury.
- The order of presentation.
- The graphs, exhibits, or documents that he intends to use.
- The manner in which the important questions will be presented and phrased.
- The areas of potential cross-examination. These will undoubtedly include questions on fees, hourly rates, and the time expended in the preparation of the report for deposition and for trial. Questions will invariably include prior experience with the plaintiff's attorney, and prior cases in which testimony was given; they will probe for the weakest areas of the case. The physician should not get into an argument with the opposing counsel. Questions should be answered directly and completely. The physician is not necessarily limited to "Yes" or "No" answers, and can explain any particular answer if necessary or appropriate.

Preparation is necessary at every step of the legal process. The plaintiff's attorney will obviously rely on the physician's medical expertise. The physician, in turn, has the right to expect that he will receive the attorney's full cooperation and assistance at every stage in the preparation of the case, and a prompt response to properly submitted bills.

Relationship With Defense Attorney

As with the plaintiff's attorney, a physician's relationship with the defense attorney will be on a number of levels.

- The defense attorney may be investigating a malpractice claim in which the physician had been one of the treating physicians, but is not involved in the litigation.
- The physician may be a defendant in a malpractice action, and the attorney has been assigned to the defense by the malpractice insurance carrier.
- The attorney is requesting the physician's assistance in reviewing a malpractice action and potentially acting as an expert witness for the defense.
- The attorney may be investigating an accident claim that he is defending, in which the physician acted in the capacity of a treating physician, and he wishes detailed information about the patient.

The attorney in all of the above cases has been retained by an insurance company. That company provides the attorney's office with hundreds of claims a year and, therefore, accounts for a substantial portion of the attorney's income. His legal responsibility is to represent his client, namely, the insurance carrier, and the physician to the best of his legal ability. With some attorneys, there may be a question as to whether the insurance company which is paying the bills is the one to whom loyalty is owed, or the physician whom he has been assigned to defend. Ideally, the loyalty should be to the person whose defense the attorney has been engaged to prepare, even if there is a conflict with the insurance company that pays for the defense. Unfortunately, this is not always the case.

A claim has been made on behalf of a plaintiff by an attorney. The defense attorney undertakes an investigation on behalf of the physician who has been sued. The defense attorney's obligation is to determine whether or not the claim is valid, as well as the nature and extent of the injuries. A further obligation is to make sure that the defendant-physician is protected, while the insurance company desires to pay the least amount of money possible in the defense and settlement of the claim.

Any current treating physician invariably will be contacted by the defense attorney, and most certainly, by the plaintiff's attorney. Each attorney will be interested in knowing the nature and extent of the injuries, and how the treating physician will be able to help him maximize or minimize the injuries. Conversations will be directed to an exploration as to the nature and extent of the claim, and whether or not there is any degree of "bloating" in the claim.

There are considerations that are important to the treating physician.

Any time an attorney asks for information about a patient, there should be a release from the patient authorizing the discussion. While releases will usually appear in routine accident cases, that is not always the case when medical malpractice litigation is involved.

In any event, any attorney can be charged for the time spent for the work involved. If the physician decides that he does not want to charge, that is his prerogative and not an obligation to the defendant-physician.

Attorneys representing defendants in medical malpractice actions, as well as claims adjusters, may abuse their position. Such an individual may have represented the treating physician in the past, or may be representing the same insurance carrier that insures the treating physician, and thereby assumes that he has certain extra rights and privileges. He does not. That individual must have authorization from the patient in order to speak to the treating physician and get a copy of his records. Once an appropriate authorization is obtained, the treating physician can then present him with all the information he requests within the limits denoted in the authorization.

An attorney representing a malpractice defendant may not always be on that individual's side. If the treating physician is a subsequent treating physician, a portion of the injury suffered may have occurred during the time that he was treating the patient. The motives of this attorney may not always be obvious. He may be considering adding the treating physician as a defendant and obtaining a "partner" for his client, the insurance company, so that the total risk will be spread out over a greater number of individuals.

When a physician becomes a defendant in a medical malpractice action, an attorney will be assigned to the defense. Under the terms of the insurance agreement, the physician must cooperate with the attorney or a representative of the insurance company, i.e., an adjuster or investigator. Cooperation means making the physician's records available for duplication, and being available for conferences in the course of preparation of the defense. Usually, the lawsuit will be for a sum that is within the limits of the insurance policy, so that there will be no fear of the physician being held personally liable for any of the damages.

There are times, however, when the verdict is in excess of the policy limits. Under those circumstances, the physician may be advised by the defense attorney and may receive a letter from the insurance carrier advising him of this potential. When this occurs, the attorney or carrier may suggest that the physician has the right, at his own expense, to secure additional counsel. Under such circumstances, the physician should consider this a mandate and obtain a personal attorney. This attorney should be experienced in handling medical malpractice (and/or negligence) cases. The defendant-physician is best advised to obtain the assistance of a plaintiff's attorney. This attorney will have no ties or obligations to any insurance companies and will be free to represent the defendant-physician's interests to the utmost. The attorney will be knowledgeable about the progress of such cases, how settlement negotiations should be handled, and when pressure for settlement should be made. The physician should not employ an attorney without negligence experience, or one who has formed the physician's professional corporation, written his will, or managed the closing on his home, unless that attorney is experienced in the area of tort liability and medical malpractice.

In addition, the defendant-physician should consult with his personal attorney as to whether he should advise the insurance carrier to make a good faith effort to settle the case for an amount up to the limits of his coverage. If the carrier does not make this effort to settle, the physician can hold the company liable for any damages assessed over the limits of his coverage.

Summary

In dealing with an attorney who requests a physician's assistance in medical negligence litigation by testifying for the defense, the physician is always on the side of the "angels". Physicians appreciate other physicians' assistance. Insurance companies and their attorneys are well aware of this fact. They may request that the physician not charge because he is helping a colleague. As a reward, the physician may be offered a reduction of his insurance premium. Any decision that the physician makes should be reached after taking into account the total amount of effort that will be requested or required, the amount of time taken from his practice, and whether or not the physician's actions will in reality be appreciated by either the attorney or insurance company. It is most likely that physicians who do not charge may be called upon frequently, but will receive no special effort or consideration when they are themselves involved as a defendant in a lawsuit.

PLAINTIFFS' ATTORNEYS

Introduction

This chapter is designed to touch upon those aspects of a house officer's life that interface with plaintiffs' attorneys. It is anticipated that after a medical school education, every resident has formulated certain opinions about medicine and the law as it relates to the medical malpractice arena. This particular chapter is not an attempt to make all of the physicians that read it plaintiff-oriented, nor is it intended to give categorical rules that should be followed in every instance. Some of these suggestions are universal. Others must be adapted and applied to the circumstances of a particular case.

Many of these suggestions may seem obvious and simplistic. Nevertheless, these basic concepts must be borne in mind and adhered to carefully, in order to avoid unnecessary legal problems.

Certainly, many of these suggestions will not result in making or breaking a case. Oftentimes, they are the "spice" that peaks the jury's interest and turns the tide against a health care professsional from a layman's point of view. Many times, the collateral circumstances surrounding the actual facts of a medical-legal case can take on special importance that may influence the ultimate disposition of that case.

Communication with the Patient

The single biggest impediment between a physician and a patient relates to a lack of proper and effective communication. Today's health care consumers believe that they have an absolute right to be fully informed and participate in decisions affecting their bodies. This is an outgrowth both of increased health consumerism, and the public's perception of a privacy right that 100 years ago may not have existed.

In the past, physicians were looked upon with a certain amount of awe, and decisions concerning a person's body and health were often left entirely to the physician's discretion. This is simply not the case today. Many patients who end up in an attorney's office do not come looking for money alone. Oftentimes, they are looking for answers to questions that they have been unable to receive from the medical profession. As medical costs and reimbursement problems pressure health care providers to speed up health care, communications with patients suffer. Many times, a patient does not even know who his or her physician is; or he or she may not know what role the physician is fulfilling. It is important to take the time to speak and communicate with the patient.

It is infrequent that a physician who has the ability to communicate with a patient is sued in a frivolous case. In addition to taking the time to speak with a patient, the physician must be careful to avoid use of medical terms that do not provide any meaningful information to the patient. The house officer should keep explanations as simple and understandable to a lay person as possible. Overly complex discussions will increase the patient's sense of frustration with the physician. Physicians often labor under the perception by the patient that they are elitist, and the use of hyper-technical terms only reinforces this belief with the lay public. If you do not speak the language of your patient, you risk placing a barrier between yourself and the patient that may come back to haunt you at a later time.

One of the circumstances wherein a health care provider can alienate a patient is when there has been a turn for the worse, or when a patient has died. This is not the time to have the chaplain or a nurse explain what happened. The physician must, as the responsible party for the patient, speak to the family and explain to them what has happened.

Medicine cannot be perceived by the patient as more of a business than a service. Otherwise, distrust will be bred, and the patient will go to other professionals to seek out answers. A health care provider should *never* deceive patients or lie to them. If mistakes have been made, the physician should not attempt to misrepresent the facts to the patient or his or her family. Such conduct could create an indefensible malpractice case; and if the matter is investigated, it may affect the physician's malpractice insurance coverage and may extend the statute of limitations in many jurisdictions. If a patient is overdosed on a medication and the health care provider is aware of this, the last thing that should be done is explain to the family that "the patient's heart just gave out", without fully informing them of the cause.

Communication with the Health Care Team

When a patient believes that the right hand does not know what the left hand is doing in the health care context, mistrust and lack of confidence is soon to follow. Physicians and the rest of the health care team must keep the lines of communication open. Many cases of malpractice occur as a result of a physician and other health care providers simply not communicating with each other.

In many locations, nurses and residents are completely overworked, and a lack of communication is often a by-product. If a nurse believes that a physician is not taking her role in the health care process seriously, or that a physician has an elitist attitude, the nurse's alienation could trigger a malpractice lawsuit. If a nurse has been alienated and makes adverse comments concerning a physician to a family, this can often result in investigations regarding the health care. Sloppiness in verbal orders between a nurse and resident who are not communicating properly can often be lethal. Time must be taken to foster a feeling by each member of the health care team that their input and work are valued by all other members of the team. The last thing a physician wants, especially a house officer, is to have a reputation among nurses that he is "unapproachable".

Oftentimes, a physician will become exasperated or unhappy when late night calls are made by members of the health care team that they believe are unnecessary. These should not be seen as attempts by the allied health care provider to bother the physician, but should be viewed as opportunities for education for that health care provider. If a call is unnecessary, the physician should communicate and explain to that person why such a call is not necessary in a given circumstance. The house officer should use tact in dealing with nurses and other paramedical personnel so that they will feel completely comfortable in calling the physician late at night. During one's career, nurses will invariably get a physician out of much more trouble than they will ever get him in. When a nurse doesn't call a physician in a difficult case, the trouble starts and a medical-legal claim may develop.

The Record is Your Friend

The medical record is absolutely your friend, not your enemy, in the vast majority of cases. Some physicians and health care providers are under the mistaken assumption that if something is not in the record that its absence will protect them. Nothing could be further from the truth. A complete, legible, and timely record will answer many more questions and help the defense of a medical claim much more often than it will help the plaintiff.

There are many ways that a physician can determine the extent of what must be put in the medical record. Everything cannot be put in every record. The medical school training a physician has received will in large part provide him with the knowledge of what needs to be included. Another source of information that should be consulted by the physician to determine the extent of medical entries would be the hospital's rules and regulations, as well as any resident's manual that is available in that particular facility. Physicians should read, follow, and know the rules, regulations, and guidelines for proper record keeping at each hospital they practice in. You can be assured that the plaintiff's counsel in a medical negligence lawsuit will have obtained that information at the time of the physician's deposition.

The record is the primary method of continuing communication between members of the health care team. The primary mission of the record is to protect the health and safety of the patient, and provide health care providers with sufficient information to continue proper care for a particular patient. Timely and complete entries are needed. Significant observations of a positive or negative nature need to be placed in the chart to provide information both for the health care team and other subsequent reviewers as to why particular decisions were made.

There is one golden rule that relates to medical record keeping. *Never, never* alter a medical record. If there is information that you believe is necessary and should be added to a chart, it should be done in a method that is provided for by the hospital's rules and regulations. Normally, this is made in the form of a late entry and marked as such with a single line being placed through an erroneous entry. If a record is obliterated or altered, this information will be found out sooner or later. There are experts in the area of document examination that have been used by the FBI for years. These individuals can review medical records to determine whether late entries have been made or changes have been made.

If it is proven that a medical record has been altered, no matter how defensible the case is, you have major problems. Credibility is everything with a jury. If a medical record has been altered, your credibility with the jury is zero. This could also affect your insurance coverage. In cases in which it can be proven that physicians altered, deleted, or destroyed medical records, the value of the cases are immediately increased.

Another important part of medical record keeping is writing legibly. Even if medical records are timely kept and complete entries are made, they are useless if they are unreadable. There are cases in which even the attending physician could not decipher his own handwriting. Medical records as the primary means of communication by the health care team become completely useless if the physicians, nurses, and other members of the team cannot read the entries.

Student for Life

In undertaking the profession of medicine, a physician has now become a student for life. Regardless of the number of years of medical school, residency, and fellowship, a physician will be a student for as long as he practices medicine. It is essential for physicians to stay current in their areas of expertise. Many lawsuits center around a particular physician's inability or unwillingness to maintain current expertise in the area of medicine he is involved in. Oftentimes, cases will revolve around a physician's failure to stay current regarding new medications and their application to various disease processes. Drug interactions and knowledge of pharmacology are a continually evolving area of medicine that will require intense study the rest of the physician's medical career. Although this may seem an obvious issue, many malpractice cases have been based upon a physician's lack of current knowledge as it relates to the use of medications.

In addition to being a student of medicine, a physican should have some basic knowledge relating to the legal system. Becoming informed on legal and insurance issues provides a physician with added knowledge that will only enure to his benefit.

Some medical schools provide a basic class concerning the legal system. Usually, this is insufficient. Seek out friends who are lawyers. Ask questions about why things happen and how a physician's actions relate to the legal system in general. Once a physician is practicing, he rarely has time to see his family, much less find the time to attend a trial. However, if a physician has the time during residency to watch a medicolegal trial, this can be an invaluable source of knowledge as to how the system works.

If a physician takes the time to learn about the legal system and how lawyers work, he is in a position to be more active in his defense should he become involved with a medical-legal claim. He also will better understand how the law impacts upon his practice through DRGs and other types of statutory control. Working actively with defense counsel is invaluable if a physician finds himself involved in a lawsuit. Although physicians should become involved in their medical-legal claims, they should have sufficient confidence to listen to the advice of their attorneys. Often, the attorney for a physician has an ability to look at a case more objectively to determine whether or not it should be resolved. A physician does not have the luxury of that objectivity if he is actively involved in the lawsuit.

Knowledge of the legal system and how lawyers work will also provide physicians with insight when they become involved in the legal system through no fault of their own. Sometimes, physicians will not become defendants in a lawsuit, but will have their depositions taken, or be served with requests for information as fact witnesses. Fighting with lawyers and being obstinate will not serve physicians or the legal system well. The so-called "conspiracy of silence" has resulted in the public and attorneys having an adverse opinion of physicians. If a physican is requested by a lawyer to provide information, records, or a deposition, then he should attempt to work with that attorney, consistent with both of their busy schedules. Lawyers armed with subpoenas are not the way a physician wants to respond to a request for a deposition.

Informed Consent

Informed consent should be obtained from patients as much for the communication factor as for legal considerations. Usually, a physician very rarely becomes involved in a bona fide medical-legal claim based solely on issues of informed consent, although it is often an ancillary element in many cases.

When properly done, informed consent can avoid the misunderstandings a patient may have when unfortunate bad results happen, despite good medical care.

This type of information must be communicated to the patient early on, so there is no belief by the patient that the physician is trying to "cover up" a bad result by late excuses. If the patient is aware that adverse results can occur, despite the best of medical care, he or she is much less likely to be surprised should a negative result occur.

Each state has different rules regarding informed consent. Physicians should make it a practice to find out from their hospital risk manager or insurance company what constitutes the proper elements of informed consent in a particular state. This can avoid problems that might otherwise occur later on.

Conspiracy of Silence

Some patients and attorneys believe that there is a conspiracy of silence among health care providers. Attempts are made to cover, protect, or avoid the issue that there may be impaired professionals providing substandard care. In the past, it has been much more of a problem; health care providers with an alcohol or drug impairment were more tolerated by the medical community. This is becoming less so today as health care providers are aware that a fellow physician with an alcohol or drug impairment may not only provide substandard medical care, but may adversely affect all physicians' insurance coverage, also.

If a fellow health care provider has an alcohol or drug impairment, fellow physicians should take steps to persuade the impaired professional to make use of programs available in all states. Oftentimes, programs dealing with alcohol or drug impairment will not adversely affect a physician, so long as he takes advantage of the sponsored programs and genuinely works through the problems.

Whether a professional has a drug problem, alcohol problem, or has committed bona fide medical malpractice, it is imperative that other health care professionals not attempt to cover up or look the other way. By protecting an incompetent or impaired physician to the detriment of a patient, physicians are only working an injustice both to the patient and the health care system. Sooner or later, these cover-ups are usually discovered, and when they are, they seriously affect the ability to defend a medical-legal claim successfully.

Information Sources

When a resident begins working in a hospital, he should immediately obtain a copy of any applicable resident's manuals that exist. Having this knowledge provides the physician with important information regarding the facilities and protocols in that particular institution. In a malpractice lawsuit, plaintiffs' lawyers will invariably obtain such documents; if the resident failed to follow hospital rules, regulations, bylaws, or protocols, he will certainly be questioned as to why these were not followed. Physicians should become familiar with these resources and use them when appropriate.

Burn-Out

One of the situations that often results in a medical-legal claim is when a physician is overworked and suffering from "burn-out". This is especially a problem for young residents who are notoriously required to work extremely long hours that affect them physically, emotionally, and psychologically. When a physician is overworked and suffering burn-out, he is more prone to make mistakes that deviate from accepted standards of care and result in injuries to patients. This is a serious problem that is only recently being addressed in some states (e.g., New York). It is no defense to a medical-legal claim for a physician to claim that he is being overworked if he has taken no steps to correct the situation.

Specialty Resources

In modern medical practice, specialty resources are becoming more available. Clinical pharmacists, nurse clinicians, midwives, and other specialists within the health care profession can be called upon in appropriate circumstances by the treating physician. Physicians should learn to utilize these resources to their fullest extent. These are methods by which health care providers can avoid stretching themselves thin and still provide optimum care to their patients. The use of such professionals on the health care team provides a higher quality product to the consumer and less likelihood of a medical-legal claim.

In the legal arena, many facilities have attorneys or other professionals as risk managers. The risk manager is a resource for a physician to use. Information outside the health care professional team can be obtained from the risk manager, which increases the ability of a physician to provide optimum care.

Conclusion

There are many ways that physicians can reduce their exposure to medical-legal claims. It should be realized by physicians that mistakes can be made that are a result of deviations from acceptable and expected standards of care. If a person runs a stop sign because he is inattentive, and the car injures someone, no one questions the right of the injured party to be compensated for his injuries. Many physicians, however, believe in their heart that there is no such thing as a medical negligence claim, and that everything in medicine is a judgment call. This is simply not the case. Without the realization that mistakes can be a result of deviations from usual standards of care, physicians will always have an adverse concept of the legal system.

All the items outlined in this chapter are situations that impact upon medical-legal claims. Some are simplistic and others more complex. Each is an observation or experience obtained from specific cases. It is hoped that these brief reminders will assist younger physicians in recognizing problems that might tend to adversely involve them in the legal system, and thereby help to avoid such a possibility.

RIGHT OF SELF-DETERMINATION

Introduction

Save for true emergencies and rare exceptions, the practice of medicine does not countenance unilateral, unfettered decision-making by physicians. Patient care takes place in a complex, interdependent environment of patient, family, hospital, government, and third-party insurers, among others. While cost and other important factors loom larger than ever, patient autonomy, privacy, and self-determination greatly override all other considerations in the decision to treat or not to treat.

Privacy — Self-Determination

It was the common law of our country that developed the concept that all individuals have the right of self-determination regarding their own bodies, a right protected by the U.S. and State Constitutions' guarantees of privacy. Flowing from that right is the notion that a *competent* individual (the patient), not the physician, any other person, or entity, decides upon a medical course of action, regardless of the wisdom of the choice, and even if the decision is likely to result in what others, e.g., the physician, would characterize as harm, provided that there is no overriding, conflicting state interest.

Competence

Of course, much depends on who is a *competent* individual. Although there are several definitions and tests used to determine competence, the most frequently applied is whether a person has the ability to understand the risks, benefits, and alternatives involving a medical course of action or inaction. Though it can be difficult to apply, this standard is consistent with the principle of the informed consent doctrine. A physician is both capable and legally authorized to make such a decision.

Right to Refuse Treatment

Relying on these principles, courts have held that competent persons have the right to refuse every imaginable form of medical intervention. Examples include the use of psychotropic medications in mental institutions, psychosurgery, ECT, behavior modification, and others. And the right is so strong that it still applies, even if the individual suffers from severe illness, and even if he or she has been institutionalized for that reason. Even if insane (legally declared mentally ill and incompetent), until and unless a patient has a *judicial determination of incompetence for the particular ability to make medical treatment decisions,* therapy (even if obviously in the patient's "best interests" from the physician's point of view) cannot be forced upon the patient without a court order.

Right to Die

Conceptually, the right to refuse lifesaving medical treatment, i.e., the "right to die", is but a simple and logical corollary of the general right to refuse treatment. But as a practical matter, acknowledging that a person can forego "necessary" therapy, knowing full well that his or her election will likely hasten or result in death, has been difficult for the American public in general, the American physician in particular, and even the courts, to accept. There are many reasons for this, not the least of which is the fact that the outcome of allowing this choice is likely to be final and irreversible - the loss of a life. Moreover, though not analogous, at first glance, condoning this right appears to resemble acceptance of suicide. Also, we hear warnings from a vocal religious and political faction that the concept moves us ever closer to that slippery slope: If people are *allowed to die,* and under some circumstances we make the decision that some unfortunate souls who are not deemed competent to decide for themselves *ought to refuse* life-sustaining treatment, then it will not be long before political, religious, and ethnic groups are victimized by social judgments regarding the value of their lives.

The Physician's Role

Further, the "right to die" concept is particularly disturbing to physicians and the medical profession. Superficially, it seems at odds with the physician's duty to support life. Of a more practical concern, physicians and hospitals fear civil liability, or even criminal prosecution, that could result if a patient is allowed to die by foregoing life-supporting therapy. Until recently, there has been a pervasive sentiment that doing less than everything possible to continue a patient's life is a violation of medical ethics. The recent pronouncement by the AMA (see below) has gone a long way to clarify that issue and assuage physicians' moral concerns. Nevertheless, these practical concerns may be more than theoretical worries. In 1984, two southern California physicians were tried for murder after withdrawing various forms of life support from their comatose post-operative patient.

Conscience Clause

The law has provided an immunity to those who refuse to effectuate a patient's moral or legal rights where to do so would violate one's own ethical beliefs. This so-called "conscience clause", construed by the courts as a right under the First Amendment of the U.S. Constitution, has been upheld so long as a mechanism is provided to ensure that the rights of the patient are not jeopardized thereby, usually by requiring that the physician or nurse relying on the "conscience clause" transfer the patient's care to another, who will carry out his or her wishes.

Nutrition and Hydration

Although in recent years, the focus has changed regarding such issues as the modalities of support that may be rejected or withdrawn, the core concept of a patient's autonomy and right to forego treatment, even refuse life-supporting treatment, and thus, the right to die, has remained the central theme. More recent cases have scrutinized whether food and water may be withdrawn from a vegetative, comatose, or dying patient. Other issues the courts have grappled with include the patient's location (for example, residing in a nursing home versus being at home or in a hospital), and whether the physician or facility can be forced to carry out the patient's treatment decision or, alternatively, force the patient to be transferred (in location, or in terms of caregiver or facility) to effectuate the right to decide.

Quality of Life

Most recent court decisions have given great deference to the *quality* of a person's life, focusing on the likelihood of a return to "cognitive and sapient life", and a person's right to privacy, effectuated by a pre-coma statement, allowed physicians to withdraw seemingly life-sustaining measures, e.g., a ventilator. Moreover, physicians were not required to go to court for an order before taking such a step. Rather, if in doubt, they could utilize a hospital ethics committee to help resolve a sticky moral or potential legal problem. The most recent decision of the U.S. Supreme Court has emphasized the need for a pre-coma utterance by the patient; otherwise, a state may forbid the withdrawal of maintenance measures.

Ethics Committees

Ethics committees are more commonplace, if not universal, especially since their existence is mandated by the JCAHO. The purpose, composition, function, and role of ethics committees regarding the difficult issues involving dying patients vary greatly in different regions and from hospital to hospital. They may exist on paper only and be quite inactive, or provide a consultative and advisory role. Occasionally, they are interventionist, set policies, and create guidelines. Some exist for the benefit of physicians and the medical staff only, while others may be available to diverse hospital personnel (such as nurses), or provide access to patients and families.

Substituted Judgment

All the cases on point have stated that an *incompetent* person does not lose the right to self-determination, and hence to refuse treatment, merely because of the incompetence. Rather, the right must simply be exercised by a surrogate using "substituted judgment". That is, the surrogate is to step into the shoes of the incompetent patient and make the choice the patient would have. In a case in Massachusetts, food and water could be discontinued for a firefighter in a persistent coma for three years, although not terminally ill, because he had stated many times before becoming ill that he would not want to be maintained on life support. The Massachusetts Supreme Court stated that this right of the patient is unconditional. The court excused the hospital from effectuating his wish because of its own moral position, necessitating the patient's transfer to another facility.

The Institution's Role

The Supreme Court of New Jersey, in upholding the removal of a patient's feeding tube in another case, later held that a skilled nursing facility did not have the right to refuse to participate in the tube's removal. New Jersey also held that another patient, who suffered from amyotrophic lateral sclerosis, could refuse a nasogastric tube, and that the hospital could not force her transfer to another facility to avoid her death by starvation within its walls.

The cases, therefore, are clear. When the patient is *competent* to make a decision, his or her right to decide is respected. Thus, in both California and Florida, patients with end-stage chronic obstructive pulmonary disease were allowed to turn the respirator off, even though their deaths were thereby assured. And the court in the California case said that the decision to refuse unwanted treatment is not medical or legal, nor at all conditional; rather, it is a moral and philosophical decision belonging to a competent adult alone. The quality of life, not its duration, is controlling.

Invasion of Privacy

This principle must be borne uppermost in the mind of a physician who would choose not to comply with a patient's wishes, or the wishes of the family or other surrogate in the case of an incompetent patient. To simply refuse to effectuate a patient's right to privacy would risk liability, and there are such cases. To avoid it, the physician has a legal responsibility and duty to either carry out his patient's desires, or to transfer the management of the case to another competent and qualified doctor who will.

Burdens v. Benefits of Life

When the patient is not competent, as in the case of a patient in an irreversible coma in a nursing home, the New Jersey Supreme Court held that a substituted judgment effectuates the incompetent's wish if that can be determined, and if it cannot, then the task is to determine what would be in the patient's best interests. This means a determination must be made as to whether the burdens of life outweigh the benefits of that life. Or, as the California court put it in determining whether the treatment is proportional or disproportionate - whether there exists a reasonable chance of providing benefits, which outweigh the burdens attendant to the treatment. Of course, in some settings, such as a nursing home, there is enough potential for coercion or abuse that a court determination will be required to decide that a patient is incompetent, or that a treatment is disproportionate.

Current Status

The common law on the right to die, as it has developed, can thus be summarized. In the case of chronically ill or terminal patients who nevertheless do not meet the criteria for defining death, the right of self-determination and the constitutional right to privacy give the patient the right to make all decisions regarding his or her own body. Of course, that right is not absolute and is measured against the state's interests in preserving life, preventing suicide, protecting innocent third parties, and safeguarding the integrity of the medical profession. Generally, for the competent individual, the patient's rights outweigh those state interests.

Parens Patriae

It is no different for the incompetent patient, except that the state must, as "parens patriae", exert its sovereign power of guardianship over persons under disability to carry out their wishes and rights in the setting of the dying patient. Generally, this is accomplished by a substituted judgment, as evidenced by written or oral pre-disability statements.

Best Interest Doctrine

When the patient *could have expressed* his or her intent while competent, but never did so before becoming incompetent, the "best interest" of the incompetent vis-a-vis treatment must be determined. When a patient has been incompetent since birth, and in some situations, when there is deemed to be a potential for abuse, the issues may require resolution by a court. Otherwise, the physicians and hospital, working and interacting with the family in good faith, do not require prior court authorization and may proceed without fear of civil or criminal liability. Thus, almost all cases dealing with withdrawal of life support have upheld the physicians' judgments not to provide life support.

Natural Death Legislation

More recently, state legislatures have addressed the issue of life support and the right to forego or withdraw it with so-called "right to die" or "natural death" legislation. Resultant acts are only extensions of the right to refuse medical treatment discussed above. These laws provide a patient the chance to do so in advance by acknowledging the moral autonomy of people to control their own lives. They also serve to define any civil or criminal liability, or immunity therefrom, for physicians and the medical profession, in case that was unclear without these laws. It is noteworthy that in addition to giving the physician protection for his compliance, they generally also provide censure and/or penalties for failure to comply or transfer patients to the care of another physician who will comply.

These laws bestow no new rights on patients, for the common law already recognized the "right to die", and decisions to forego or withdraw treatment are and have been made constantly by the physician with his or her patient and/or family. Moreover, whereas the common law demands only that a patient be competent to make treatment decisions, these state laws may be quite burdensome and require the patient to be terminally ill or dying, or that death be imminent, or "artificial means of life support" be involved. Most of the acts impose onerous procedural requirements that must be complied with for the patient's directive to be valid, including waiting periods, the use of particular forms and documents, placement of the documents in specal locations (e.g., the medical record), renewal requirements and revocation procedures, special requirements for patients in extended care facilities, number and qualifications of witnesses, etc. The physician, patient, and family must be cognizant of special applications of these laws to pregnant women, minors, and incompetents. Attention must also be paid to the effect of validly executing a directive under one of these state laws, whether the physician must follow the directive or has the power to refuse, the effect of the document, if any, when improperly executed or ineffective for some other reason, penalties for non-compliance, any effects on life or health insurance, and so forth. In short, the law of the particular state involved must be studied and applied.

It should be noted that such right to die acts have now been enacted in 42 states, and cannot be ignored. They do not represent, as some critics have alleged, euthanasia. As a matter of fact, most of them bar any positive act to shorten life. Nor, by complying with the state death act, is the patient committing, or the physician assisting, a suicide.

State Legislative Acts

Physicians must also be aware of other types of legislation that affect patients in the setting of terminal care for the dying patient. Some states (e.g., New York) have enacted laws providing detailed procedural requirements for issuing "Do Not Resuscitate" orders. If, but only if, a physician follows the mandated procedures, he or she is assured of civil and criminal immunity. Of course, hospitals are being required by the JCAHO and licensing bodies to have "Do Not Resuscitate" (DNR) or no-code policies for accreditation, so a physician may be constrained to follow some procedural mandates, even if his or her state has not yet enacted pertinent legislation. Also, some states (e.g., Oklahoma) have directly and specifically addressed such ethical issues as withholding food and water. Oklahoma's "Hydration and Nutrition For Incompetent Patients Act" has stringent requirements for withholding, and requires the physician to assume the patient would wish to receive food and water.

Ethical Guidelines

Physicians will want to be familiar with *ethical guidelines* dealing with foregoing or withdrawing treatment as well. Though lacking the force of common or statutory law, such pronouncements can guide the physician, and also help establish the standard of care (and thus diminish the threat of civil liability). The recent pronouncement by the AMA's Council on Ethical and Judicial Affairs has had particular impact on physicians and their care of dying patients. It stresses respect for the patient's dignity, compliance with the patient's wishes, and establishes that it is not unethical to discontinue life support in the situation of irreversible coma, even if death be imminent. The guidelines go on to say that even food and water can ethically be withheld, and that if a physician disagrees with these precepts, he or she can ethically follow his or her conscience, as long as the patient is not abandoned.

Ethical guidelines of local professional associations can have important impact as well, especially when developed in a joint effort with the local bar association. A good example is the "Guidelines For Discontinuance of Cardiopulmonary Life Support Systems", drawn up jointly by the Los Angeles County Medical Society and the Los Angeles County Bar Association. The guidelines reiterate the common law, stress the preservation of the patient's dignity and enhancement of patient comfort, state that a physician may discontinue life support and may refuse to participate in life support withdrawal and arrange to transfer the patient's care to another qualified doctor. They also specifically enumerate the situations when a physician can discontinue life support without prior court approval: (1) Brain death is established; (2) The patient has executed a valid directive under the Natural Death Act; and (3) In an irreversible coma when the family concurs, the patient has not indicated contrary desires, and certain procedural details have been satisfied.

It should be stressed that although a physician must be aware of such national and local ethical guidelines, they are no more that that - guidelines. They do not have the force and effect of law. The two southern California physicians prosecuted for murder learned this lesson when they adhered to the LACMS/LACBA's guidelines in withdrawing all life support, including food and water, from their comatose patient in 1984. At the very least, however, such guidelines evidence the local standard of care, and therefore, protect the adherent from civil liability.

Living Will

One of the most helpful things for both the physician and the patient, as well as the family and others, to effectuate the right to die and to refuse treatment is the existence of a written directive, setting forth the patient's wishes. Such documents take variable forms and are of varying complexity and legal effect. For example, millions of Americans have signed a simple, widely distributed, one page "Living Will". In many states, these have an advisory effect only, and do not carry the authority of law. In such states, medical personnel could (in good faith) ignore or disdain the "Living Will", without threat of liability. Nevertheless, the document would be of some value as it evidences the patient's wishes and state of mind before becoming incompetent and unable to otherwise express his or her desire to forego life support and medical treatment.

Durable Power of Attorney

Of much greater significance is the Durable Power of Attorney for Health Care. In California and other states, this is a legal document recognized by the state through legislation which allows a competent adult to appoint a surrogate decision-maker, in advance, for use in future health care decisions when he or she might be unable to express his or her own wishes. In contrast to the "Living Will", the durable power is legally enforceable like a directive under the Natural Death Act; unlike that document, it is not difficult to validly execute. When the issue of life support or other treatment comes up, and the principal is unable to decide or speak, the appointed attorney for health care may decide and speak for him or her in accordance with the instructions and sentiments expressed in the document, and if unclear or there is no guidance therein, the attorney must act in the principal's best interests.

Although the Durable Power of Attorney for Health Care provides the best means of assuring the patient's right to die and to refuse treatment are respected, if he or she should become incompetent, it is not perfect. The attorney may make decisions the physician believes the patient would not have made had he or she retained decision-making capacity. Unless specified to be shorter, the power's duration is seven years, and presumably, it must then be renewed. There are provisions for revocation and qualifications to be an attorney or a witness which are provided in the Act. If the physician acts in "good faith" regarding the authority of the attorney to make decisions and the likelihood that the attorney really reflects the principal's wishes, he or she may act upon the attorney's authority and enjoy civil and criminal immunity.

Surrogacy

There are several unique circumstances regarding the refusal of treatment and the right to die that demand special comment. Several medical situations involve some incapacity or disability that render the patient unable to make a treatment decision, and hence, require a surrogate to decide and speak for the patient. Of course, we have already analyzed this situation extensively regarding the dying or terminally ill incompetent, who nevertheless retains the right to refuse treatment. A surrogate effectuates the right, either by exercising a Durable Power of Attorney if one exists, or by complying with pre-stated written (e.g., a "Living Will") or verbal wishes. If neither exists, caregivers or courts may have to determine the incompetent patient's prior attitudes from family, friends, or by other means.

Organ Donation

When organ transplantation is involved, the potential donor and/or potential donee may be incompetent for a variety of reasons. The toughest situation occurs when both are, usually because they are children and the issue is whether the parents may decide to refuse a donation, perhaps against medical advice, or to force transplantation to the possible detriment of the potential donor, for example. The outcome, and the parents' (surrogates') authority to make the treatment decision, or to refuse the treatment, perhaps resulting in the death of the potential donee, may depend on the jurisdiction, what type of legal test it uses, the characteristics of the incompetent, etc. Incidentally, the right to refuse, and not be forced to come to the aid of another, applies in the transplantation situation, even if the refusing potential donor is related to the potential donee and is the only medically possible donor who could save the recipient's life. In such a case, in effect, there is a right to decide that another will die by exercising the right to privacy and to refuse medical treatment.

Disabled Infants

A very special situation wherein the surrogate decision-maker, usually the parents, may be foreclosed from refusing medical treatment for an incompetent minor concerns handicapped infants, usually newborns. In 1985, Congress enacted legislation, setting up the offense of withholding medically indicated treatment from a disabled infant with a life-threatening condition, except in circumstances of chronic irreversible coma, or where the treatment would be futile and merely prolong dying, or be inhumane. The regulations under this law have been criticized as injecting uncertainty into a situation in which the law has historically given the parents great, though not absolute, deference. In the past, and in general, the parents as surrogates have exercised the right to refuse treatment and the right to die for these disabled infants, but the new law would seem to alter the usual equation, so the physician working with defective newborns must be alert to these new federal regulations.

Fetal Rights

Under some circumstances, a patient, and if incompetent, that patient's surrogate, loses the right to refuse treatment and the right to die. For example, the state may order a retarded young woman sterilized, and neither she nor her proxy may be able to refuse this "treatment". And all states treat the pregnant comatose, hence, incompetent, woman differently by stating in their legislation and/or their common law that she cannot refuse life-sustaining therapy. Apparently, because of its interest in the potential life of the fetus, the state may refuse to allow her to die while carrying a viable fetus. In some jurisdictions, courts have taken away the competent woman's right to refuse the substantial bodily invasion of a Cesarean section in order to save the baby. However, other jurisdictions have held the contrary.

Suicide and Euthanasia

Finally, it should be mentioned in passing that although there is a "right to die" stemming from the right to refuse medical treatment, there is no right to perform an affirmative act to take one's own life (suicide), or to cause another to die, even if that may seem morally humane under the circumstances (euthanasia).

In a recent dramatic case in Michigan, a physician, who had utilized a device that he had designed to assist a woman in committing suicide, has been enjoined from using this device in the future.

RISK MANAGEMENT
AND QUALITY ASSURANCE

In health care, both risk management and quality assurance are vitally important at a number of levels.

Responsibility for Hospital Quality of Care —
Hospital Staff

Within the hospital, each individual physician staff member has social responsibilities associated with the general quality of health care. As a member of the hospital staff, he or she is responsible for the protection of all patients, not just those under his or her individual care. A portion of this general staff responsibility relates to the behavior of one's fellow physicians. In some states, this is enforced by the so-called "snitch laws". These laws provide penalties for any physician who observes a lapse of conduct by a fellow physician and fails to report it. The various state laws specify what sort of lapses are to be reported and the form of reporting, which is usually to a hospital committee or directly to the licensing board.

Failure to report aberrant or deviate behavior can lead not only to sanctions by state agencies and hospital boards, but also to liability suits by injured parties against the hospital, the staff, and individual physicians. When a Sacramento, California, surgeon admitted that he had operated repeatedly under the influence of amphetamines, the injured patients sued the other physicians on the staff for their failure to stop him from committing this malpractice. The hospital was forced to pay damages to the permanently crippled victims on the basis of collective medical staff responsibility for the actions of one of its members.

Similarly, the 1989 lawsuits filed against Dr. James Burt, the Dayton, Ohio, "Love Surgeon", named 82 other physicians as co-defendants for their alleged failure to prevent him from performing his unique and medically unrecognized "vulvo-vaginoplasties". There is no allegation here that the other staff physicians ignored such things as drug abuse; rather, it is their having allowed such novel surgical procedures to take place. Dr. Burt's operation was not generally recognized, and therefore, the suits charge, the staff should have taken positive action to prevent his continued practice upon patients within the hospital.

This responsibility can arise directly; that is, by observing that a fellow physician is abusing controlled substances or alcohol, or by personal observation of negligence or deviation from accepted practice. However, it is more likely to arise indirectly as a member of one of the many review committees responsible for the hospital's quality of care.

Risk Management

Within hospitals, risk management committees are most frequently headed by the hospital administrator and have representatives from a number of divisions of the hospital, including the medical staff. Obviously, the composition of the committee is dependent upon the size and type of hospital. Risk management committees are involved in protecting the hospital against liability suits for mishaps suffered by patients, employees, and/or visitors outside of the realm of medical care. These committees are usually concerned with protection from fire hazards, falls from beds, injuries suffered in the course of transferring patients from one place to another, etc.

Orders/Medications

Occasionally, risk management committees will also be involved with the problems of inappropriate care, particularly medications and physicians' orders. These latter concerns will more closely involve a physician, since many of these problems come about from the misinterpretation of the physician's orders, written or oral, by the nursing staff and in their transmission to the pharmacy. Other errors, of course, come about through misunderstandings by the pharmacy in filling orders, or by the nursing staff in administering the medications.

For example, it is easy, but legally inexcusable, to confuse Disipramine with Disopyramide. When a physician is imprecise about either the name of the medication or its dosage, he or she is difficult to defend in any malpractice action. Statements such as "Well, the nurse should have known that I meant this drug instead of the one which she actually gave" are of little avail if the names sound alike or one's writing is indecipherable by the jury, as well as by the nurse.

Furthermore, imprecision about decimal points has resulted in incidents when ten times the appropriate medication was given. It is difficult to believe that nursing personnel would meticulously give ten single doses to a patient all at the same time, in order to carry out their misperception of the dose. However, it has occurred, and when it does, the physician is named in the liability suit, as well as the nurse and the hospital. It is usually the risk management committee which attempts to cut down on these inter-professional miscommunications.

Medical Records

The liability aspects of medical records may be the province of the risk management committee, or of a separate records committee. For either one, the hospital staff member finds that what is written at the time of an event is taken legally to be what actually happened. It is almost impossible later to disavow the written statement made just after the event. The assumption is that one's memory is best when it is freshest. Similarly, if it was not recorded, the presumption is that it did not happen. Much of the regulation of medical records sounds and feels like the mindless harassment of the busy practitioner by the nitpicking, paper loving bureaucrat. Some of it may be. However, the failure to check one's own records and be sure that one's colleagues watch their own is the path to large settlements of non-meritorious lawsuits, which have been rendered indefensible by careless mistakes. Juries are hostile to hospital errors and those who make them.

As an added caution, the physician must be sure that the nursing notes do not do him or her in. Whether or not a physician responded to a call in the middle of the night is an integral part of many cases with bad results when it comes down to the physician's memory against the nurses' notes - the physician is not likely to win the jury's confidence. The physician must be certain that his or her response was recorded. Also, the physician must be sure that the nurses have not described the patient in different terms than the physician's perception of the patient's condition. A notation of "severe pain" or "heavy bleeding" needs to be matched by the physician's note with his or her adjectives, or else the failure to take strong measures will look like neglect. The need for comprehensible progress notes and a firm warning against going back to "correct" the physician's records are important enough to be repeated over and over.

Quality Assurance Committees

Depending on the size and organization of the hospital, there are a variable number of committees devoted to quality assurance. Quality assurance usually is concentrated on the medical care delivered in the hospital. Some committees are quite localized in their forms, such as tissue committee, tumor committee, surgical suite, intensive care unit, etc. Others are more generalized and look at across-the-board quality assurance issues.

The most common methods of review involve, in general, some form of screening, usually by computer, which identifies outliers. These outliers are the physicians with an increased number of post-operative wound infections, unplanned returns to surgery, returns to the hospital within 30 days of dismissal, excess nosocomial infections, hospital mortality, etc.

This screening sets aside for further review the unusual patterns of practice. It is imperative that committee members distinguish sharply between issues of quality of care, such as a high Cesarean rate, and those of cost control, such as keeping a patient in the hospital after the diagnosis-related group (DRG) length of stay for a patient's diagnosis has expired. The latter may be of more concern to the hospital administrator, but emphasis on saving the hospital money is a different concern than that of protecting quality, which is of more importance to the patient and to the practicing physician. Quality assurance is a professional responsibility.

In addition to looking for outliers by using computers, the various quality assurance committees usually are shown patient charts that have been regarded by some observers as demonstrating patterns outside the usual parameters of practice. Frequently, these are charts of patients who died in the hospital — a mortality conference. However, it may be more subtle; for example, a pattern of increased use of transfusions or of antibiotics by a physician, as compared with his or her peers.

No matter how charts are brought before the committee, whether by computer screening for selected indicators of quality, by mortality, by report, or by complaint, the committee must decide whether that individual physician's practice is within the accepted guidelines of care.

The fact that a physician's method of practice is unusual does not, of itself, prove that it is wrong. Raw statistics will identify the outliers, but, of themselves, do not demonstrate inadequate performance. In fact, they will often show that the best physician in the hospital has some of the worst outcomes. The reason, of course, is obvious enough after looking at the charts. The excellent physician gets only the sickest patients referred to him or her, and the poor outcomes are not unusual once the severity of the illness is taken into account. To the contrary, some of the worst physicians have superb outcome statistics because they operate only on patients who are well and would have recovered nicely without the operation in the first place. The first physician should be complimented; the second physician should be chastised, and hopefully rehabilitated, just the reverse of the initial impression from the first scanning of the printouts. Only medical practitioners, and often only fellow specialists, can make this type of sophisticated judgment. This requires peer review.

Peer Review

When sitting on hospital committees having to do with quality assurance, which include the credentialling and/or privileges committees, a physician is passing judgment upon one's fellow staff members. This peer review is always somewhat difficult. It is made much more difficult when one is attempting to peer review a competitor and/or a friendly colleague. In large departments of large hospitals, it is usually possible to get a relatively impartial review. In smaller departments in smaller hospitals, the number of physicians involved is so small that each is a friend, or, unfortunately, an adversary of all his or her other fellow specialists. Almost inevitably, they are economic rivals as well. In these cases, it is essential that peer review be done by physician experts from outside the hospital. Good faith peer review is vital to maintain a high quality of care in a hospital; but bad faith review, such as occurred in the *Patrick v. Burget* case recently heard before the Supreme Court, will lead to heavy financial penalties for the physicans involved. The use of membership on the credentialling, privileges, and other quality assurance committees as the means for preserving the economics of one's practice is not only unprofessional and unethical, it is also quite apt to lead to an unhappy experience in court. Fortunately, some specialty societies and the American Medico-Legal Foundation are willing to furnish expert reviewers from out of the area.

Credentialling

It may seem ridiculous overkill to require a committee to assure the hospital that a physician really is a physician. Unfortunately, as high as 10% of persons applying to U.S. medical schools and physicians applying to one of the larger specialty boards have used false credentials. Applicants to hospital staffs have also been found much too often to have fudged in their statements of qualification. It is, therefore, necessary to be certain that everyone attempting to join or continue on the staff is everything that he or she says. Again, physicians, with appropriate clerical assistance, are the best qualified to judge both the credentials needed for their own hospital and the validity of the documentation.

Privileges

Granting privileges to be active in certain departments or to perform certain procedures is the essence of peer review. While specialty board certification is a help, it is not a panacea. Certification by one of the 23 member boards of the American Board of Medical Specialties (ABMS) is a good start. However, the fact that someone has finished several years of residency without any serious demerits or black marks, and then passed a cognitive examination does not, by itself, prove that he or she is fit to operate in the surgical suite, for instance.

On the other hand, some physicians have acquired considerable skill in a field without obtaining formal certification, and they should be allowed to exercise this skill. This is particularly true of the approximately 50 fields of sub-specialty certification currently recognized by the ABMS, a number which is expanding rapidly.

The effect of the acceptance by a specialty certifying board of a new sub-specialty certificate upon currently practicing hospital staff members in that field can be troublesome. Most see no reason to take time off from their practice long enough to get the requisite formal educational training for the certificate when they already consider themselves — and often are — proficient in that sub-specialty. This can pose a delicate problem for a staff committee.

The granting of privileges is further complicated by the presence of over 100 specialty boards which are not recognized by the ABMS. What privileges do the diplomates of these boards deserve? Some are well-regulated and capable of evaluating skills, while others are little more than mail order diploma mills.

All of this means that certificates cannot substitute for observation by peers. Certificates can mask substance abuse, senility, disease, and dishonesty. To protect the public, the hospital, and one's own professional integrity, the physician committee member must make personal observations and judgments about another physician's performance. In order to make judgments about performance, the committee member needs standards against which to match the observations.

Joint Commission on Accreditation of Health Care Organizations (JCAHO)

The Joint Commission accredits hospitals, and thereby establishes many of the rules which hospitals must follow in quality assurance. In the past, the Joint Commission has concentrated on the process; that is, it looked to see if the medical records were completed, that the committees had been meeting and keeping minutes, etc. Recently, it has begun to look at measuring outcomes. This entails reviewing whether the quality assurance committees assess the work of the physicians within the hospital, and measuring that assessment against some objective indicators of performance. Since hospitals are unlikely to survive without Joint Commission accreditation, it is increasingly essential that quality assurance committees not only exist, but that they function effectively, are able to prove that they are effective, and that they use definitive standards.

Practice Standards

When in the course of peer review, committee members are forced to make judgments about the practice of other physicians, they must measure the practice against some objective standards to be effective. Simply comparing how another physician practices with the way one does things him or herself is not good enough. There are often a number of different methodologies by which to accomplish a desired therapeutic result. One physician may achieve success through a procedure which another does not or cannot use. This does not prove that either is right, but simply that there must be room for flexibility, and certainly, for innovation in the setting and implementation of standards. However they are developed, these standards must be applied uniformly to all of the staff members.

Standards have at least two steps. The first is *technology assessment,* which allows experts to draw conclusions as to which procedure is best for a given diagnosis. For instance, an analysis of well-performed clinical trials can determine whether it is usually better to use surgery, radiation, and/or chemotherapy to treat a given stage of carcinoma. This function is performed by clinical researchers and specialty society leaders. It results in nationally accepted guidelines.

The *quality assurance* comes into play when the peer review within the hospital assesses both whether the individual physician selected the proper procedure for that diagnosis, as identified by the technology assessment, and if so, whether he or she applied it properly. For instance, if surgery is the preferred method of treatment, whether the physician performed the surgery correctly.

In studying this phenomenon, one authority looked at a large, multi-institution study of the relative merits of using surgery and radiation to treat a given cancer. The conclusion of the survey was that surgery was superior. However, in looking at the individual hospital results, the authority found that in those hospitals which followed the radiology protocol precisely, the results from radiation were superior to those from surgery. The technology of surgery was not superior to that of radiation for that condition. It was the fact that the surgery was performed according to the experimental protocol, and that the radiation was not what led to the disparity of results in favor of surgery.

The lesson is that members of a hospital committee must not only determine which approach is better, but whether the physician carried out that approach adequately.

Standards for which procedure is best in a given set of circumstances and general guidelines for carrying it out are best when produced by the specialty societies. After an initial reluctance, in past years the specialty societies have increasingly been willing and have begun to develop positive "policies", "parameters", or "guidelines". This is not cookbook medicine with a single set of steps to be followed meticulously, but rather a description of the outer limits of what should be acceptable practice. Within these outer limits, different types of approaches are acceptable if they are performed competently. The main role of the physician on the hospital staff peer review committee is to assure the hospital that the physician being reviewed actually performed the appropriate procedure in an appropriate way. It is usually not the reviewing physician's function to determine what type of procedure is best for a given diagnosis in a particular specialty. That should be ascertained by the specialty society clinical guidelines.

Experimentation

Practice standards should allow for both flexibility and innovation; however, they do not allow the individual physician to experiment on his or her patients without having had the protocol for experimentation reviewed by others. These others may be as distant as a federal agency such as the Food and Drug Administration, or as near as the hospital's research and/or ethics committees. Certainly, the patient must be fully informed and in agreement with the fact that an experimental treatment is being used. The use of unproven techniques which have not been accepted within medicine is professionally irresponsible and legally hazardous.

Individual Physician —
Patient Safety

In the largest study of the causes of medical malpractice, performed by the National Association of Insurance Commissioners and partially funded by the Council of Medical Specialty Societies, the medical reasons for 75,000 claims were reviewed. Each specialty looked to the misadventures which had led to malpractice claims within that specialty. A couple of the general ones are worth mentioning. Some of the most common causes of professional liability claims are the missed diagnoses of cancer and myocardial infarction.

Cause for Suits

An all too frequent scenario is the patient who visits a physician with a question about a lump in her breast. Some form of examination is done, whether it be palpation, mammography, needle biopsy, etc., but no definitive diagnosis is made. Presumably, the patient is told to return, but there is inadequate recording of this fact, and the patient does not return. When that patient subsequently is found to have cancer, it may be possible that this cancer arose in a different lump, or that the failure to return is all the patient's fault, but the physician is usually helpless to defend him or herself in court. The patient will say that she was never told to return and, despite the physician's fervent protestations, the patient will almost always be believed by the jury. The failure to follow up on a patient with possible cancer with aggressive and documented efforts to get her to return is hazardous to the health of the patient and the malpractice insurance of the physician.

The misdiagnosis of myocardial infarction is usually in an emergency room, and ordinarily involves a man with chest pain, for which there is some other logical diagnosis such as esophagitis, chest wall injury, etc. The patient is not followed long enough for definitive signs, EKG, and/or laboratory evidence to appear, but he is sent out to suffer an extension of the infarction, which may be fatal, and which then leads to a subsequent indefensible liability claim.

Another common error is to order a laboratory test, and then fail to be certain that one knows the result. The patient is admitted to the hospital for a procedure requiring only a short stay and a routine chest x-ray and laboratory work are ordered. After the patient has gone home, or at least after the physician has last reviewed the chart, a report with an abnormality indicating a previously unknown, asymptomatic condition, unrelated to the procedure, is returned and filed. It may be a coin lesion, hyperglycemia, abnormal calcium, etc. Later, the patient returns with advanced clinical manifestations of the disease, which have been accentuated by the failure to diagnose the pathologic condition sooner. When the previous chart is reviewed again, the attending physician is helpless. If the physician is not going to review the results of a test, he or she should not order it. If the physician does not need the test, he or she should not order it. If the physician does need it, he or she should order it, and then be sure that he or she received and reviews the results.

Out of Hospital Practice

A recent trend in malpractice cases has been an increased number from out of the hospitals. In 1984, 92% of the total indemnity paid in California came from hospital cases. Since that time, there had been a steady decline until 1988 when only 65% of total indemnity was represented by hospital located cases. Since these statistics represent only the large verdicts in excess of $50,000.00, the decline is striking. It also indicates the increased need for quality assurance in ambulatory facilities, imaging centers, and, of course, the physician's own office.

Unfortunately, in these areas, quality assurance techniques lag well behind those in hospitals. Whereas the national inspection of hospitals was begun during World War I by the American College of Surgeons, the evaluation of ambulatory clinics has only occurred in the last few years. This means that the responsibility for quality assurance within one's office is largely on the shoulders of the individual physician. Those physicians who work within larger clinics, HMO's, and other structured practice arrangements will find some form of quality assurance system, although the quality is unfortunately variable.

Dr. David Axelrod, the New York State Ccmmissioner of Health, has advocated systems of quality control, which include looking at individual physicians' offices. There is a good chance that the idea will spread, and that quality assurance systems for out of hospital practice will become mandatory.

The best protection for the office-based physician is good medical records, and obviously, to practice acceptable medicine and be able to prove it. Continuing medical education and recertification are methods of demonstrating one's knowledge of appropriate practice.

Conclusion

The constant assessment of one's own practice and the practice of one's associates in and out of the hospital is both a professional responsibility and a legal necessity. The objective monitoring of medical care in one's community is vital for patients and physicians alike.

IV.
GOVERNMENTAL

GOVERNMENT REGULATIONS — FEDERAL

Peer Review Immunity

In 1986, Congress passed the Health Care Quality Improvement Act (HCQIA), having concluded that federal attention was needed to deal with the increasing occurrence of medical malpractice, and also to restrict the flow of incompetent physicians from state to state. Congress believed that this nationwide problem could be remedied through effective professional peer review, but also realized that the threat of money damage liability under federal laws, including treble damage liability under federal antitrust law, would unreasonably discourage physicians from participating in effective professional peer review. Congress emphasized that there was an overriding national need to provide incentives and protections for physicians engaging in peer review. (See Section 402 of the Health Care Quality Improvement Act of 1986.)

In Section 412 of the Act, Congress stipulated the standards for professional review actions which must be applied in order to immunize a physician from antitrust liability. The individual state is not required to opt into Section 412; some may not because they believe that their own state laws provide ''better'' immunity protection. *Physicians are advised to consult their local medical society or hospital attorney about a particular state's relationship to federal law.*

National Practitioner Data Bank Provision

In addition, there were concerns that incompetent or impaired physicians could migrate from state to state to avoid disciplinary action. The Act contains two major provisions; one granting limited liability for peer review activity by professional bodies, and the other establishing a National Practitioner Data Bank for the reporting of ''adverse'' information concerning health care practitioners. The HHS contracted with Unisys to establish and run the Data Bank. The Secretary of HHS established an executive committee, which is to provide guidance to Unisys in the establishment and operation of the Data Bank.

The final regulations pertaining to the Data Bank were published in October of 1989. The regulations became effective when the actual operation of the Data Bank became operational in the early Fall of 1990.

The articulated purpose of the statute is to restrict the ability of incompetent physicians to move from state to state without disclosure or discovery of a physician's previous damaging or incompetent performance. The overall goal is to improve the quality of medical care by creating an environment in which impaired or incompetent health care practitioners can be weeded out.

The statute sets forth three general areas for which information must be reported to the Data Bank. They are as follows:

1. Payments made on behalf of health care practitioners for medical malpractice suits or claims;

This part (B) of the HCQIA is not optional. Section 421 requires that a medical malpractice action or claim (settlement or partial settlement) must be reported

to a designated central Data Bank. The information shall include the name of
the physician or licensed health care practitioner for whose benefit the payment
was made, the amount of the payment, the name (if known) of any hospital at
which the physician or practitioner is affiliated or associated, a description of the
actual admission and injuries or illnesses on which the claim was based, and such
other information as the Secretary determines is required for appropriate interpretation of information reported under this section. Hospitals shall be required to
obtain information about members of the medical staff from the central Data Bank
every two years. Physicians should understand that they have an ethical duty to
participate in peer review in order to assure that standards of care are applied
in a reasonable manner, and to assure that the physician undergoing peer review
receives a fair assessment of his medical practice.

2. Adverse licensure actions taken by state licensing boards; and

3. Adverse actions taken against health care practitioners relating to clinical
privileges.

All provisions of the Act are applicable to physicians and dentists. Reporting
is voluntary for various allied health care practitioners who hold clinical privileges,
insofar as reporting limitations on privileges is concerned. The Act is mandatory
for allied health care practitioners, insofar as reporting requirements are concerned
for medical malpractice payments. The Act does not apply to licensure actions
for allied health care practitioners.

Controlled Substance Regulations

Physicians must be forever mindful that enforcement agencies, both federal
and state, have increased their surveillance of physicians who may be prescribing
controlled substances illegally. A prominent, scholarly, and excellent physician
was heavily fined because he did not know about a Drug Enforcement Administration Regulation [21 CFR (s) 1306.05], which states:

"All prescriptions for controlled substances shall be dated as of, and signed
on, the day when issued and shall bear the full name and address of the patient,
and the name, address, and registration number of the practitioner. A practitioner may sign a prescription in the same manner as he would sign a check
or legal document. Where an oral order is not permitted, the prescription shall
be written with ink or indelible pencil or typewriter and shall be manually signed
by the practitioner. The prescription may be prepared by a secretary or agent
for the signature of a practitioner, but the prescribing practitioner is responsible in case the prescription does not conform in all essential respects to the
law and regulations. A corresponding liability rests upon the pharmacist who
fills a prescription not prepared in the form prescribed by these regulations.
An intern, resident, or foreign-trained physician, or physician on the staff
of a Veteran's Administration facility, exempted from registration under Section
1301.24 (c), shall include on all prescriptions issued by him the registration
number of the hospital or other institution and the special internal code number
assigned to him by the hospital or other institution as provided in Section
1301.24 (c), in lieu of the registration number of the practitioner required by
this section. Each written prescription shall have the name of the physician
stamped, typed, or handprinted on it, as well as a signature of the physician."

A physician should not allow patients or health care persons to convince him
or her to "be a nice guy" by writing a post-dated prescription for a controlled

substance drug. A patient could be a policeman.

According to the Food, Drug & Cosmetic Act, an approved drug may be labeled, promoted, and advertised by the manufacturer only for those uses for which the drug's safety and effectiveness have been established and approved by the FDA. On the other hand, in the 1983 PDR (37th edition), Jack E. Angel, publisher, pointed out that the FDA had announced that the Act does not limit the manner in which a physician may use an approved drug. Once a product has been approved for marketing, a physician may prescribe the drug to treat disease or patient populations that are not included in approved labeling. Thus, the FDA implies that "accepted medical practice" could include drug use that is not reflected in approved drug labeling.

When a physician decides to prescribe a drug for indications outside those uses for which the drug's safety and effectiveness have been established, or when a physician decides to use a contraindicated drug because there are no other alternatives, the *rationale* for deviating from established recommendations *must be documented,* and agreement by a second physician would appear to be prudent.

GOVERNMENT REGULATIONS — STATE AND LOCAL

General Law Regarding Health Department Regulations

By virtue of the police power inherent in the status of being a sovereign governmental entity, each state is obligated to exercise the clear duty of promoting the general welfare by preserving the public health. Of all the purposes of government, no duty is considered to be more important. Accordingly, this inherent power is plenary in scope, and the duty to provide for and protect the public health is imperative, an obligation which cannot be surrendered. In order to carry out this fundamental duty of creating and enforcing health regulations, the state exercises its fundamental power by legislation, including the delegation of such power to lower levels of government, i.e., to state agencies and other subordinate governmental subdivisions such as counties, cities, and local boards of health.

The details of organizational structure vary from one state to the other in terms of the legal and administrative relationship of the lower governmental subdivision to the state government. It is, therefore, necessary to be familiar with the specific arrangement in the jurisdiction in which one practices medicine. Such minor differences in form, however, do not significantly alter the legal efficacy of the delegation of local health power. In many states, the local health departments/agencies conduct their daily activities pursuant to the general law, independently of the state health department. Typically, even though the state agency has authority to intervene in the operation of the local department when special conditions warrant (e.g., major emergencies or poor local management), the primary supervisory responsibility resides in the local department. The local board of health is established with a mandate to follow state health law in the formulation of local codes pertinent to a given locale.

In those instances where state law is not preempted by federal law, the public policy of the state is expressed via an enabling statute in general terms by declaring the intention to establish a program to detect, prevent, and control communicable diseases. The reason why the legislative language is couched in such broadly worded prescriptions is clear: the technical knowledge and ongoing advancements requiring expertise in the regulation of public health are clearly beyond the scope of the legislature. Detailed regulations and implementation of the mandated programs are left to the appropriate administrative agencies with experts on their staff. In this way, legislation affords the necessary flexibility to meet the public health needs and to keep up concurrently with state-of-the-art technological advances and technical standards.

Typically, the local boards of health are invested with broad power to establish necessary prescriptions (whether in the form of regulations, rules, bylaws, or ordinances) for the protection of the health of the relevant community. Such delegated power includes wide-ranging authority to ordain procedures for the determination of facts necessary to enforce both the statutorily enacted laws and the derivative, substantive rule decreed at the local level. As an example, one facet of the exercise of such extensive power involves the virtual plenipotentiary capacity of local boards to designate specific diseases as being contagious or infectious. In other words, the statutory provisions are general in scope, allowing considerable leeway for the specific methods and details to be worked out by local authority. In construing legislative enactments which delegate such comprehensive power, the lower level and appellate courts of the respective states interpret the legislation liberally, but apply the rule of strict construction when confronting issues pertaining to the infringement of a citizen's common law rights.

The state statutes vary to some extent, but all generally provide for the protection of the public health by mandating that specific individuals report designated contagious/infectious diseases to a state authority. For example, Kentucky Revised Statute (KRS) 214.010 provides:

"Every *physician* shall report all diseases designated by regulation of the Cabinet of Human Resources as reportable which are under his special treatment to the local board of health of his county, and every *head of family* shall report any of said diseases, when known by him to exist in his family, to the local board or to some member thereof in accordance with the regulations of the Cabinet for Human Resources." (Emphasis added.)

In turn, the legislation also provides for the adoption of regulations by the highest level cabinet or department within the state's organizational structure in an effort to prevent the spread of disease:

"When the Cabinet for Human Resources believes that there is a probability that any infectious or contagious disease will invade this state, it shall take such action and adopt and enforce such rules and regulations as it deems efficient in preventing the introduction or spread of such infectious or contagious disease or diseases within this state, and to accomplish these objects shall establish and strictly maintain quarantine and isolation at such places as it deems proper." (KRS 214.020)

The regulations promulgated by the state and local agencies, by virtue of their purpose to promote the general welfare, are generally sustainable in courts of law with respect to requirements that individual citizens and other legal entities adhere to them. This judicial approach applies so long as such regulations are construed to be reasonable, impartial, and not violative of public policy. As in any case of the legislative enactments involving invocation of the state's police power, constitutional limits on the exercise of such power always obtain. Ultimately, the courts must determine the constitutionality of a statute or administrative regulations, balancing the exercise of the police power against constitutional guarantees providing for due process of law and equal protection of the laws.

Subordinate to the legislative enactments, then, the next tier of rule-making exists at the level of the highest state agency/cabinet, which implements the general law by establishing administrative regulations.

Specific Requirements for Reporting Communicable Diseases

In order to ensure uniformity of definition and methods of control with respect to communicable diseases, most state level administrative regulations incorporate by reference a generally accepted treatise in the field. For example, many states adopt the definitions of communicable diseases and methods of control outlined in punctilious detail in the 1975 edition of the booklet, *Control of Communicable Diseases in Man,* published by the American Public Health Association. Copies of this publication are required to be on file and available for public inspection in various health agencies within the state's hierarchy relating to the regulations of public health.

The administrative regulations further require that any physician actively practicing in the state or any other health care providers must report all epidemic and communicable diseases to the local health agency/department. For these purposes, a communicable disease is defined as "any illness due to a specific infectious agent or its toxic host which is capable of being transmitted to a susceptible host". The standard of care upon which to adjudge the issue of whether a "communicable disease" has been diagnosed is that practice accepted generally among physicians deemed to be within reasonable medical probability. In those rare instances involving reports by non-physicians, the "reasonable man" standard is invoked, i.e., that under the circumstances, the individual acted reasonably and prudently in (a) determining that a given host has a communicable disease, and (b) taking steps to report such disease. State statutes also provide for penalties in cases of failure to report. Any physician failing or refusing to comply with the reporting statute is subject to a monetary fine, which increases on a daily basis for each day of continued neglect or refusal. Repeated failure to report is deemed to be sufficient cause for revocation of a physician's certificate or license to practice medicine, pursuant to the established policies and practices of the jurisdiction's board of medical licensure. Non-physicians are also subject to similiar fines in cases of willful failure or refusal to report.

Beyond those reporting requirements, the administrative regulations typically require other legal entities, such as licensed hospitals (or the person in charge of such hospital) or licensed laboratories (or the person in charge of such laboratory), to report *mutatis mutandis* to the appropriate local authority the diagnosis of a communicable disease in any hospitalized patient, or the detection of any positive microbiologic or serologic tests indicative of the presence of any infection as defined by regulations.

The specified reporting period varies, depending upon the type of infection. Typically, the following diseases or conditions must be reported on a case-by-case basis within 24 hours of diagnosis of the disease:

Animal Bites (or within 12 of attendance)
Anthrax
Botulism (Foodborne)
Campylobacteriosis
Cholera
Diphtheria
Encephalitis
Gonococcal Infections
Hepatitis (Viral)
Measles (Rubeola)
Meningitis and Other Diseases Caused by *Haemophilus influenzae* Type B
Meningitis Caused by *Neisseria meningiditis*
Meningococcemia
Pertussis (Whopping Cough)
Plague
Poliomyelitis
Rabies (Human)
Rubella
Rubella, Congenital Syndrome
Salmonellosis
Shigellosis
Syphilis, Primary, Secondary, Congential, and Other Infection
Trichinosis
Tuberculosis
Typhoid Fever
Yellow Fever
Yersiniosis

The following diseases or conditions are to be reported individually within seven days of diagnosis:

AIDS (HIV Infection)
Amebiasis
Ascariasis
Botulism (Infant)
Brucellosis
Chancroid
Chlamydia Infections
Giardiasis
Gonococcal Infections
Granuloma Inguinale
Herpes Simplex (Genital)
Histoplasmosis
Hookworm
Kawasaki's Disease
Lead Poisoning
Legionnaire's Disease
Leprosy

Leptospirosis
Lyme Disease
Lymphogranuloma Venereum
Malaria
Meningitis (Caused by any
    organism other than *H. meningiditis*
    or *H. influenzae*)
Mumps
Psittacosis
Q. Fever
Reye's Syndrome
Rocky Mountain Spotted Fever
Syphilis
Tetanus
Toxic Shock Syndrome
Tularemia
Typhus

Chicken pox (varicella) and influenza are to be reported collectively by the number of cases and county of residence on a weekly basis.

The following diseases/conditions are to be reported individually within three months of diagnosis:

Asbestosis   Silicosis
Coal Worker's Pneumoconiosis   Mesothelioma

Some jurisdictions now require reporting of all malignancies, particularly of the breast.

Information contained in each report, as required by regulation, generally includes the following information: patient's name, address, date of birth, race, and county of residence; hospital number and attending physician; date of onset and name of disease; pertinent clinical, laboratory, and epidemiological information.

Confidentiality

Special consideration is given by regulation to those cases of sexually transmitted diseases, also defined by regulation, and which typically include syphilis, gonorrhea, chancroid, granuloma inguinale, genital herpes, acquired immune deficiency syndrome (AIDS), non-gonococcal urethritis, mucopurulent cervicitis, and chlamydia infections, including lymphogranuloma venereum. In this category of reportable cases, confidentiality is deemed by regulation to be essential for the proper administration and operation of sexually transmitted disease (STD) control activities, so that all such reportable information is required to be provided in the form of a reidentifiable code number assigned to the patient in lieu of the patient's name and address. Access to such reports is limited to the patient's personal physician and authorized health department personnel, with release of such information to others only upon written consent of the patient.

Forms

With regard to the exact form of the report, each state and local health agency has available and provides a variety of printed forms containing in great detail slots and classification data for rapid and efficient completion of the report. Virtually all such forms for a given reportable disease are uniform on a national basis, prepared at the federal level by the Department of Health and Human Services, Public Health Service, Centers for Disease Control, Atlanta, Georgia. For house officers, such forms are readily available through the hospital's infection control department.

Liability of Public Health Officers

The question of liability of public health officers employed by and working in the various state agencies is different from that involving the private physician, including the house officer undergoing residency training in an accredited hospital program. The power delegated to public health officials must be exercised in a reasonable and legitimate manner. Further, the law requires that there must be a reasonable relationship between the method adopted to prevent the spread of a contagious disease and the actual danger of contagion associated with that disease. When these public officials perform their acts in good faith, they are not personally liable for injuries resulting from errors in judgment or the exercise of discretion. However, they are not free from liability in instances where it is established that they acted beyond the scope of their authority, or with a degree of negligence so great as to constitute malice. Examples of liability for personal misfeasance or malfeasance in the performance of such duties include the unreasonable and arbitrary destruction of property designated as a nuisance, or false imprisonment of an individual with a contagious disease by quarantining the individual in an unreasonable manner when no menace to public health, in fact, existed. These issues are typically determined by a jury at trial. In sum, the delegated power to regulate health in order to detect, prevent, and control communicable diseases must be exercised in a reasonable manner by means reasonably related to such detection, prevention, and control.

Authority of Public Health Officers

The local health agency may elect either to adopt fully the administrative regulations promulgated by the state agency, or to establish sets of regulations tailored to the locale, or to rely upon regulations generated at both levels, which are invoked in combination to regulate public health. Regardless of the level of generation and promulgation of health regulations, such rules are generally upheld by courts if the rules are construed to be reasonable and substantially related to promote the public health, or even tend to do so. In the absence of express legislation prohibiting such action, local health agencies may, in the exercise of their authority, act summarily to make determinations and take actions, the failure by delay of which may imperil the public health. For example, such agencies may not need to give advance notice or conduct a hearing prior to such action.

Potential Legal Issues Affecting the House Officer in Diagnosing and Reporting Communicable Diseases

Legal issues arising out of the legislative mandate to report communicable diseases as it relates to the house officer are generally limited. Each hospital or health institution with accredited residency programs has, as a general policy, a set of published regulations and directives, which delineate the definitions of the relevant concepts and the obligations of the physicians with regard to the process of reporting communicable diseases. Typically, as part of the general hospital policy, each institution will have established an intramural infection control division as part of its organizational structure. The experts in that department are trained and directed specifically to coordinate and effectuate the hospital policies in the area of disease control. Each house officer should, therefore, be familiar with those policies and official reporting mechanisms designed by the infection control department. Failure to follow the institutional policies constitutes a prima facie violation at law and subjects the violator to either administrative disciplinary measures or legal action, as particularized in the state statutes.

As it applies to all members of the public, including physicians, the general principle is well-established that any individual negligently exposing another to a communicable disease, which that person so exposed subsequently contracts, is liable in damages. The degree of care necessary to prevent contraction of a given disease is dependent upon the nature of the disease and the danger of communicability. An element of proof in such cases includes establishing that the alleged offender, in fact, knew of the presence of the disease. As this relates to physicians, including house officers, all such medical personnel are required by law not to act negligently (below the accepted standard of care) in any way. This requirement applies to both diagnosis and reporting, the failure of which engenders the likelihood of causing the spread of the infectious disease. Enforcement of state laws, departmental regulations, and rules of the local health agency, however, lies beyond the scope of the private physician's duties.

Blood Transfusions

Another area relating to state regulations for public health, as it affects the house officer, is exemplified in a new section of a Kentucky Statute (KRS 214.450 et seq.) relating to blood transfusions. In essence, the statute provides that no blood may be transfused to any human donee without first ruling out by appropriate testing the presence of any blood borne sexually transmitted or communicable disease, including the human immunodeficiency virus. Elaborate details for labeling and transfusing blood (and blood products) are spelled out in this statute and are geared to the prevention of tranfusing untested blood, in the absence of an emergency situation. Knowing violation of the statute subjects the alleged violator to felony prosecution. The house staff physician, as an employee of the health facility and part of the health care provider team, therefore, must adhere to all institutional policies with regard to the labeling and transfusion of blood in a manner free of negligence, so as to avoid potential criminal prosecution. As a general rule, adherence by the house staff officer to the intramural regulations and policies serves as a defense and insulates him or her personally from legal actions.

Compliance with Statutory Language

With regard to the diagnosis of a limited number of specified diseases, the postgraduate resident must be aware that, regardless of what he may have been taught, certain definitions and methods pertaining to a given diagnosis are elaborated in administrative regulations relating to communicable diseases. Although such terms generally represent well-established criteria within the medical community, failure to incorporate these concepts into the physician's diagnostic considerations may subject the physician to claims of negligence and medical malpractice. As examples, "induration" of skin and the tuberculin "skin test" employed in the diagnosis of tuberculosis, or such terms as "Anti-Hbs", "HBsAg", or "HBV Negative", are spelled out equivocally in such regulations. For purposes of diagnosis and the reporting of diseases relating to these definitions, the house staff physician must ensure that his understanding comports with the statutory language.

In another vein, the house officer must be aware of regulatory language mandating that certain categories of patients be treated with special regard to that condition. For example, in drawing a specimen of blood from a woman known or suspected to be pregnant, the physician must not only properly label the specimen container, but also "identify the specimen as being from a pregnant woman". Such requirements apply, even if there is no clinical suspicion that the pregnant woman harbors a communicable disease.

Consideration of that specific disease in question also has legal implications. Certain disease conditions, e.g., tuberculosis, are frequently referred to specifically by name in state statutes, which impose specific special obligations on the physician. Such statutory language may be couched in mandatory ("shall") or permissive ("may") terminology. For example, any person, including the physician, having "reasonable cause to suspect" that an individual has communicable tuberculosis, and further, has failed to comply (as a "recalcitrant tuberculosis patient") with the statutory provisions imposing a legal duty on the patient to take steps to prevent the spread of the disease, may submit an affidavit to courts of various levels to that effect. If the affiant acts in good faith, he or she is held harmless and free from further legal action, and moreover, is entitled to legal representation afforded by various state agencies, should a legal action arise as a result of the affidavit.

Minors

Another area of potential legal liability involves the treatment of minors. Each state by statute defines the age of majority for different purposes, buttressed by volumes of judicial interpretation as to the meaning of "minority" in relation to the rights and duties of the minor and his parents or legal guardian/custodian. Even though the statutorily expressed policies in this regard may vary among the respective states, the house officer needs to be cognizant of certain problem areas. Using Kentucky law as an example, the relevant statute (cf. KRS 214.185) provides for the diagnostic examination of a minor by a physician, requiring only the consent of the minor, for the purpose of diagnosing and treating a venereal disease. Although the legal status of minority does not affect the requirement to report a diagnosed communicable disease as discussed previously, it is generally permissible by statute to conduct the necessary examination, collect the appropriate specimens, and make the indicated diagnosis, all without consent, not to mention notification, of the adult(s) responsible for the minor. In such cases, no criminal or civil liability devolves upon the physician, except for the usual instances which also apply to the adult population, i.e., negligent act or omission by the physician in diagnosis or treatment. Representations may be given by the minor that he or she is legally entitled to give such consent when, in fact, he or she is not. If the physician relies upon such representation in good faith, however, his or her actions in diagnosing and treating the communicable disease are not subject to criminal or tort liability on the basis of a subsequent claim of lack of effective consent. Finally, even upon the minor's stated objections, the physician is authorized by statute to inform the parents or legal guardian of the minor that treatment of the venereal disease is needed or was given, if, in the good faith judgment of the professional, such information would favorably affect the minor's health.

Privacy

Finally, beyond the area of direct patient care and contact, house officers engaged in research or epidemiological studies and the submission of papers for publication are advised to familiarize themselves with the statutes of their jurisdiction requiring strict confidentiality, a principle deemed inviolate in the control of sexually transmitted diseases. In essence, dissemination of such information is severely limited, and in the absence of a specific individual's legally obtained consent, release of any medical or epidemiological data identifying (by name or other means) an individual diagnosed as having a sexually transmittable disease is impermissible.

NOTES